"Lisa has revolutionized meal prep to be approachable, fresh, and easy, and it has everything you need to make healthy eating a breeze, from the best storage containers to how to extend the life of your most finicky produce to the simplest way to whip everything together for a delicious weeknight meal. You'll be inspired to reorganize your pantry, stock your freezer, and take a trip to the farmers' market!"

—**EMILY MARIKO,** TikTok creator

"Lisa's gorgeous cookbook will teach you the tips and tricks to make meal prep your superpower! With *Downshiftology Healthy Meal Prep,* no matter what life throws at you, a quick and wholesome meal is minutes away."

—**MICHELLE TAM,** *New York Times* **bestselling cookbook author and creator of** *Nom Nom Paleo*

"Lisa's recipes are legit, and she does not mess around. Her cookbook delivers healthy recipes that are not only easy to make, but they're packed with whole-food ingredients you can feel good about."

—**BOBBY PARRISH,** author and creator of *FlavCity*

"Lisa's approach is thoughtful, practical, and doable! This isn't just a cookbook but a resource for meal planning. Every time I open the book, I'm inspired to eat healthier and meal prep for my family."

—**NATASHA KRAVCHUK,** creator of *Natasha's Kitchen*

"Lisa is the queen of meal prep on social media! And now she's bringing her passion and expertise to this book to inspire and help you save time in the kitchen, eat a variety of colors, nutrients, and flavors, and reduce the stress of what to make for dinner!"

—**YUMNA JAWAD,** creator of *Feel Good Foodie*

"Lisa had me hooked in the first few pages when she explained that meal prep is like having a buffet bar in your fridge—seriously, who wouldn't love that?! Not only are Lisa's meals completely doable and craveable, but her book is also an amazing resource for how to prep, store, freeze, and reheat an incredibly wide variety of foods."

—**JENN SEGAL,** *Once Upon a Chef: The Cookbook* and *Once Upon a Chef: Weeknight/Weekend*

DOWNSHIFTOLOGY
Healthy
Meal Prep

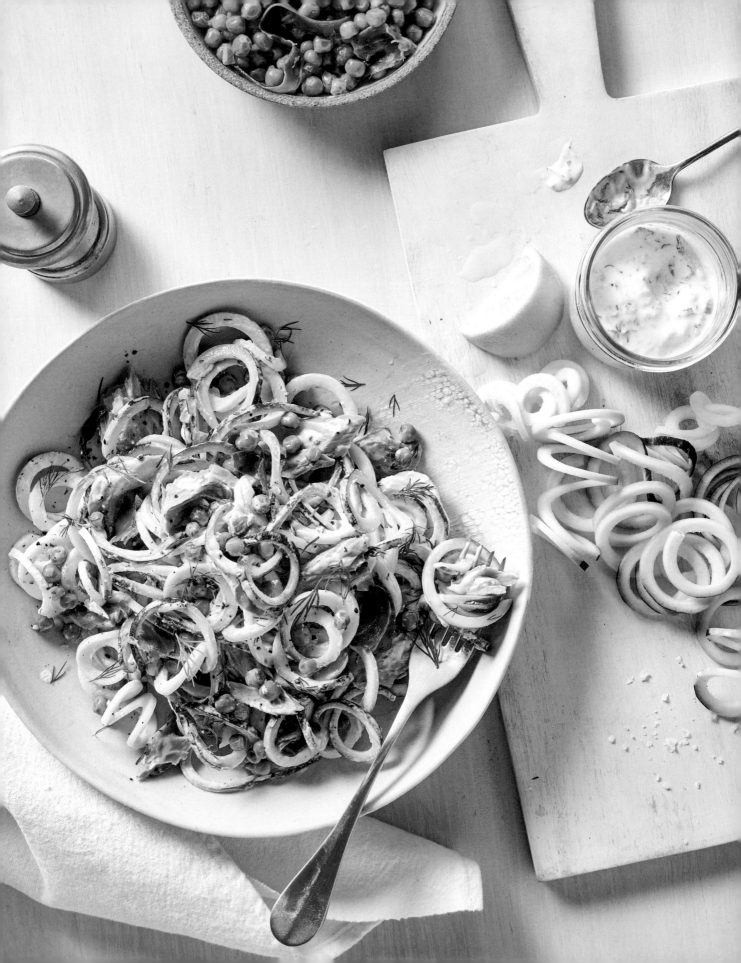

DOWNSHIFTOLOGY
Healthy
Meal Prep

100+ Make-Ahead Recipes and
Quick-Assembly Meals

Lisa Bryan

PHOTOGRAPHS BY REN FULLER

Clarkson Potter/Publishers
New York

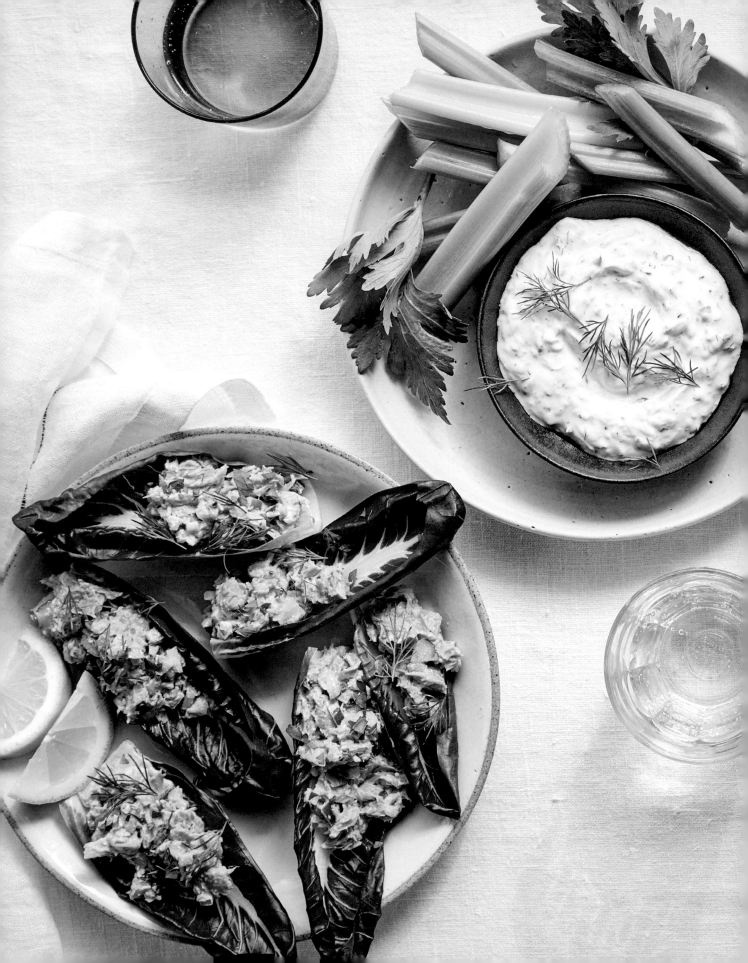

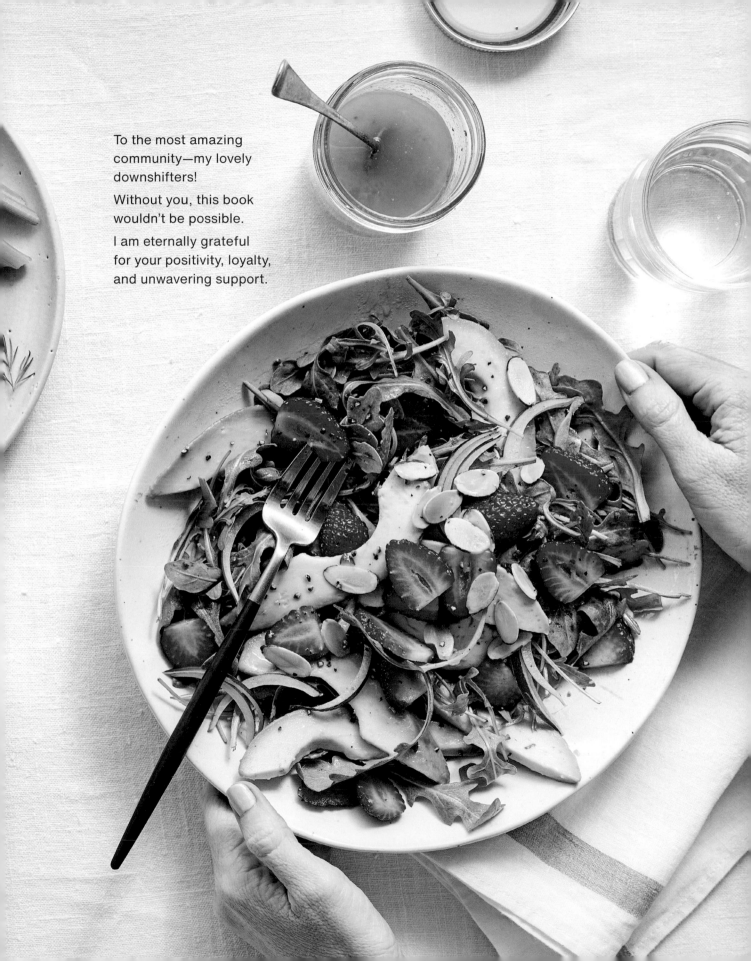

To the most amazing community—my lovely downshifters!

Without you, this book wouldn't be possible.

I am eternally grateful for your positivity, loyalty, and unwavering support.

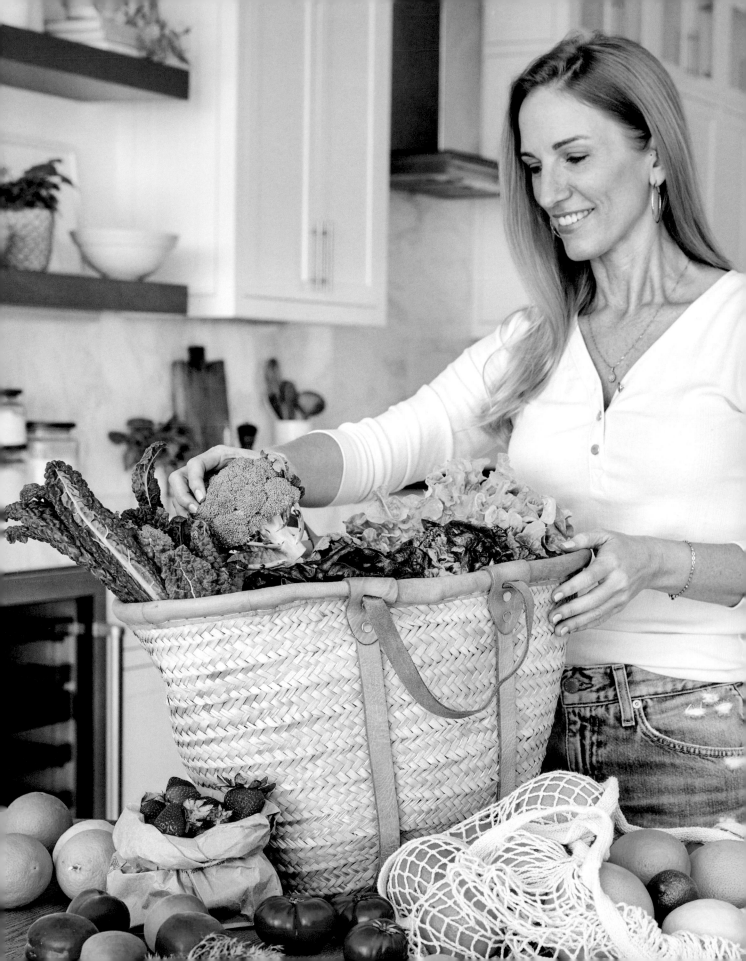

contents

introduction

I'll be honest, I never imagined that one day I'd write a cookbook. But then again, I also never imagined that I'd create a food blog or plaster my face across YouTube videos for millions of people around the world to see. Life is funny that way, isn't it?

When I first started Downshiftology, my goal was humble and simple—to inspire people to eat more vegetables, to cook from home more frequently, and to ditch processed food. I'm not a professional chef (or even a trained chef for that matter). I'm a former burned-out corporate gal who struggled to balance life and healthy eating while dealing with several autoimmune conditions and an overly sensitive gut. I'm an introvert, albeit a chatty one, who reluctantly started my YouTube channel to appease a few blog readers who asked for tutorial videos, and then I chuckled to myself at how silly it was for a forty-something to be starting a YouTube channel (I mean, I was double the age of the average YouTuber!).

Somewhere along the way, though, my moderate, mostly anti-inflammatory, and certainly not-perfect approach to eating clicked with a few of you, and then a few more, and before I knew it, what started out with me saying, "Oh, I'll just toss a few recipes on a website and cobble together a few videos" turned into my full-time job.

my wellness journey

I thought I was generally healthy for most of my life. Which kind of makes me laugh now, considering my diet was the "standard American diet," full of processed food, fast food, sugar, and hard-to-pronounce ingredients. I was fairly active and assumed that because I was not overweight, I was healthy. Never in a million years did I correlate food and lifestyle with health.

In my twenties, my main nourishment came from fast food and processed food, with McDonald's double cheeseburgers and Taco Bell Mexican pizzas always at the top of my list. I was also quite the sugar fiend and had a massive addiction to anything sweet and sugary, like candy, cakes, and pastries. I even thought about opening a bakery for a while!

In my thirties, my career progressed and I climbed the corporate ladder as an executive for healthcare companies. High levels of stress, long hours, and reduced sleep were now added to my lifestyle mix. Without really realizing it, I had become the quintessential type A corporate workaholic, grabbing coffee and snacks while running between meetings.

At this same time, mysterious symptoms were increasingly appearing. I had seasonal allergies for the first time in my life, gastrointestinal issues, and dry patches of skin on my legs and face. I suffered from dizziness and fainting episodes, as well as hormonal imbalances. But it was the massive fatigue that really got me. I'd go to bed at 8 p.m., sleep for ten hours, and still be tired the next day.

I visited several doctors and underwent lots of testing but was told that other than low blood pressure, I was the epitome of good health. I received inhalers for the asthma and corticosteroids for the skin issues and was sent on my way. But deep in my core, I knew something was off. So I became a late-night Google-oholic and began connecting the dots myself. At the age of thirty-five, I received my first autoimmune diagnosis—celiac disease. From there, other diagnoses rolled in one after the other—Hashimoto's, psoriasis, and endometriosis—all within two years! As you can imagine, my world was flipped upside down.

the importance of real food and lifestyle

After I was diagnosed with celiac disease, I did just about everything wrong. I thought the easiest way to eat gluten-free would be to raid the entire gluten-free section of Whole Foods. So I dropped two hundred dollars on gluten-free packaged food the week after I was diagnosed.

Instead of feeling better, I actually felt worse for several months. And I triggered candida and SIBO (small intestinal bacterial overgrowth) because the packaged food contained massive quantities of sugar and unique, gluten-free starches that my body wasn't used to. My other symptoms also flared up, and I felt absolutely deflated. Wasn't going gluten-free supposed to make me feel better?

Desperate, I researched everything I could about autoimmune disease, nutrition, gut health, and the mind–body connection. I also began working with a functional medicine doctor who forced me to evaluate what I was putting into my body and how I was living my

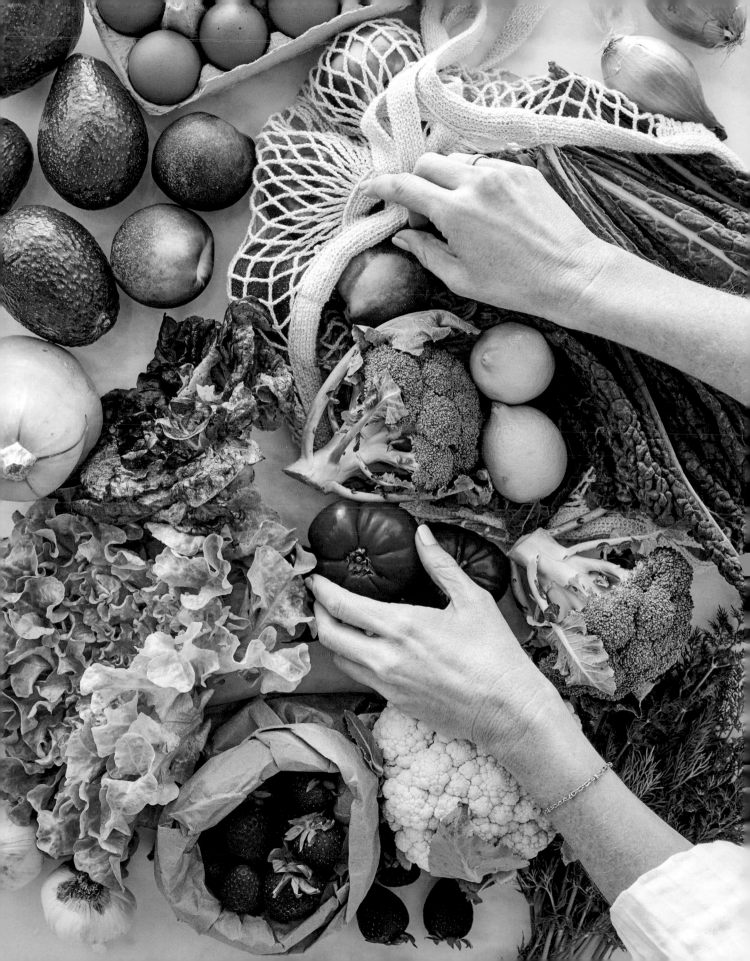

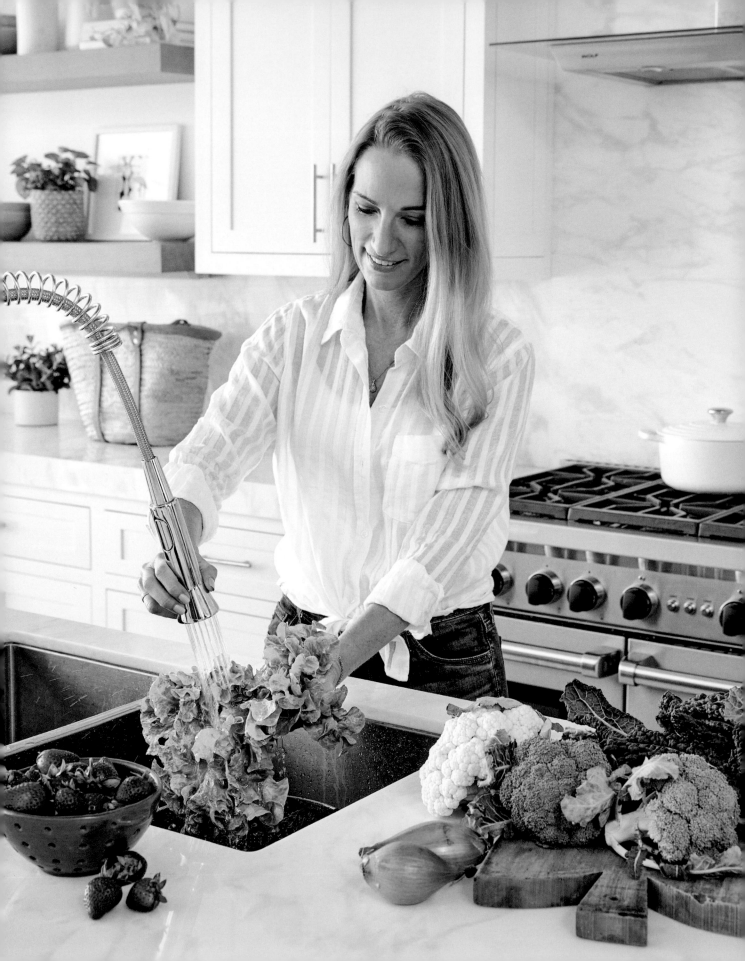

life. Long story short, I stopped eating processed foods and started eating whole, nutrient-dense foods, and I *finally* started to feel better!

Through trial and error, I eventually learned my body's unique triggers and began to reverse the autoimmune symptoms that had piled up. Within a year, simply through nutrition and lifestyle changes, virtually all my autoimmune symptoms disappeared—which I thought was nothing short of miraculous.

Today, a decade later, my wellness journey continues with just small tweaks here and there, because that simple, back-to-basic approach that I started with has proven to be the most sustainable. But just in case you think I've got this healthy thing 100 percent figured out, let me remind you that I still have challenges (hello, "the mena"—aka perimenopause). That's why I'm all about progress over perfection and just doing the best I can day by day!

where meal prep fits in

When I changed my diet, I began meal prepping to prevent food waste. People always assume cooking for one person *must* be easier than cooking for a family. I mean, how hard can it be to whip up a single portion of something? Well, the truth is, it's actually difficult to scale down recipes to just a single portion, *and* I also couldn't eat the fresh produce I purchased fast enough. Spinach, berries, and zucchini were all going moldy in my fridge, and my potatoes were wildly sprouting to the point that it looked like I had a farm in my pantry. I was wasting food *and* money.

So I decided to do something different. I started prepping individual ingredients to create quick-assembly meals. First, I roasted a sheet pan of sweet potatoes and put them into a single container. Then I cooked some wild rice and put that into another container. I baked a couple of chicken breasts, shredded them, and stored them in a third container. I diced up a raw red onion, so I'd have to cry only once a week rather than every day of the week and placed that in yet another container. When I took a step back and looked at what I had done I was blown away! Not only was it fast and easy to prep individual ingredients, but I now had this astounding *buffet bar* in my fridge. I could combine those individual ingredients with other fresh foods like avocados, cherry tomatoes, nuts, and seeds, and when I added a sauce or dressing, I was able to create delicious and flavorful meals throughout the day in less than five minutes.

I originally shared this meal prep concept on my YouTube channel several years ago, and it absolutely went viral! Needless to say, my approach resonated with many of you, and I'd wager that's how many of you discovered Downshiftology.

But as much as I love individual ingredient meal prep and quick-assembly meals, it's not the only way I prepare meals. I'm a staunch believer that in order to build sustainable healthy habits, you need variety—in colors, nutrients, and flavors. That's why my weekly meal-prep routine also includes big-batch and freezer-friendly recipes such as soups and stews, as well as stir-fries, casseroles, and even breakfast items, like chia pudding, that will last for months in the freezer. Between quick-assembly and storage-friendly recipes, I'm now covered with an assortment of healthy food that can be easily assembled or quickly reheated, with very little effort.

The recipes in this book, like my diet, are 100 percent gluten-free. I also typically avoid refined sugar, and most dairy, though I do enjoy yogurt and a little cheese here and there. So while you may notice sprinkles of feta or goat cheese on recipes, know that it's optional and you can make every recipe in this cookbook dairy-free. I'm all about healthy with a dash of comforting normalcy. That's also why you'll find a dessert chapter—something not found in most meal-prep cookbooks. I'm a fan of healthier sweet treats that can be portioned into smaller bites and nibbles to satisfy sugar cravings in a balanced way. Balance is key, both on the plate and in life—it's the Downshiftology way!

As you flip the pages of this book, I hope you'll be inspired to get back to basics and embrace the versatility of whole food ingredients. My motto with Downshiftology is to "take life down a notch," and what better way to start than with a new approach to healthy eating, thinking about meal prep in an entirely new way, and giving yourself permission to switch directions to a simpler path (it's never too late and you're never too old). I'll be over here cheering for you, along with the entire community of downshifters!

xo
Lisa

IS PREPPED FOOD LESS NUTRITIOUS?

This is one of the most common questions I get. And my short answer is this—yes, slicing and dicing fruits and vegetables ahead of time can cause them to lose a small amount of nutrients. Fat-soluble vitamins may oxidize, and water-soluble vitamins can leech out (for instance, when celery is stored in water). But (and this is a biggie) opting for healthy prepped food, even with a small amount of nutrient loss, *is still better for you* than the alternative—grabbing takeout or eating unhealthy convenience food. So it's best to keep it in perspective. As long as you're prioritizing whole foods, you're doing a great job!

a sample day of meals

For each of these meals, it takes about five minutes to warm up a few ingredients or slice and dice a few veggies, then assemble. It's not the monotonous meal prep you may be used to (ahem, rice, chicken, and veggies for five days straight), and you can serve it up faster than you can order from Uber Eats (and obviously, it's far healthier). In my meal prep world, a day may look like this:

BREAKFAST

Leftover **Balsamic Roasted Mushrooms** (page 235), and **Garlic Sautéed Beet Greens** (page 262) with a jammy, **soft-boiled egg** (see page 65) on top.

LUNCH

A macro bowl with **Lemon Herb Rice** (page 243), fresh baby spinach, and diced veggies (tomatoes, cucumber, and red onion), topped with **Mediterranean Lamb Meatballs** (page 167) and a dollop of **Tzatziki** (page 253).

DINNER

Reheated **Roasted Chicken with Fennel, Pear, and Onion** (page 179) on a mound of **Garlicky Root Vegetable Mash** (page 247).

DESSERT

Reheated **Ginger Roasted Stone Fruit** (page 287) topped with a few spoonfuls of yogurt and **Homemade Granola** (page 106).

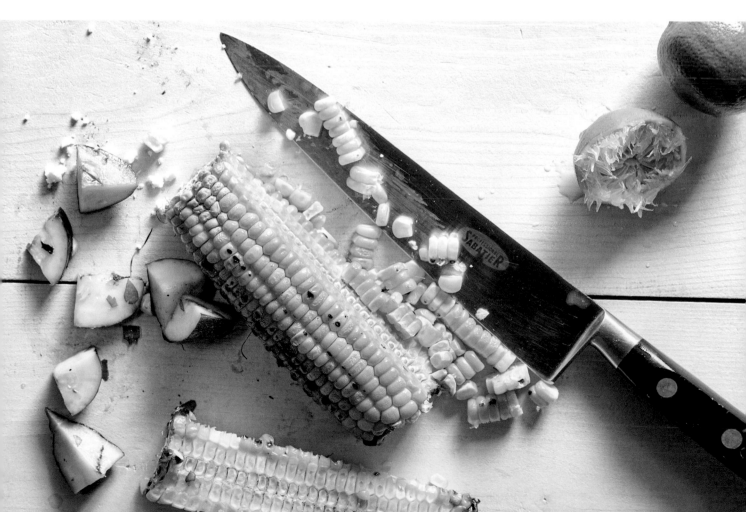

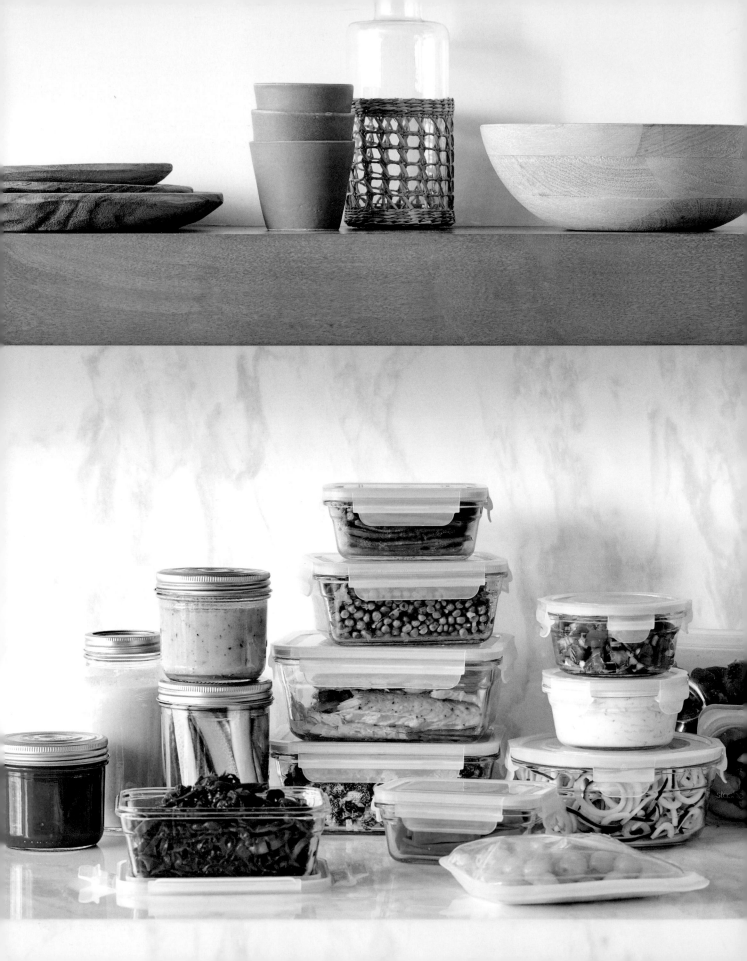

meal prep containers

An essential for weekly meal prep is good storage containers. You've got to have a method to store 'n' stack all that make-ahead food! So what makes a good container? One that is durable and reusable, can be used for both cold storage and reheating, and is nontoxic.

My favorite containers are all made from glass and silicone. When you're storing food, and more importantly when you're reheating food, it's critical to stay away from plastic, which can leech harmful chemicals into your food.

glass

I have a variety of glass jars that I've accumulated over the years from brands such as Weck, Le Parfait, Ball, Anchor Hocking, and Kerr. I use them for storing everything from homemade cashew milk to chia pudding, soups, almond butter, and overnight oats. They're also great for storing dry goods in the pantry.

When it comes to storing larger food items, I use Glasslock containers, but Pyrex is great as well. I'll use these larger containers (you can buy them round or rectangular in shape) to store sliced chicken, roasted vegetables, meatballs, flaked salmon, stir-fries, spiralized zucchini noodles, and pretty much 80 percent of what I meal prep.

No matter which brand you invest in, just make sure the glass is tempered (making it extra durable) so it can be used in the fridge, freezer, microwave, and oven.

silicone

There are many options for silicone bags and storage containers nowadays, but two brands I love are Stasher and Souper Cubes.

Stasher bags are great for meal prep because they can usually fit in those nook and cranny spaces in your fridge and freezer. They're also perfect for travel and on-the-go snacks, like homemade granola and energy balls. These bags are TSA compliant because you can see what's inside, and they're lightweight, which makes them easy to pack in your carry-on luggage.

Souper Cubes are silicone trays that come in a variety of sizes, perfect for freezing everything from mini cubes of fresh herbs in oil to perfectly portioned soups and appetizer servings of hummus. You can leave the food item frozen in the silicone tray (there's a lid), or you can pop it out when frozen, stack in the freezer in a freezer-safe bag, and make the silicone tray available for your next meal!

the freezer is your friend

On social media it often looks like I have an endless supply of ready-to-go meals coming out of my freezer. And to be honest, it's not smoke and mirrors—it's because I really do! I'll often whip up a big-batch meal when ingredients are on sale and then freeze leftovers to use for months. Then, when I'm exhausted and don't feel like cooking, I can simply reheat a meal. It keeps me on the healthy train and *away* from the munchie snack shelf in my pantry. Here are a few tips for getting the most out of your freezer:

Double a Recipe: It's really no additional work (or additional dirty dishes) to double some recipes (for example, soups and stews), so plan ahead and cook extra for the purpose of freezing and reheating in the future.

Cool Food Before Freezing: You don't want to put steaming hot food into storage containers and then place those in the freezer. Not only will they thaw surrounding items in the freezer, but you'll have ice crystals form on your food as the steam freezes. Likewise, don't let food hang out on the counter too long before freezing, as bacteria thrives at room temperature.

Freeze in Usable Servings: Instead of packing a recipe into one large storage container, divvy it up into smaller containers before freezing. This can make it easier to store in smaller freezers and also makes reheating for one or two people a breeze!

Liquids Expand: If you're freezing a recipe with water, broth, or other liquids, don't forget that liquids expand when frozen and can shatter glass storage containers. Always leave a little headspace at the top of storage containers for expansion.

Label It: I've been guilty of forgetting to label my frozen meals, which leads to a guessing game of "name that blob" while it thaws. To prevent mystery food in your freezer, use painter's tape or masking tape to label the storage container with the item and date. Especially the date!

Freeze Away: I've indicated on each individual recipe how long you can store that meal, but you'll likely notice a theme—I typically list three months for storing items in the freezer. Sure, you can store some items longer than that, but I've found that at three months my food is still tasty upon reheating—with no freezer burn—and it doesn't somehow get lost in the back of my freezer.

10 pieces of kitchen equipment I can't live without

1 **Stainless-steel pans.** These are the workhorses in my kitchen. I've had my All-Clad set for over twenty years—it's definitely been worth the investment.

2 **High-powered blender.** I have a slight (okay, more than slight) obsession with my Vitamix. Every week I whip up ultra-creamy soups, easy dips, homemade nut milks, the most indulgent desserts, and, of course, green (and brown) smoothies.

3 **Chef's knife.** This is essential for meal prep and cooking in general—it makes easy work of slicing, dicing, and breaking down every ingredient imaginable. I have a Zwilling Pro knife block set, but at the very least, grab yourself a really good chef's knife.

4 **Cutting board.** What goes along with a sharp knife? A high-quality cutting board! I love my extra-large walnut John Boos cutting board. It's what you see me using in every YouTube video.

5 **Cast-iron braiser.** This incredibly versatile, 3.5-quart hefty pan with large handles and a domed lid is my favorite stovetop-to-oven pan. I have both Le Creuset and Staub.

6 **Cast-iron Dutch oven.** Can you get through a winter without a Dutch oven? Hmm . . . it's questionable. I have several sizes but use my 5.5-quart round Dutch oven most often (if you're a bigger family, you may prefer a larger one).

7 **Commercial-grade sheet pans.** They're thicker than standard sheet pans, super durable, and hold your heaviest foods without bending. I use half- and quarter-size sheet pans most often.

8 **Magnetic measuring spoons.** They stick together, which means I don't have to rummage through my drawer to find a missing spoon size when I'm in the middle of a recipe. So functional!

9 **Stainless-steel garlic press.** The perfect gadget for adding fresh garlic to a recipe fast. I've got an OXO press that accommodates several garlic cloves—there's no such thing as too much garlic!

10 **Spiralizer.** I've had my Paderno spiralizer for nearly a decade, and it was the best twenty-dollar investment. It's also the fastest way to slice up (and sneak in!) veggies throughout the week.

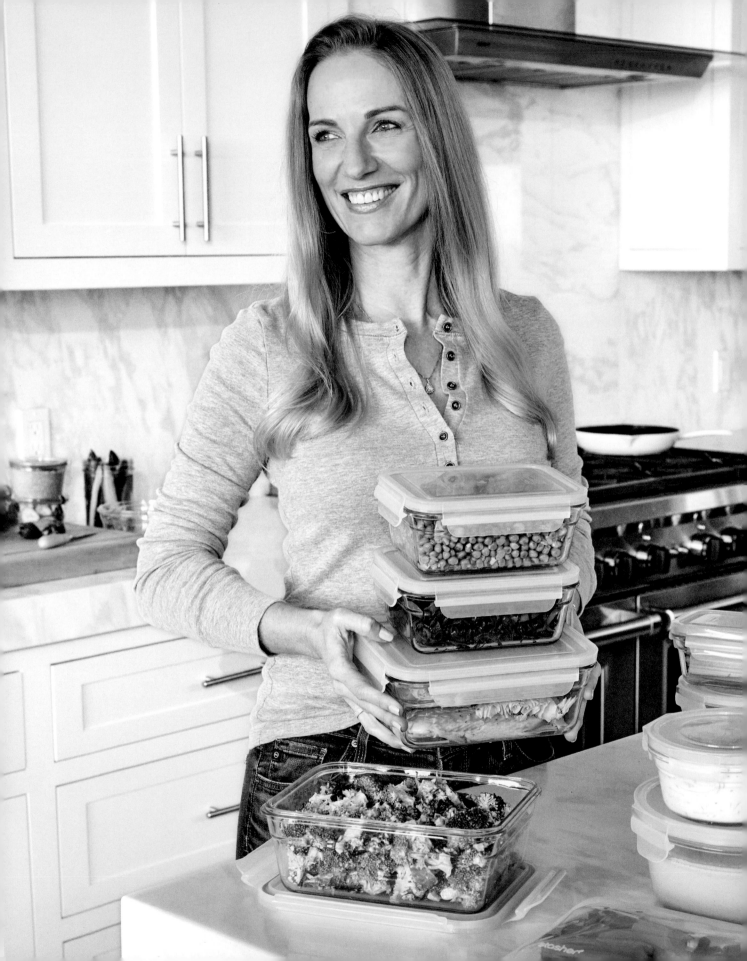

ready to eat?
here's how to thaw properly

Kudos to you for having a stash of ready-to-go homemade meals in your freezer. But just as important as freezing meals is learning how to unfreeze them. Here are some tips for properly and safely thawing your soups, stews, chicken breasts, meatballs, and other dishes before reheating.

1. Move It to the Fridge: While it may be tempting to take a frozen serving from the freezer and plop it straight in the microwave, it's always best to move that frozen serving to the fridge first and let it thaw overnight. Not only will it reheat faster once it's thawed, but it will also minimize the risk of adversely changing the texture of the food (this is key with frittatas and egg muffins).

2. Heat It Up: In terms of which reheating method is best (stove, oven, or microwave), it's really up to you. I always recommend reheating the food the same way it was originally cooked for the best texture. So if you're reheating potato wedges, opt for the oven to help them stay crispy. But if you're in a rush and not fussy, of course the microwave will work.

3. Zhuzh It Up: To give frozen and reheated meals that *fresher* feeling, garnish with fresh herbs, diced avocado, or crumbled feta; spritz with a little lemon juice; splash with water or broth to thin anything that may have thickened a bit too much; add a dash of seasoning; or drizzle a sauce (especially useful if you feel your meal may have dried out a bit upon reheating). You get the idea!

individual meal prep ingredients

Want to create that coveted buffet bar *in your own fridge*? Awesome. First things first: It all starts with learning how to prep and store individual ingredients in a way that makes them most usable throughout the week. Take zucchini, for example, one of my favorite vegetables. It can be spiralized and stored in the fridge (for salads or egg nests), sliced and frozen (for smoothies or stews), or grated and frozen (for zucchini bread and other baked goods). So many possibilities!

Today, you can buy pre-chopped vegetables (and even spiralized vegetables) at the grocery store, and while convenient, you'll save money and have a fresher starting point if you chop and spiralize them yourself, so I highly recommend doing so.

In this chapter, I break down the veggies I meal prep most often *and* answer the questions I'm asked daily across social media—how to select the best ones, how to meal prep them, and what to do with them once they're sliced/diced/spiralized/grated (consider it a sneak peek into the next chapter for quick-assembly meals). Also in this chapter? Tips for storing starches, proteins, and herbs—because herbs make everything better, and how frustrating is it when your cilantro starts wilting two days after buying it? On page 59, you'll learn how to fix that!

asparagus

One of my favorite indicators that "spring has sprung" is the bundles of local asparagus that line the supermarket shelves and farmers' market stalls. Fresh green stalks are the norm, but you may also find white or purple varieties. (Fun fact: I attended a weiße spargel—"white asparagus"—festival in Germany during college.) Some people think asparagus tastes like broccoli, green beans, or artichokes, so feel free to sub it in for any recipes that include those ingredients.

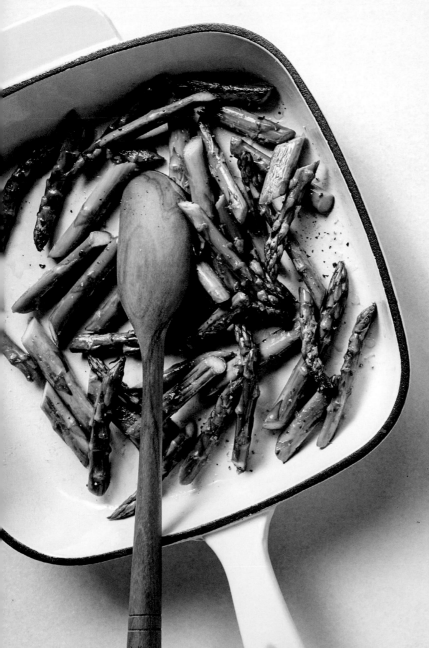

pick the best ones

You'll notice that asparagus varies in thickness, from super thin to fairly thick. Choose spears based on how you plan to use them. Thin ones are great for a quick sauté. Thick ones work best for roasting, grilling, or steaming, and medium spears can go either way. The most important thing is that the tips are firm, not floppy or wilted.

how to store

Keep asparagus dry and unwashed. Then treat it as you would a bunch of flowers, by trimming the ends and placing the bundle upright in a container filled with 1 inch (2.5cm) of water. Store in the fridge for 2 to 3 days. Wash and trim off the woody ends before cooking.

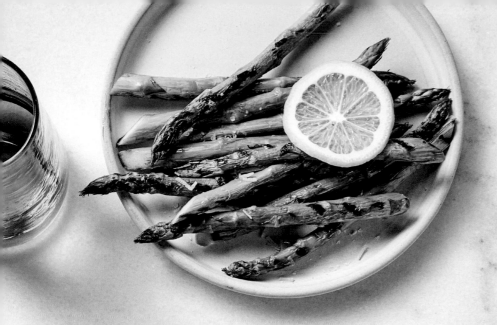

ways to prep and use

Sauté: Heat olive oil in a pan and sauté the asparagus for 8 to 10 minutes. Season the asparagus with salt and pepper. Store in an airtight container in the fridge for 3 to 4 days. To use, warm and top with prosciutto, a poached egg, and shaved Parmesan for breakfast, or serve as a side at dinner.

Roast: Preheat the oven to 425°F (220°C). Toss the asparagus with olive oil, salt, and pepper. Spread the spears on a baking sheet and roast for about 10 minutes. Store in an airtight container in the fridge for 3 to 4 days. Enjoy as a side dish with roasted chicken and mashed potatoes or chop it up into a macro bowl with shrimp or tuna.

Grill: Preheat a grill to medium-high heat. Toss the asparagus with olive oil, salt, and pepper. Grill in a vegetable basket until bright green and cooked through, about 3 minutes. Store in an airtight container in the fridge for 3 to 4 days. Warm the asparagus and add a squeeze of fresh lemon juice or balsamic glaze before serving with grilled salmon or chicken.

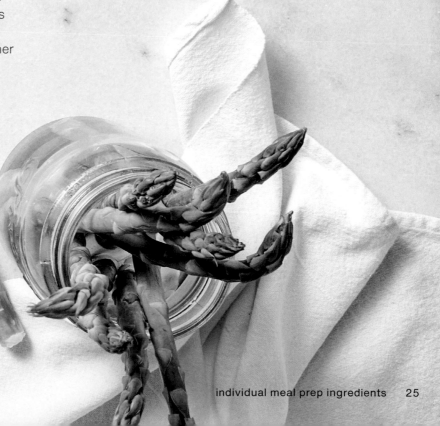

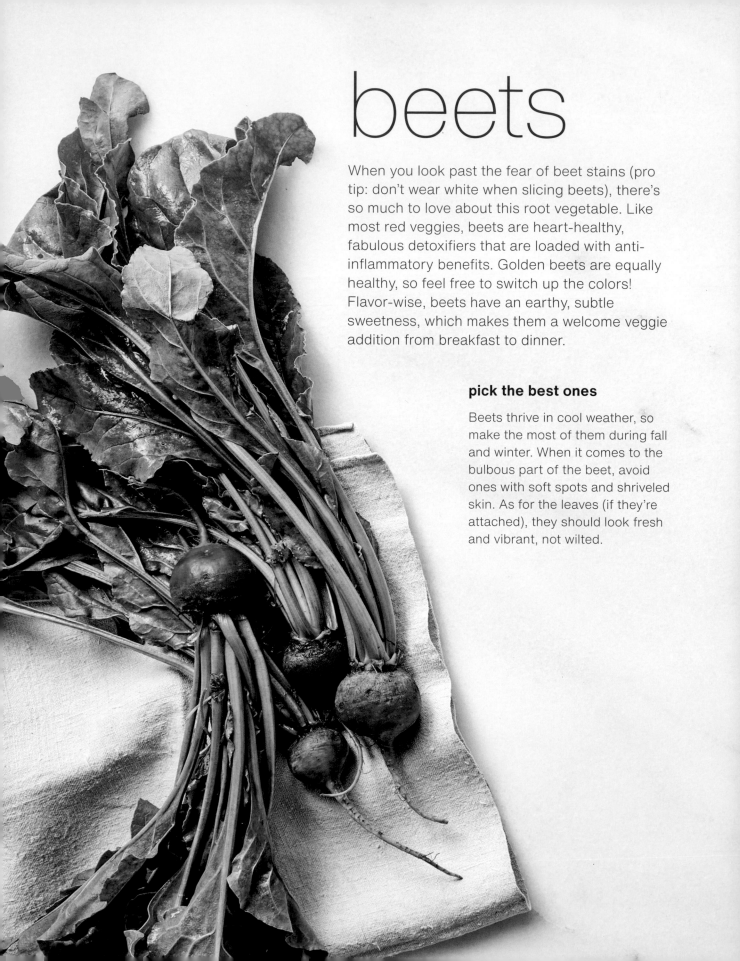

beets

When you look past the fear of beet stains (pro tip: don't wear white when slicing beets), there's so much to love about this root vegetable. Like most red veggies, beets are heart-healthy, fabulous detoxifiers that are loaded with anti-inflammatory benefits. Golden beets are equally healthy, so feel free to switch up the colors! Flavor-wise, beets have an earthy, subtle sweetness, which makes them a welcome veggie addition from breakfast to dinner.

pick the best ones

Beets thrive in cool weather, so make the most of them during fall and winter. When it comes to the bulbous part of the beet, avoid ones with soft spots and shriveled skin. As for the leaves (if they're attached), they should look fresh and vibrant, not wilted.

how to store

If the beets have their stems, cut them off, leaving an inch or two attached. Then store the beets in a plastic bag (be sure to squeeze the air out) in the crisper drawer in your fridge for 2 to 3 weeks. If you plan to use the stems and leaves, like in my Garlic Sautéed Beet Greens (page 262), store them separately in an airtight container in the fridge for 2 to 3 days.

how to meal prep and use

Spiralize: After removing the stems, cut a little bit off each end of the beet to create a flat surface, then peel and spiralize. Store in an airtight container in the fridge for 3 to 4 days. In a pan over medium-low heat, sauté spiralized beets with a little olive oil, then add them to a warm salad. You can also bake them into a Spiralized Beet Frittata (page 105) or turn them into egg nests by cracking a raw egg on top, and cooking the egg to your liking.

Roast: Preheat the oven to 425°F (220°C). After removing the stems, place the beets in a baking dish. Drizzle with olive oil, cover the baking dish with a lid or aluminum foil, and roast for 50 to 60 minutes. Peel and then slice them into quarters. Store in an airtight container in the fridge for 4 to 5 days, or in the freezer for up to 3 months. Warm them up and serve as a side dish, blend them into a Roasted Beet Hummus (page 258), or make them the star of a Roasted Beet Salad with Pistachios (page 147).

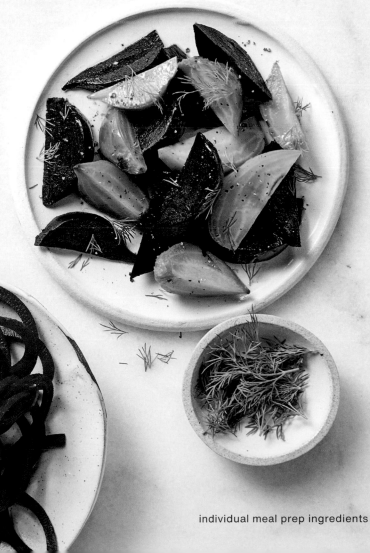

bell peppers

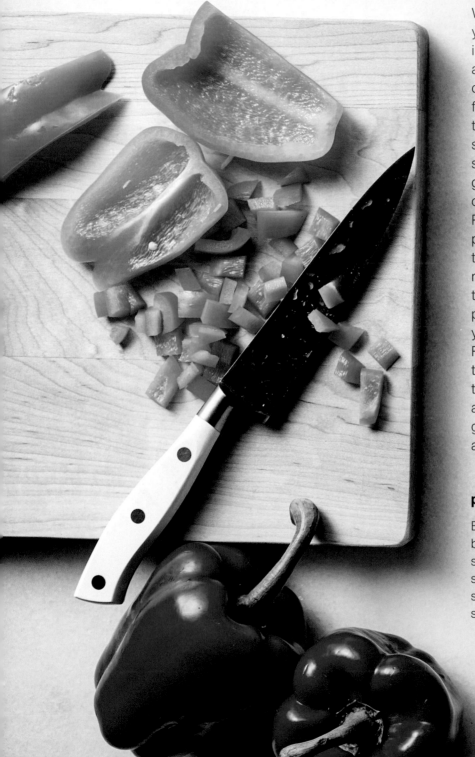

When I think of the ultimate year-round meal-prep ingredient, bell peppers are a personal favorite. When cut into strips they're ideal for dipping, and when diced they're perfect for topping salads or stirring into egg scrambles. They are also great for stuffing—just check out my Breakfast Stuffed Bell Peppers (page 97). All bell peppers start out green and then change color as they mature and ripen. If allowed time on the vine, green bell peppers turn into vibrant yellow, orange, and red ones. Red bell peppers, because they're more ripe, have twice the amount of vitamin C as green bell peppers (this gives them a higher price tag as well).

pick the best ones

Bell peppers should be firm, with bright coloring and shiny smooth skin. Avoid those with wrinkly skin. In terms of flavor, red is the sweetest, and green will have a slightly more bitter taste.

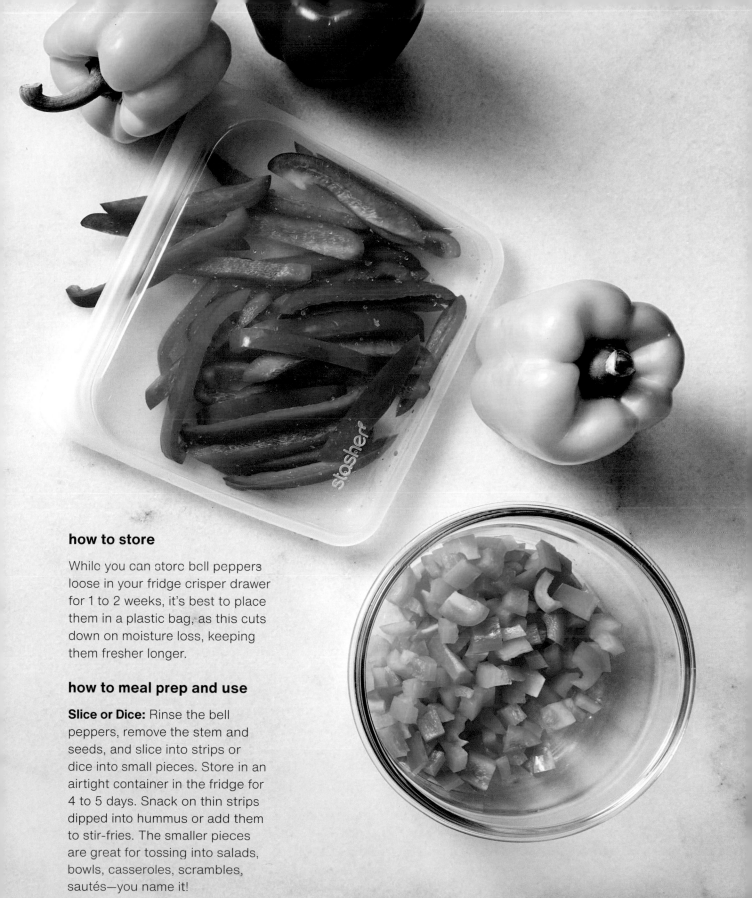

how to store

While you can store bell peppers loose in your fridge crisper drawer for 1 to 2 weeks, it's best to place them in a plastic bag, as this cuts down on moisture loss, keeping them fresher longer.

how to meal prep and use

Slice or Dice: Rinse the bell peppers, remove the stem and seeds, and slice into strips or dice into small pieces. Store in an airtight container in the fridge for 4 to 5 days. Snack on thin strips dipped into hummus or add them to stir-fries. The smaller pieces are great for tossing into salads, bowls, casseroles, scrambles, sautés—you name it!

broccoli

For multiple years running, broccoli has secured the spot as America's favorite vegetable (followed by corn and carrots, if you're curious). It's also brimming with vitamin C, fiber, and antioxidants. A cup of broccoli even has more vitamin C than an orange! That's why it's almost always prepped in one form or another in my fridge. And bonus: Broccoli rice is oh so sneaky—its smaller form goes virtually unnoticed in many recipes. Perfect for getting kids to eat more greens!

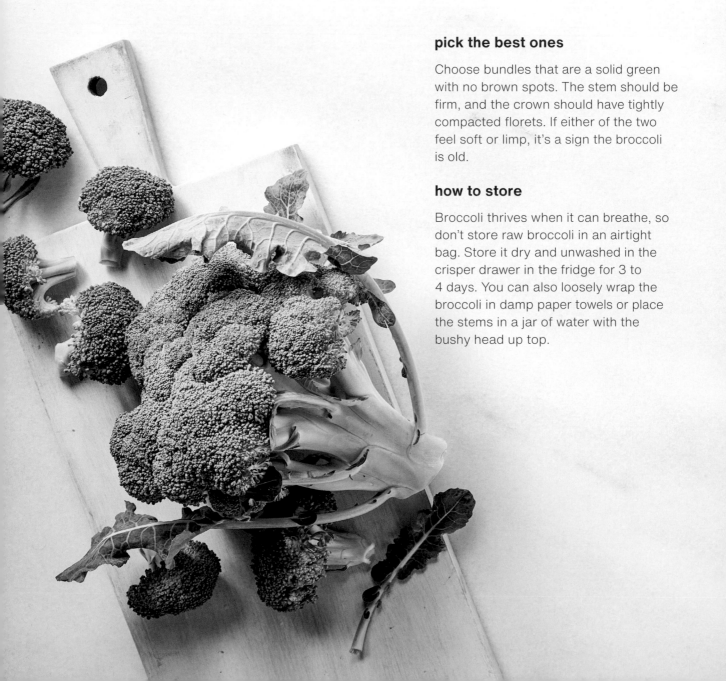

pick the best ones

Choose bundles that are a solid green with no brown spots. The stem should be firm, and the crown should have tightly compacted florets. If either of the two feel soft or limp, it's a sign the broccoli is old.

how to store

Broccoli thrives when it can breathe, so don't store raw broccoli in an airtight bag. Store it dry and unwashed in the crisper drawer in the fridge for 3 to 4 days. You can also loosely wrap the broccoli in damp paper towels or place the stems in a jar of water with the bushy head up top.

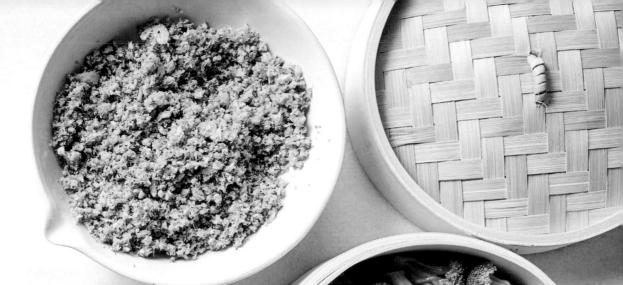

how to meal prep and use

Raw: Cut the broccoli florets into bite-size pieces and wash them in a colander. Store in an open bag or container, on top of a damp paper towel, for 4 to 5 days in the fridge. Raw florets make for a great healthy snack with a homemade dipping sauce, like Tzatziki (page 253).

Steam: Bring a pot filled with 1 inch (2.5cm) of water to a boil. Place a steamer insert in the pot and add the florets. Reduce the heat to medium, cover tightly with a lid, and steam for 5 to 6 minutes. Store in an airtight container in the fridge for 3 to 4 days. Enjoy cold or warm, add to a grain bowl with chicken and quinoa, or toss into a salad.

Roast: Preheat the oven to 425°F (220°C). On a baking sheet, toss the florets with olive oil, minced garlic, salt, and pepper. Spread them out into an even layer and bake for 20 minutes, until the edges are slightly crispy. Store in an airtight container in the fridge for 3 to 4 days. Make a green breakfast bowl with roasted broccoli, roasted sweet potatoes, avocado slices, red onion, and a poached egg.

Rice: Place the florets (and pieces of the stalk) in a food processor and pulse until they're broken up into tiny rice-size pieces. Quickly sauté for 3 to 4 minutes with olive oil, diced shallot, and garlic. Store in an airtight container in the fridge for 3 to 4 days. Add broccoli rice to breakfast scrambles or make broccoli fried rice with sautéed carrots, peas, garlic, ginger, green onions, eggs, salt, and pepper.

brussels sprouts

The key to enjoying Brussels sprouts is knowing how to cook them. Most of us remember eating bland and flavorless boiled sprouts as kids (and likely avoided them for years or decades after). But trust me, they're incredibly tasty when thinly shaved into a salad or roasted until the edges are crispy and caramelized. And if they remind you of baby cabbages, that's because they're both members of the brassicas family. They're loaded with fiber, vitamins, and minerals, similar to other cruciferous veggies.

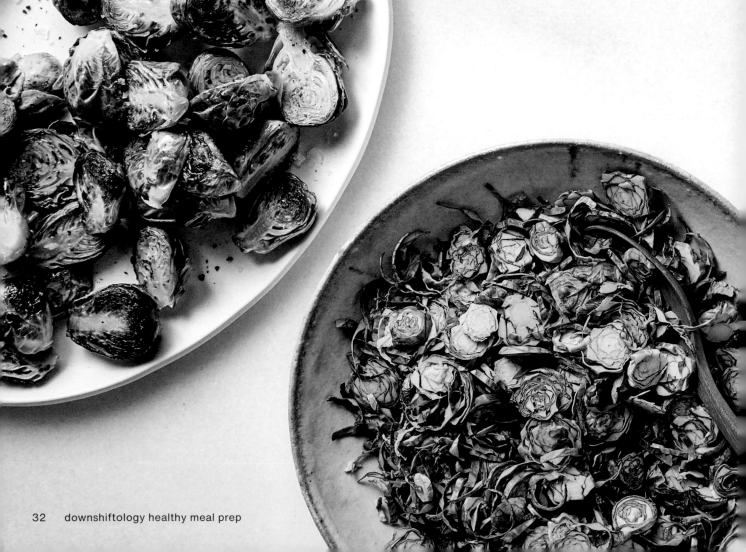

pick the best ones

Depending on the season, you can find Brussels sprouts on the stalk or loose, as individual sprouts. They'll stay fresh longer on the stalk, but if you can't find them that way, not to worry. Just make sure they're firm when you give them a squeeze with the leaves tightly compacted and bright green. Avoid any with yellowing or wilted leaves.

how to store

Store the sprouts loose or on the stalk in the crisper drawer of your fridge for about a week. If they're still on the stalk, stick the end of the stalk upright in water to keep them fresh even longer.

how to meal prep and use

Shave: Wash the sprouts, trim off the stem, and thinly slice with a knife or mandoline. Store in an airtight container in the fridge for 2 to 3 days. Make a shaved Brussels sprouts salad with sliced apples, cranberries, diced red onions, and a lemon vinaigrette, or mix them into a morning egg scramble for added greens.

Roast: Preheat the oven to 425°F (220°C). Cut off the ends of the sprouts and slice them in half. Place them and any loose leaves onto a baking sheet, and toss with olive oil, salt, and pepper. Roast for 25 to 30 minutes, until the edges are caramelized. Store in an airtight container in the fridge for 3 to 4 days, or in the freezer for up to 3 months. Enjoy alongside any protein option, such as pulled pork or chicken. You can also top them on a grain bowl with rice, roasted chickpeas, grated carrots, and diced avocado.

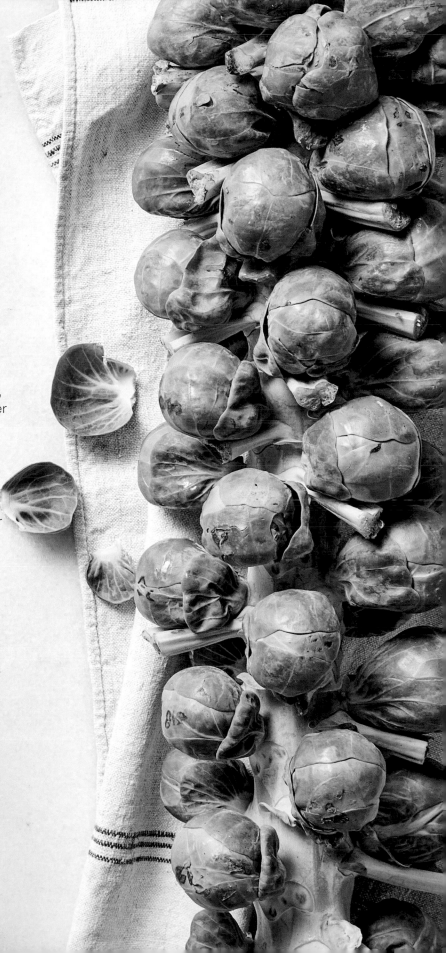

butternut squash

The beauty of winter squash is that it lasts a long time in your kitchen. In fact, its name refers to the length of time it can be stored (all winter long!), not that it grows in the winter. I love butternut squash for it's sweet, nutty, and buttery flavor. It becomes beautifully caramelized when roasted, though it's also great as a vegetable mash. It can be a bit intimidating to prep, but it does get easier with practice!

pick the best ones

Look for a squash that's a solid beige color and blemish-free. The outside should be hard and firm. If you feel any soft spots, it may be past its prime. It should also feel heavy for its size, which is also an indication of freshness.

how to store

Store in a dark, dry, cool part of your kitchen (such as your pantry or cupboard) for several months until you're ready to use it.

how to meal prep and use

Roast: With a vegetable peeler, peel the skin, cut the squash in half lengthwise, scoop out the seeds, then cut into small cubes. Preheat the oven to 400°F (200°C). On a baking sheet, toss the cubes with olive oil, salt, and pepper. Roast for 40 to 45 minutes, tossing the cubes halfway so all edges get caramelized. Store in an airtight container in the fridge for 3 to 4 days, or in the freezer for up to 3 months. Toss into a salad with leafy greens, chopped dates, crumbled goat cheese, and a drizzle of lemon vinaigrette. Add it to a grain bowl with wild rice, chopped kale, dried cranberries, and a drizzle of tahini sauce.

Mash: Peel the skin, cut it in half lengthwise, and scoop out the seeds. Preheat the oven to 400°F (200°C). Brush the inside with olive oil and season with salt and pepper. Place the squash cut side down on a baking sheet and roast for 40 to 45 minutes. Scoop out the flesh and mash with butter or a little milk. Store in an airtight container in the fridge for 3 to 4 days, or in the freezer for up to 3 months. Serve it up as a side dish to any protein option, just as you would mashed potatoes.

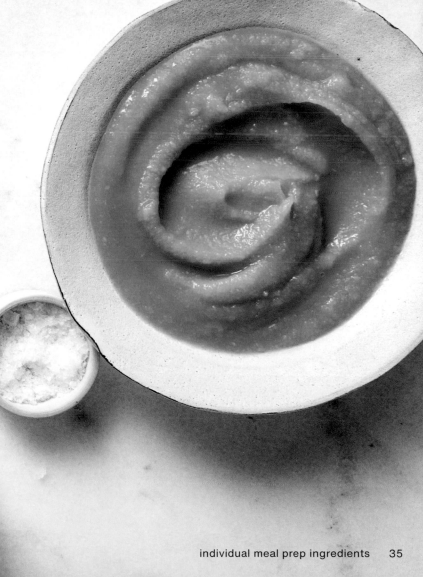

cabbage

A head of cabbage is humble, inexpensive, and a meal-prep winner, as it has a relatively long shelf life—it will keep in the fridge for several weeks. Translation: If you struggle with your veggies going bad before you can enjoy them, cabbage is your best friend. There are also several varieties of cabbage to choose from, including red, green, Napa, Savoy, and more. No matter which variety you choose, cabbage will add a delicious crunch to salads, tacos, and wraps. It can be sautéed until buttery soft and added to macro bowls or served up as a side dish. It really is the unsung hero of meal prep!

pick the best ones

Choose a cabbage that is large, firm, and fairly heavy for its size. Its leaves should be tightly compacted, showing a bright hue, especially the red ones. Just watch out for signs of cracking, bruising, or yellowing.

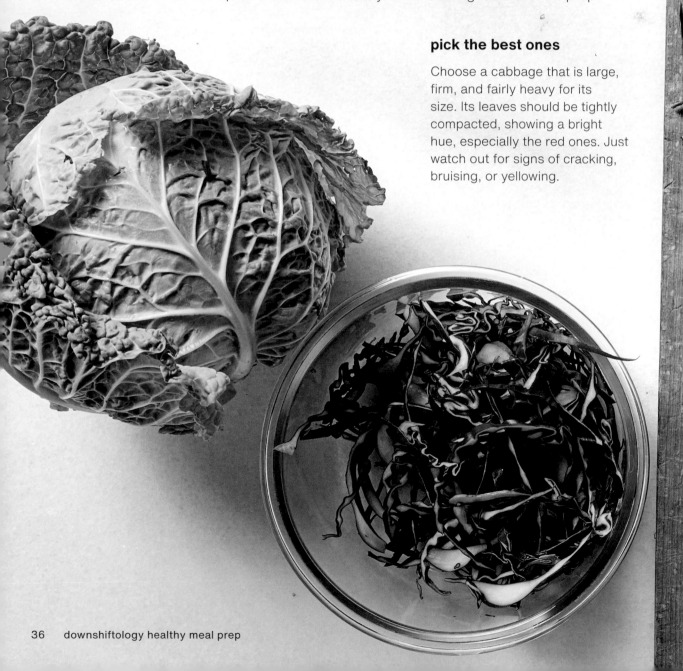

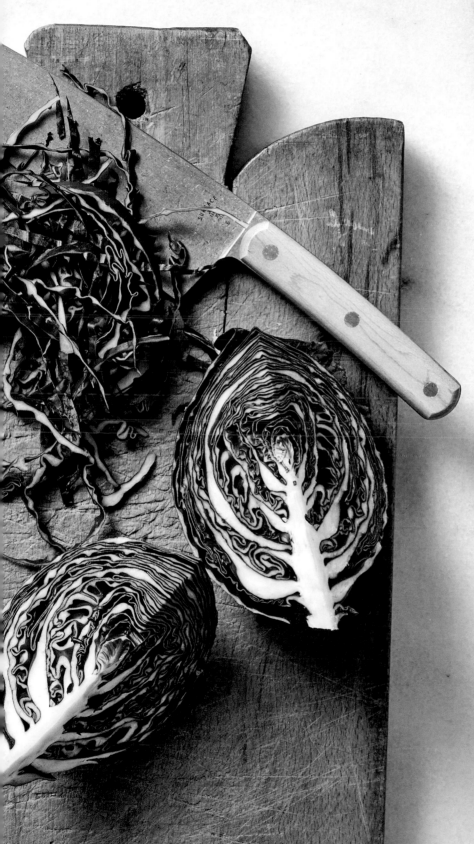

how to store

Store a whole cabbage in the crisper drawer in the fridge for up to 2 months; halved (or quartered), a cabbage will keep for several weeks in a bag.

how to meal prep and use

Shred: Chop the cabbage into quarters (through the stem), remove the core, then thinly shred with a knife. You can also use a spiralizer to create even, thin strips from a whole cabbage in an instant. Store in an airtight container in the fridge for 4 to 5 days. Toss it into a slaw with chopped bell peppers, shredded carrots, cilantro, green onions, and a sesame vinaigrette.

Sauté: Heat olive oil in a pan and sauté sliced onions for a minute or two. Add minced garlic, stir, then add shredded cabbage and sauté for 12 to 15 minutes, until soft and caramelized. Season with salt and pepper. You can also follow the recipe for Sautéed Red Cabbage on page 248. Store in an airtight container in the fridge for 4 to 5 days, or in the freezer for up to 3 months. Warm and enjoy as a side dish with baked salmon or add it to a ground beef stir-fry with a soy garlic sauce.

cauliflower

Cauliflower, like its cruciferous relative broccoli, is a powerhouse veggie with unique compounds that may reduce the risk of several diseases. It's incredibly versatile and naturally low in carbs and can easily be transformed into rice, hummus, sauces, steaks, and so much more. Some may say that cauliflower is a bit bland and boring, but I love to think of it as an adaptable base for building any number of flavor profiles. With some seasonings and aromatics, this veggie truly shines!

pick the best ones

Look for heads that are firm with packed florets. Make sure they are free of brown spots and show no signs of softness. Also, if the surrounding leaves are fresh, you've likely found a cauliflower that's been recently harvested.

how to store

Keep raw cauliflower loosely wrapped in a plastic bag in the crisper drawer in the fridge for 4 to 5 days. Before eating or cooking, just cut off the florets and give them a good rinse.

how to meal prep and use

Roast: Preheat the oven to 425°F (220°C). On a baking sheet, toss the cauliflower florets with olive oil, minced garlic, salt, and pepper. Spread them out into an even layer and bake for 20 minutes, until slightly crispy on the edges. Store in an airtight container in the fridge for 3 to 4 days, or in the freezer for up to 3 months. Layer into a tortilla with smashed black beans, green onions, avocado slices, pico de gallo, cotija cheese, and a squeeze of lime juice.

Mash: Bring a pot filled with 1 inch (2.5cm) of water to a simmer. Place a steamer insert in the pot and add the florets. Cover tightly with a lid and steam for 6 to 8 minutes. Meanwhile, sauté minced garlic in a little olive oil in a separate pan. Add the sautéed garlic and oil to the drained cauliflower, along with 1 to 2 teaspoons of finely chopped herbs, such as thyme, rosemary, and chives. Season with salt and pepper, then mash. Store in an airtight container in the fridge for 3 to 4 days, or in the freezer for up to 3 months. Add a dollop of butter and serve up the cauliflower as you would mashed potatoes.

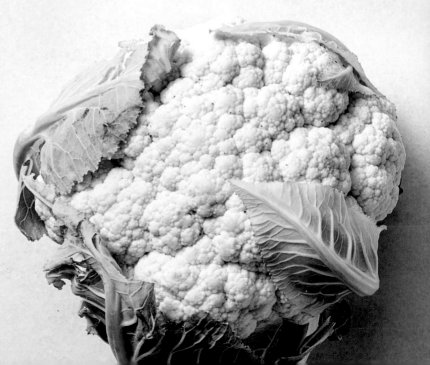

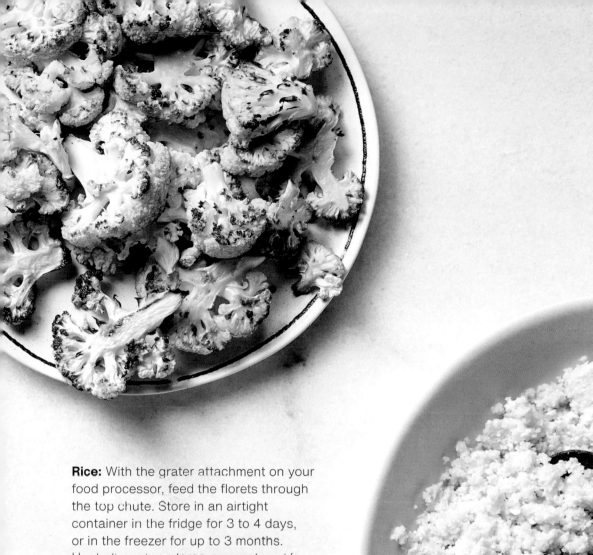

Rice: With the grater attachment on your food processor, feed the florets through the top chute. Store in an airtight container in the fridge for 3 to 4 days, or in the freezer for up to 3 months. Heat olive oil in a large pan and sauté diced onion for a few minutes, until translucent. Add the riced cauliflower to the pan and sauté for 5 to 7 minutes. Season with salt and pepper.

Freeze: Blanch florets in a pot of boiling water for 1 to 2 minutes. Chill in an ice-water bath, drain, and pre-freeze on a baking sheet for 1 to 2 hours. Once frozen, toss into a freezer bag. Store up to 3 months in the freezer. Toss into smoothies for a healthy veggie boost. The florets can also serve as a replacement for frozen bananas to help thicken smoothies.

carrots

In my quest to add more color to every meal, carrots have become a meal-prep regular. They're full of fiber, vitamin A, and beta-carotene (which imparts that lovely orange hue), and they're great for bone health, thanks to their calcium and vitamin K content. Carrots also have a natural sweetness, which makes them perfect for snacking raw, although I think they're extra delicious when roasted and slightly caramelized.

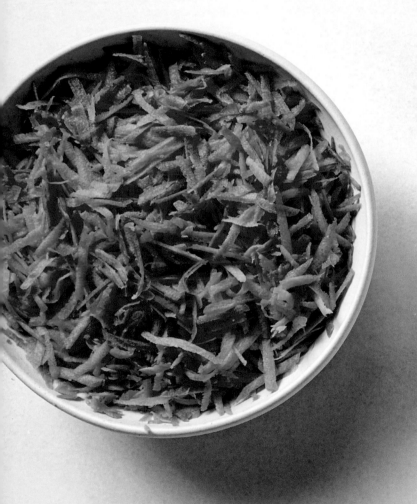

pick the best ones

Grab a bundle of carrots that have an even color throughout with no signs of deterioration toward the crown. And if you're buying ones with tops, make sure the greens are vibrant and strong, not wilted.

how to store

While the green tops are edible, make sure to trim them off before storing. The greens will continue to pull moisture out of the carrots until they're separated from the root. To store the greens, wrap them in a damp paper towel in a separate plastic bag. To store the carrots, fully submerge them in a container of water and store in the fridge for a week or more. Just replace the water every couple of days when it starts to look cloudy.

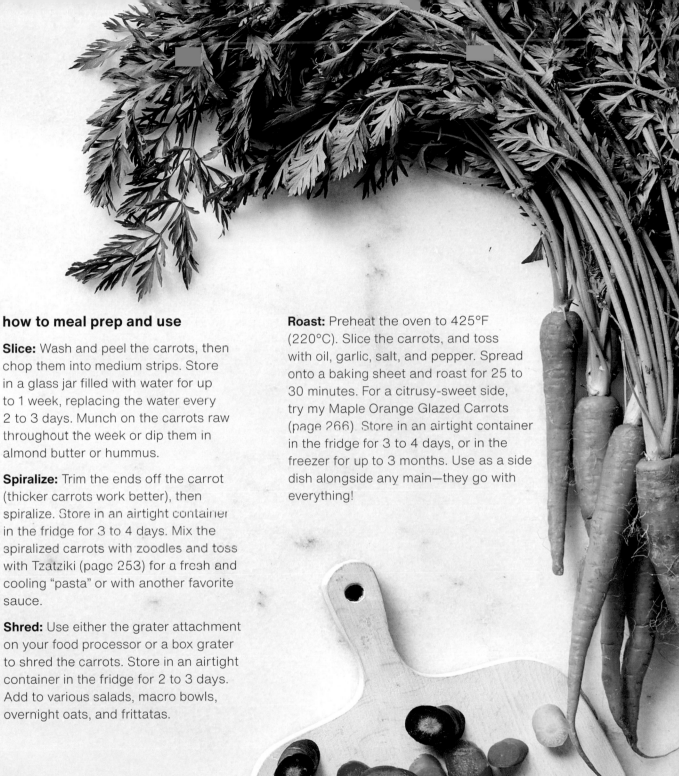

how to meal prep and use

Slice: Wash and peel the carrots, then chop them into medium strips. Store in a glass jar filled with water for up to 1 week, replacing the water every 2 to 3 days. Munch on the carrots raw throughout the week or dip them in almond butter or hummus.

Spiralize: Trim the ends off the carrot (thicker carrots work better), then spiralize. Store in an airtight container in the fridge for 3 to 4 days. Mix the spiralized carrots with zoodles and toss with Tzatziki (page 253) for a fresh and cooling "pasta" or with another favorite sauce.

Shred: Use either the grater attachment on your food processor or a box grater to shred the carrots. Store in an airtight container in the fridge for 2 to 3 days. Add to various salads, macro bowls, overnight oats, and frittatas.

Roast: Preheat the oven to 425°F (220°C). Slice the carrots, and toss with oil, garlic, salt, and pepper. Spread onto a baking sheet and roast for 25 to 30 minutes. For a citrusy-sweet side, try my Maple Orange Glazed Carrots (page 266). Store in an airtight container in the fridge for 3 to 4 days, or in the freezer for up to 3 months. Use as a side dish alongside any main—they go with everything!

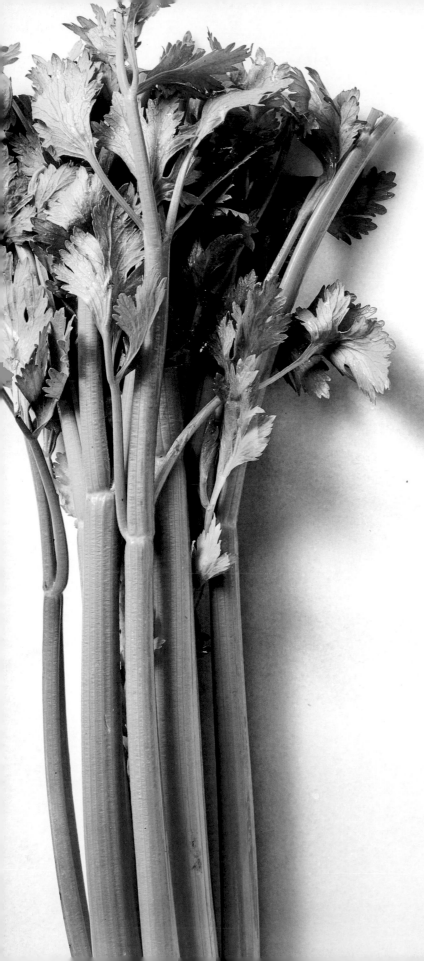

celery

Light and crisp, celery is an easy ingredient to grab when you're in need of a refreshing snack. Celery is also a key ingredient in mirepoix soup bases, casseroles, and, of course, tuna salad—it's a great flavor enhancer! But if you find yourself using a few ribs of celery, then wondering how to store the rest before they go limp, I've got you covered.

pick the best ones

For the freshest celery, choose firm, bright green ribs that are tightly packed. The greener the celery, the more intense the flavor! Watch out for any bunches that have wilted leaves, soft spots, or show signs of yellowing. If you really want to get creative, buy celery with the leaves still attached, then pick them off and use them as you would tender herbs or dry them for later use in dishes like stews.

how to store

Ditch the plastic supermarket bag (which promotes spoilage) and wrap the celery in damp paper towels before wrapping again in aluminum foil—this will lock in moisture. Store in the crisper drawer in the fridge for 1 to 2 weeks.

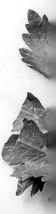

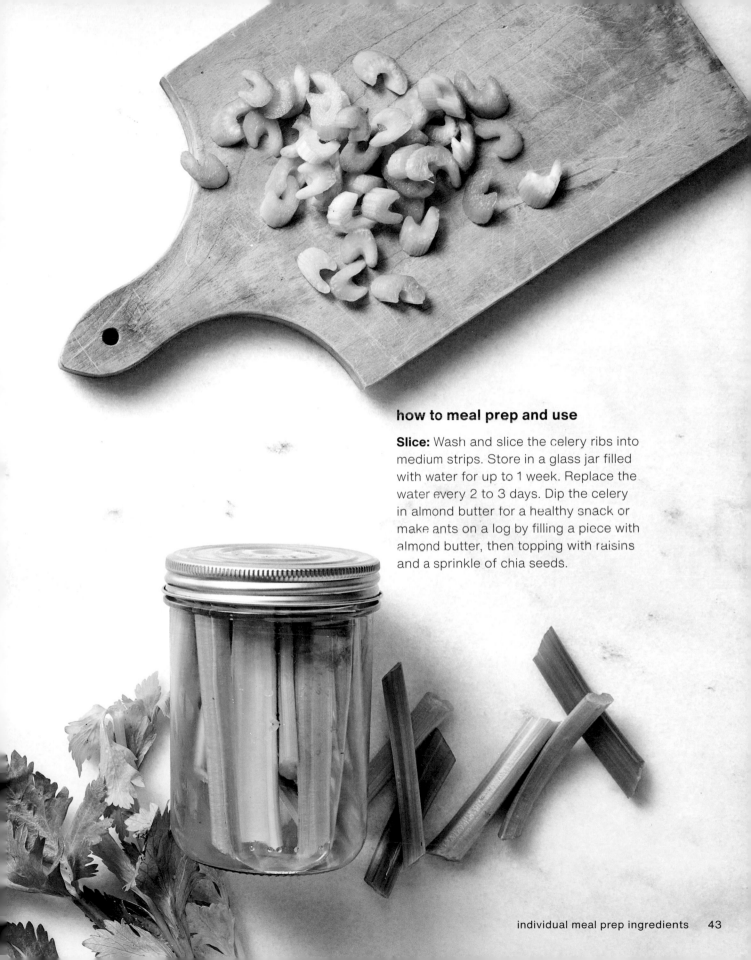

how to meal prep and use

Slice: Wash and slice the celery ribs into medium strips. Store in a glass jar filled with water for up to 1 week. Replace the water every 2 to 3 days. Dip the celery in almond butter for a healthy snack or make ants on a log by filling a piece with almond butter, then topping with raisins and a sprinkle of chia seeds.

cucumber

Cucumbers, whether they're garden cucumbers, English cucumbers, or Persian cucumbers, are known for their crisp, refreshing crunch. They're exceptionally hydrating, and during the summer months they take center stage on crudités platters, in garden-fresh salads, and in veggie wraps. But when they're not stored properly, they can become limp and lackluster in the fridge and lose their excellent snappy texture. So here's how to keep your cukes perfectly crunchy!

pick the best ones

Look for unblemished cucumbers, avoiding those with browning or soft spots, which are an indication that the cucumber is overripe or starting to rot. You may have to take an extra-close look if the cucumber is wrapped in plastic.

how to store

Garden cucumbers are generally coated in a food-grade wax, which allows them to keep in the crisper drawer in the fridge for up to a week. If you buy English cucumbers, remove the plastic wrap, then give them a rinse. Persian cucumbers usually have no coating or wrap, so just rinse them. Once clean, wrap the cukes in dry paper towels to absorb moisture, then tuck them whole into an open plastic bag. They'll stay good for up to a week in the crisper drawer in the fridge.

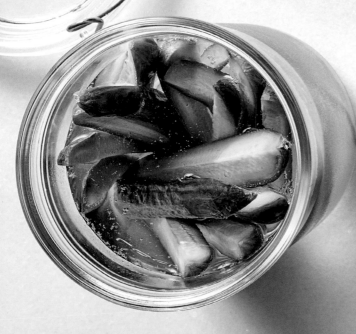

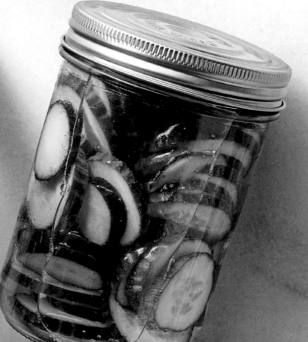

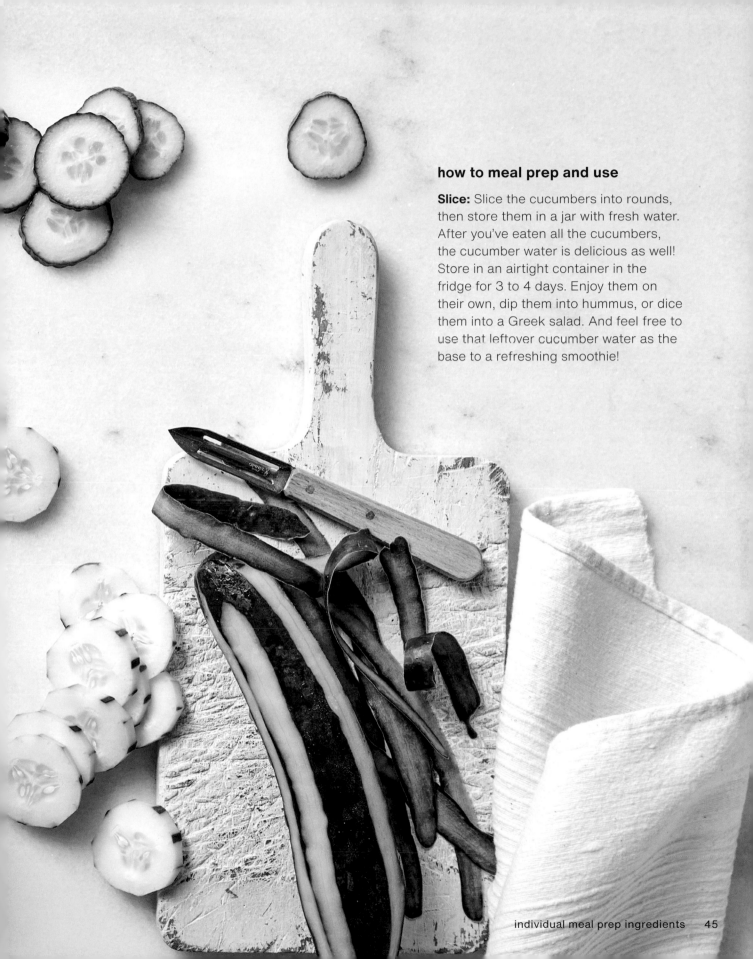

how to meal prep and use

Slice: Slice the cucumbers into rounds, then store them in a jar with fresh water. After you've eaten all the cucumbers, the cucumber water is delicious as well! Store in an airtight container in the fridge for 3 to 4 days. Enjoy them on their own, dip them into hummus, or dice them into a Greek salad. And feel free to use that leftover cucumber water as the base to a refreshing smoothie!

garlic

"I love garlic" is an understatement. It's my holy grail allium vegetable that I add to almost everything and anything. Aside from its irresistibly pungent yet mildly nutty taste, it's my favorite anti-inflammatory ingredient and immunity booster. In other words, it's a good idea to keep peeled and pureed garlic ready to go!

pick the best ones

Give the bulbs a light squeeze to make sure none of the cloves are soft or dry. They should feel firm for the most part. If they're sprouting, they're getting old.

how to store

As with onions, keep your bulbs stored in your pantry or other cool, dry place so they don't rot or sprout from any direct sunlight. They'll keep for weeks this way.

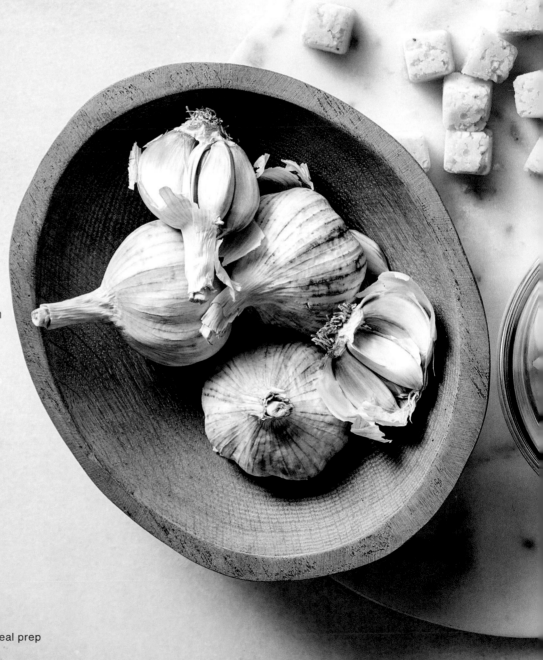

how to meal prep and use

Whole Peeled: Remove the individual cloves from the head and peel them. To expedite the peeling process, add the cloves to a cocktail shaker or jar with tight-fitting lid and shake vigorously. The skin should come right off! Store in an airtight container in the fridge for up to 1 week, or in the freezer for up to 3 months (note that the texture will be a bit more spongy when frozen and thawed). Mince or chop them straight into sautés without having to worry about peeling them.

Frozen Puree: Peel a whole bunch of individual cloves, place them in a food processor, and blend into a puree. Use a cookie scoop to mound them on a sheet pan or place them in a small ice cube tray, then freeze. Once firm, transfer them to an airtight container in the freezer and store for up to 3 months. No need to thaw before using, just add them straight to whatever you're making!

kale

Kale has a stellar reputation for being one of the healthiest greens. And good news—that reputation is well deserved as it truly is one of the most nutrient-dense plant foods out there. But what you may not know is that kale is a cruciferous vegetable—yes, it's a sibling to cabbage, broccoli, cauliflower, and Brussels sprouts. In terms of taste, opinions vary widely. Some love this hearty green, while others think its strong earthy flavor is too bitter. If you fall into that latter category, remember that tossing roughly chopped kale into cozy soups and quick sautés will mute its flavor while still giving you a hefty dose of antioxidants and vitamins.

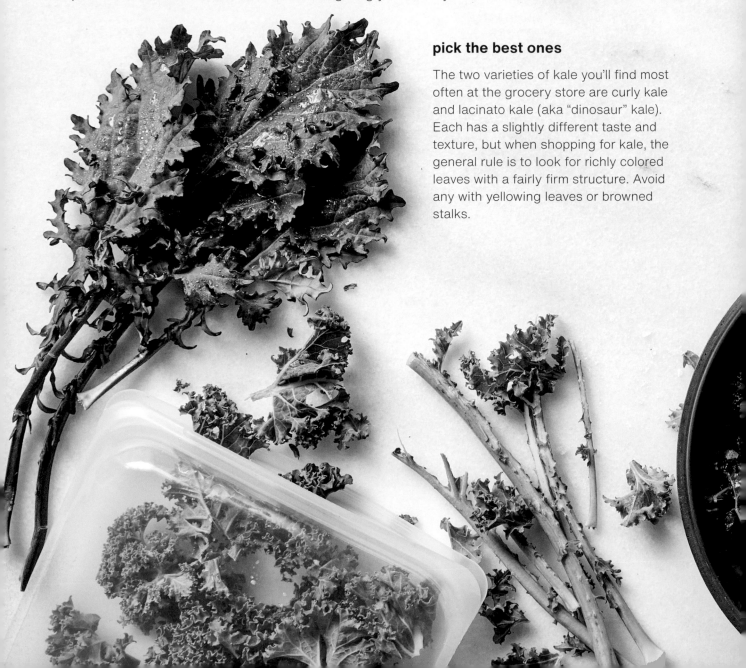

pick the best ones

The two varieties of kale you'll find most often at the grocery store are curly kale and lacinato kale (aka "dinosaur" kale). Each has a slightly different taste and texture, but when shopping for kale, the general rule is to look for richly colored leaves with a fairly firm structure. Avoid any with yellowing leaves or browned stalks.

how to store

Kale is a sensitive green that will last longest if you keep it dry and away from moisture. I recommend wrapping it in some paper towels, then placing it in a bag in the crisper drawer in your fridge. It will keep up to a week.

how to meal prep and use

Chop: Remove the leaves from the stem, then chop them into smaller pieces before storing raw. Just remember to give the kale a good rinse in a colander before using it. Store in an airtight container in the fridge for 3 to 4 days. Think of this as your own version of packaged chopped kale. Make a salad out of it or add it to almost any meal for an extra veggie boost.

Sauté: Heat olive oil in a pan, add minced garlic, and sauté for 30 seconds. Add chopped kale and sauté it until slightly wilted, about 5 minutes. Season with salt and pepper. Store in an airtight container in the fridge for 3 to 4 days. Add it to a loaded protein bowl, eat it with a breakfast plate topped with fried eggs, or enjoy it as a power-packed side dish to a meaty main.

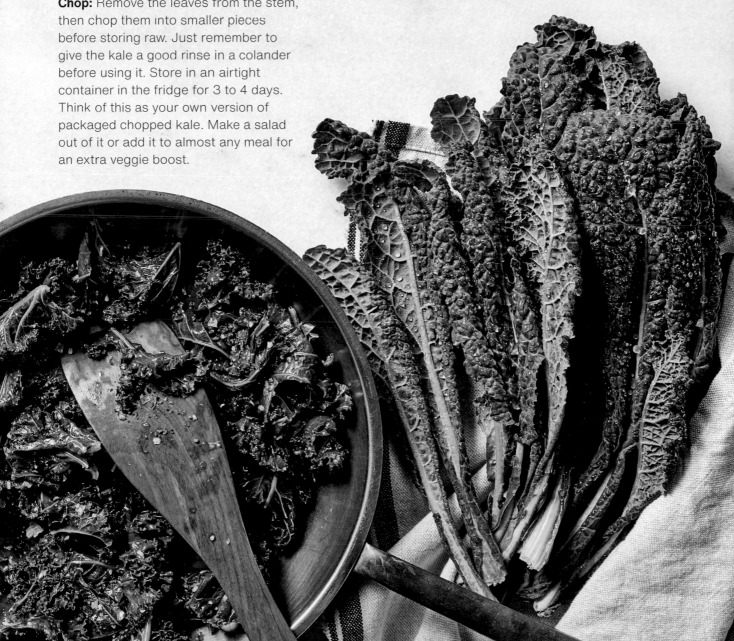

onions & shallots

If you follow me on YouTube, you know that I *always* cry when chopping onions. It's a given—tears are just going to stream down my face! Although I've tried many tips and tricks over the years, I find the best solution is to simply meal prep onions ahead of time (that way I have to cry only once a week). Diced onions last for up to a week in the fridge, which means I can easily add them to breakfast, lunch, and dinner throughout the week.

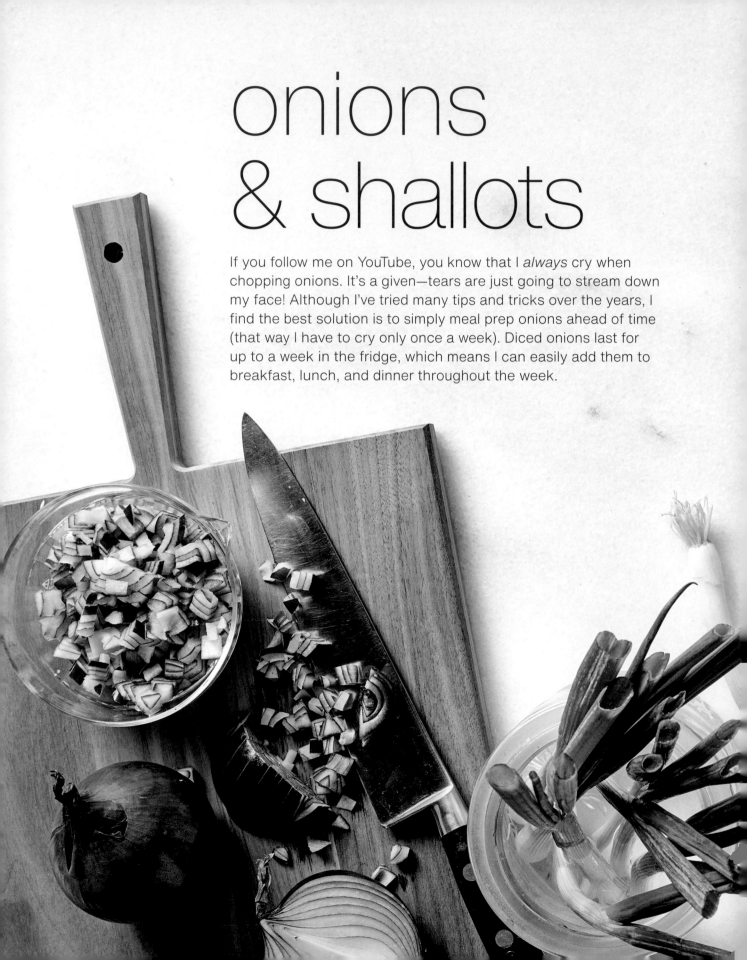

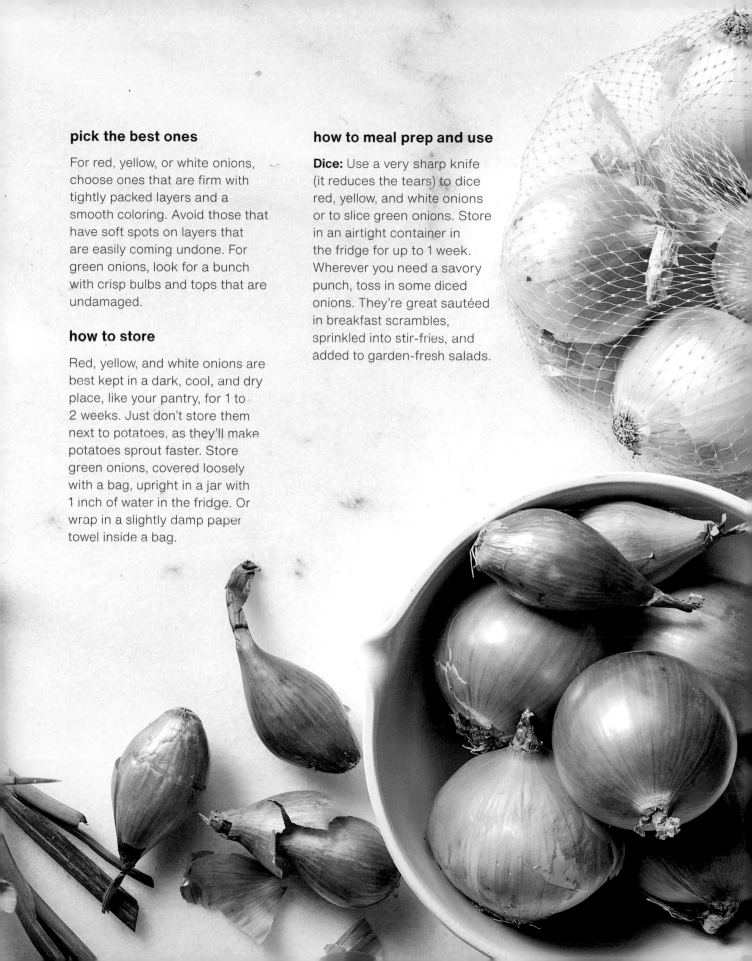

pick the best ones

For red, yellow, or white onions, choose ones that are firm with tightly packed layers and a smooth coloring. Avoid those that have soft spots on layers that are easily coming undone. For green onions, look for a bunch with crisp bulbs and tops that are undamaged.

how to store

Red, yellow, and white onions are best kept in a dark, cool, and dry place, like your pantry, for 1 to 2 weeks. Just don't store them next to potatoes, as they'll make potatoes sprout faster. Store green onions, covered loosely with a bag, upright in a jar with 1 inch of water in the fridge. Or wrap in a slightly damp paper towel inside a bag.

how to meal prep and use

Dice: Use a very sharp knife (it reduces the tears) to dice red, yellow, and white onions or to slice green onions. Store in an airtight container in the fridge for up to 1 week. Wherever you need a savory punch, toss in some diced onions. They're great sautéed in breakfast scrambles, sprinkled into stir-fries, and added to garden-fresh salads.

spaghetti squash

While I have no problem with carbs, I do try to avoid the processed ones (like store-bought gluten-free spaghetti) as much as possible. And what's the best way to do that? Swap in veggies! Spiralized veggies are a great spaghetti replacement, but Mother Nature created a veggie that needs no spiralizer—spaghetti squash! After a pop in the oven, spaghetti squash magically turns into delicate, angel hair–like pasta strands that are low in calories and contain a ton of fiber and vitamins. It may not fool you completely, but its impressive nutritional profile will one-up any type of store-bought noodle.

pick the best ones

Choose a spaghetti squash that's a uniform yellow color and heavy for its size. Avoid any that have cracks or soft spots, are extra shiny (which means it was likely picked too early), or don't have a stem.

how to store

Like most winter squash, they're best kept in cool and dry places, such as your pantry, for up to 2 months.

how to meal prep and use

Roast: Preheat your oven to 400°F (200°C). Slice the squash in half lengthwise and scoop out the seeds. Coat the inside with olive oil, salt, and pepper, then roast cut side down on a baking sheet for 35 to 45 minutes. Let it cool slightly before using a fork to scrape and fluff the insides to create long, thin strands. Store the stands in an airtight container in the fridge for 3 to 4 days. You can also freeze it! If freezing, it's best to first drain the squash "noodles" in a colander over a bowl for several hours in the fridge, to remove extra moisture before freezing. Sauté it with kale, garlic, and toasted pine nuts for an abundant side dish. Looking for a main? Use it as a pasta replacement and top with a Bolognese sauce.

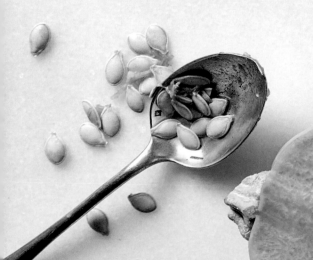

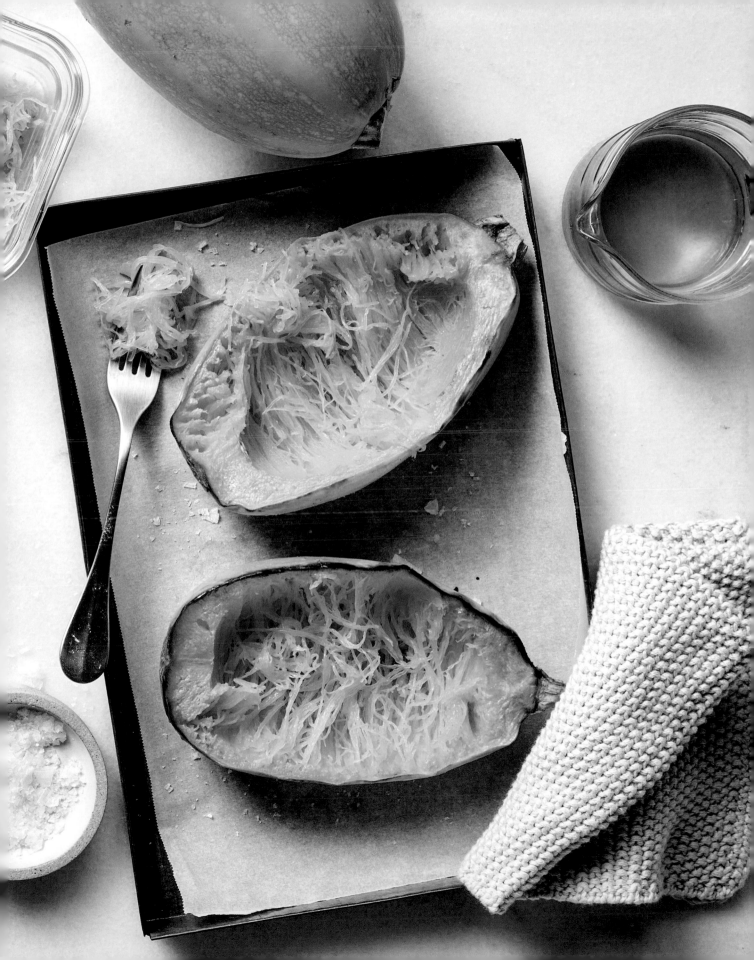

sweet potatoes

Don't get me wrong, I'm a lover of all sorts of potatoes. But a spud that's abundant in nutrients, is ultra-creamy, and has a hint of sweetness? Count me in! Sweet potatoes have a natural carb-y coziness to them (especially during the fall and winter months), and they're incredibly versatile in a wide variety of recipes. So grab a bunch and feel free to roast, spiralize, or mash them—no matter which cooking method you choose, they're sure to fill you up and add a welcome pop of orange to any meal.

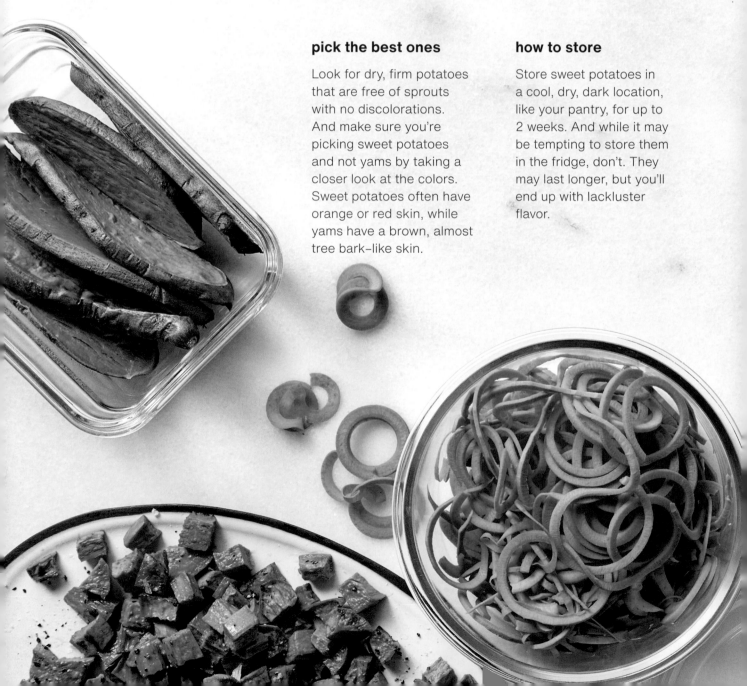

pick the best ones

Look for dry, firm potatoes that are free of sprouts with no discolorations. And make sure you're picking sweet potatoes and not yams by taking a closer look at the colors. Sweet potatoes often have orange or red skin, while yams have a brown, almost tree bark–like skin.

how to store

Store sweet potatoes in a cool, dry, dark location, like your pantry, for up to 2 weeks. And while it may be tempting to store them in the fridge, don't. They may last longer, but you'll end up with lackluster flavor.

how to meal prep and use

Spiralize: Peel the sweet potato, slice a little bit off each end to create a flat surface, then spiralize. Store in an airtight container in the fridge for 4 to 5 days. These hearty noodles can be cooked into egg nests, tossed in a warm salad, or even baked into a casserole (see page 214).

Roast: Preheat the oven to 425°F (220°C). Peel and cut the potatoes into ½-inch (1.3cm) cubes and toss them with olive oil and spices on a baking sheet. Roast for 30 minutes, or until the edges are caramelized. Store in an airtight container in the fridge for 4 to 5 days. Toss into a breakfast hash with scrambled eggs and leafy greens; whip up sweet potato tacos with shredded cabbage, guacamole, and cilantro; or layer in a hefty salad with kale, black beans, and avocado.

Mash: Peel the potatoes, dice into chunks, and cook in a pot of boiling water for 20 to 30 minutes. Drain and place in a large bowl. Season with salt and pepper, add butter and milk for an extra-creamy texture, and then mash. Store in an airtight container in the fridge for 3 to 4 days, or in the freezer for up to 3 months. Serve as a creamy side to chicken, steak, or pork. They're also a great holiday side to accompany turkey or baked ham.

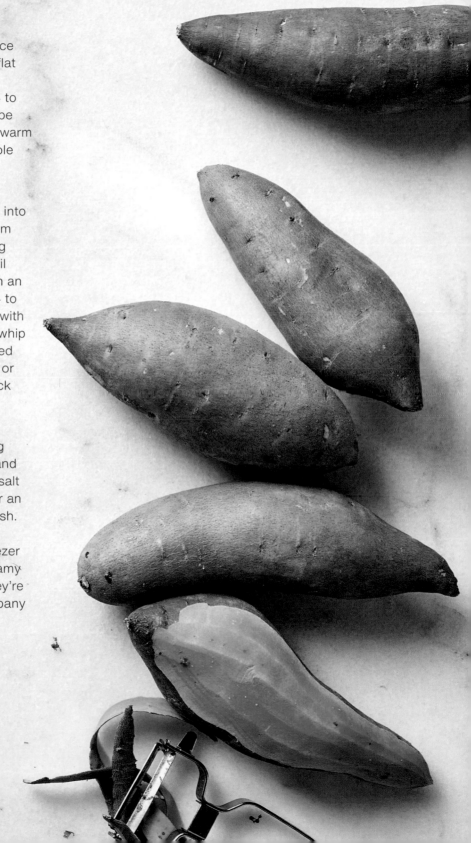

zucchini

If there's one thing to know about me, it's that my love for zucchini *runs deep*. Zucchini is one of the most versatile vegetables (you can bake it, grill it, spiralize it, and blend it), it's hydrating (with a 95 percent water content), and it can miraculously replace pasta in so many dishes (swap zoodles in for spaghetti and long, thin slices of zucchini for pasta sheets). With its mild flavor, it really lets other ingredients shine, making it the undisputed champ when you're looking for a stealth veggie to sneak into a wide variety of recipes.

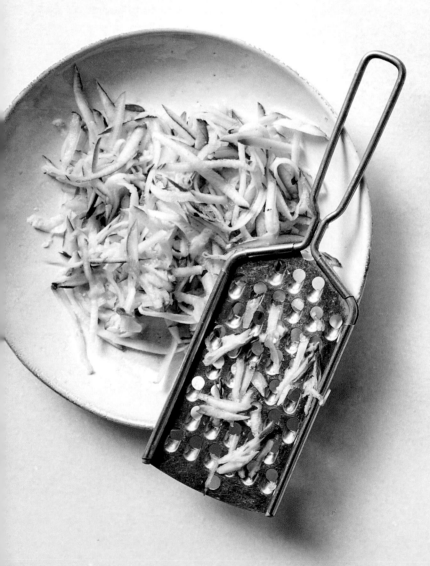

pick the best ones

Zucchini can grow to be gargantuan, but bigger is not always better. Those extra-large ones have more seeds and more moisture and will spoil more quickly. Younger zucchini is naturally sweeter, has thinner skin, and is better for meal prep. Look for zucchini that is bright green with no blemishes, about 6 inches long and 1 to 2 inches in diameter.

how to store

Store zucchini dry and unwashed in your fridge crisper drawer. If it's in a bag, make sure one end of the bag is open to promote circulation, as the key to keeping it fresh is keeping it dry. You can even pat it down with a paper towel to remove any extra moisture. Zucchini will last about a week in the fridge before it starts to shrivel and go bad.

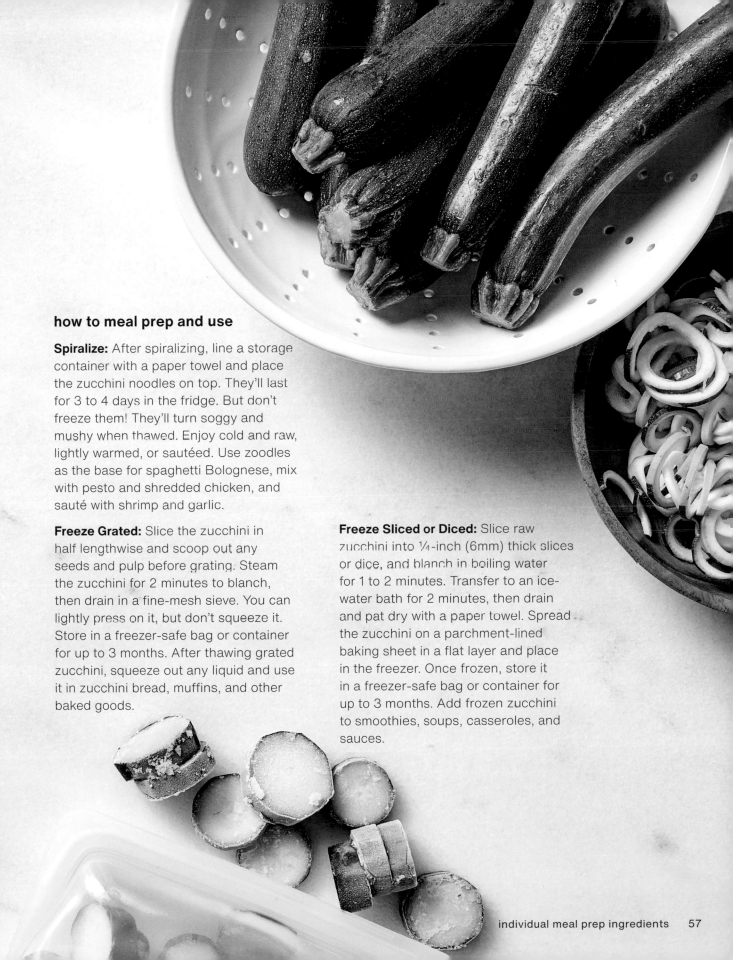

how to meal prep and use

Spiralize: After spiralizing, line a storage container with a paper towel and place the zucchini noodles on top. They'll last for 3 to 4 days in the fridge. But don't freeze them! They'll turn soggy and mushy when thawed. Enjoy cold and raw, lightly warmed, or sautéed. Use zoodles as the base for spaghetti Bolognese, mix with pesto and shredded chicken, and sauté with shrimp and garlic.

Freeze Grated: Slice the zucchini in half lengthwise and scoop out any seeds and pulp before grating. Steam the zucchini for 2 minutes to blanch, then drain in a fine-mesh sieve. You can lightly press on it, but don't squeeze it. Store in a freezer-safe bag or container for up to 3 months. After thawing grated zucchini, squeeze out any liquid and use it in zucchini bread, muffins, and other baked goods.

Freeze Sliced or Diced: Slice raw zucchini into ¼-inch (6mm) thick slices or dice, and blanch in boiling water for 1 to 2 minutes. Transfer to an ice-water bath for 2 minutes, then drain and pat dry with a paper towel. Spread the zucchini on a parchment-lined baking sheet in a flat layer and place in the freezer. Once frozen, store it in a freezer-safe bag or container for up to 3 months. Add frozen zucchini to smoothies, soups, casseroles, and sauces.

herbs

If there's one ingredient that I can't live without, it's fresh herbs. Not only do their green leaves elevate any meal's presentation, but their concentrated flavor—even just a tablespoon or two!—also makes everything taste *extra* special. What's more, herbs are rich in anti-inflammatory and antioxidant properties thanks to polyphenols (compounds with remarkable health benefits).

As you're cooking through the recipes in this book, pay close attention to how each herb is used. The more you use them, the more you'll know when and where to add one, two, or even a combination of herbs to create sensational meals. The only drawback with fresh herbs? They can wilt, brown, and go slimy-yuck if not stored properly. So here's a few tips for helping fresh herbs extend their shelf life—and these tips apply to bunches purchased at the market or just snipped from your garden.

tender herbs

These have soft leaves and stems and are more fragile than woody herbs. They work great as garnishes and are usually added toward the end stage of a recipe because of their delicate nature. These include basil, cilantro, chives, dill, mint, and tarragon.

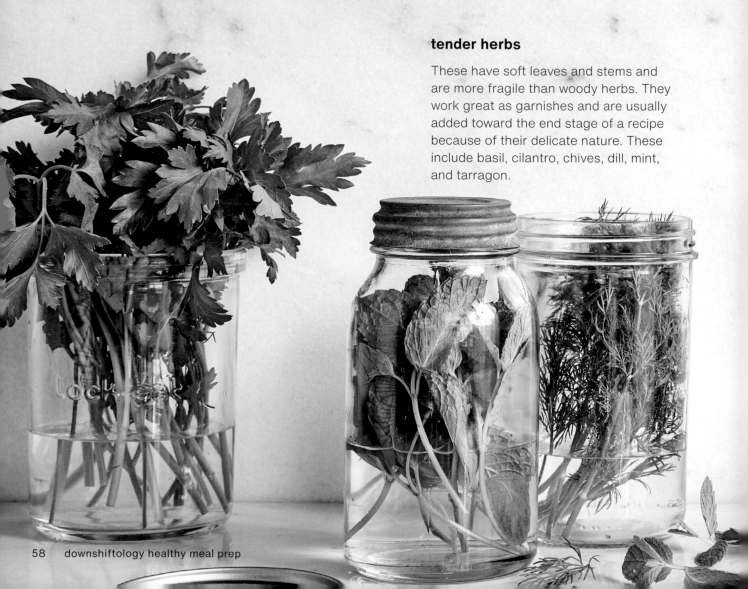

How to Store: Lightly rinse tender herbs, then spin them dry in a salad spinner or gently blot them with a paper towel. Trim the ends, remove any wilted leaves, and place them in a jar with 1 inch (2.5 cm) of water (like a bouquet of flowers). If your jar isn't tall, loosely cover the leaves poking out of the top with a plastic bag. If using a taller jar, simply screw on the lid, then place the herbs in the fridge (except basil—basil is best stored on the counter at room temperature). Trim the stems occasionally and change the water every few days. They'll stay good for 2 to 3 weeks.

woody herbs

These have tougher stems and are more hardy. They're typically added earlier in the cooking process so they can infuse meals, and depending on the recipe, they may even be removed before serving (like bay leaves from a pot of soup). They include bay leaves, marjoram, oregano, rosemary, sage, and thyme.

How to Store: Lightly rinse woody herbs, then spin them dry in a salad spinner or gently blot them with a paper towel. Loosely roll them up on a clean paper towel and place them in a silicone or plastic bag. Store in the fridge, where they'll keep for 2 to 3 weeks.

substituting dry herbs for fresh herbs

Dried herbs work best in foods that are cooked; they're not great in salads or used as garnishes. Because dried herbs are more potent than fresh herbs, you'll need to use less of them—about a third of the amount. So, for reference, 1 tablespoon fresh herbs = 1 teaspoon dried herbs.

freezing fresh herbs

One of my favorite kitchen hacks is to chop up fresh herbs and freeze them in an ice cube tray with a little bit of olive oil or butter. You can make herb blends and even add minced garlic, salt, and pepper for a homemade compound butter. The oil and butter help preserve the herb flavor, and these cubes make cooking a breeze. Just add them to mashed potatoes and veggies, or top them on a perfectly cooked steak.

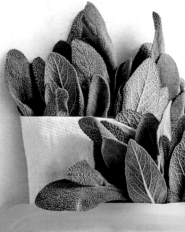

grains & pulses

Pantry staples like rice, lentils, and black beans are not only shelf stable (which means you likely have them on hand), they're also cost effective and a great way to bulk up healthy meals. Grains make for solid, adaptable bases, such as quinoa bowls with roasted veggies. I love to let a bed of rice soak up all the savory goodness from saucy mains. Pulses, such as chickpeas, lentils, and beans, on the other hand, are mighty sources of protein and fiber, which help keep you nice and full. Simply add black beans to a quick-and-easy taco salad, or serve white beans with shredded chicken, roasted sweet potato, and massaged kale in a power bowl.

how to meal prep and store grains

Once cooked, spread out the grains on a large, rimmed baking sheet so that they cool faster (this is key to prevent bacteria from forming). When they are completely cool, pack them in airtight containers. Grains will stay good in the fridge for 3 to 4 days, or in the freezer for up to 3 months.

how to meal prep and store pulses

Once cooked and drained, cool completely, then store in an airtight container in the fridge for 4 to 5 days, or in the freezer for up to 3 months. If you prefer using canned beans and lentils, simply rinse and drain them, then store in an airtight container.

how to use frozen grains and pulses

Good news—the texture of previously frozen grains and pulses is nearly identical to just cooked! Thaw grains and pulses in the fridge overnight for quick reheating, or you can add them frozen to stir-fries, curries, and soups!

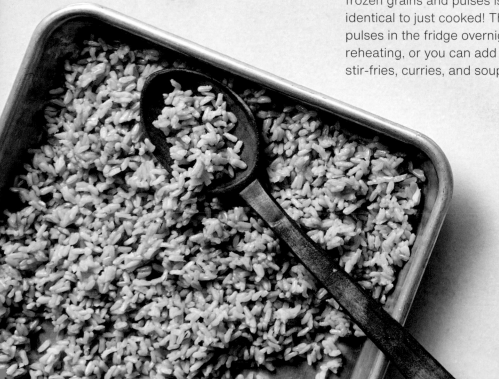
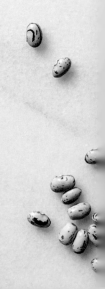

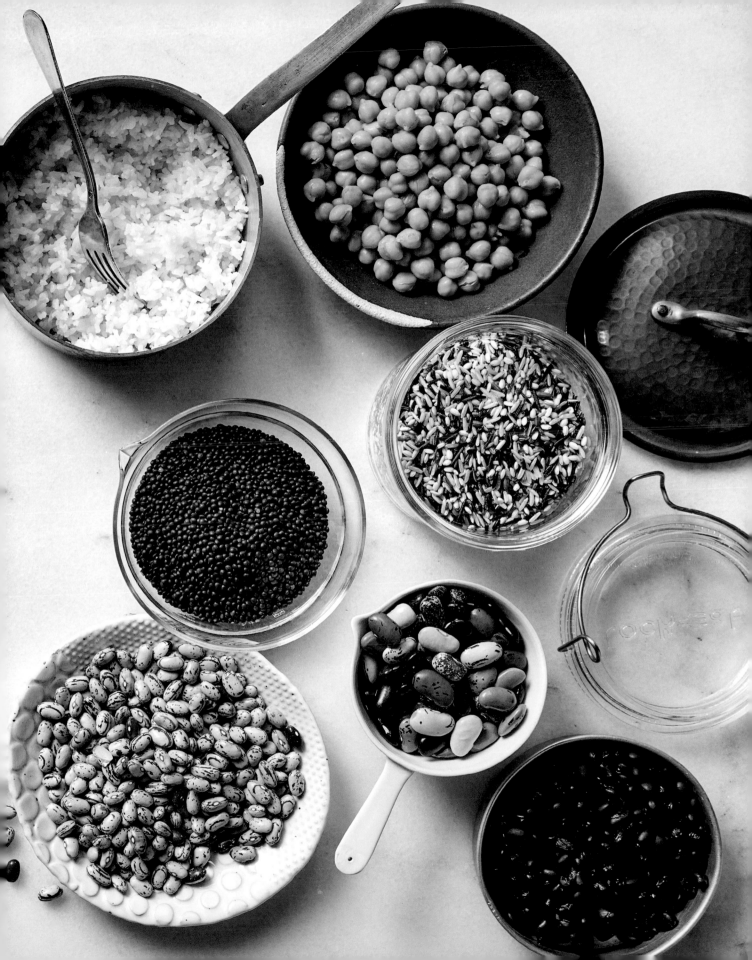

meat & seafood

Let's be honest, boneless skinless chicken breasts are often considered the default meal-prep protein, but it's certainly not the only meaty protein you can cook ahead of time and store. Juicy pulled pork is a personal favorite for topping on grain bowls, leafy green salads, and sautéing into a breakfast hash. Ground beef is astonishingly versatile and often underrated as a meal-prep option, and yes, you can even pre-cook salmon, shrimp, and other seafood (though there are a few tricks).

Any animal protein—such as chicken, turkey, beef, pork, fish, and shrimp—can be cooked simply with just a little seasoning or dry rub, knowing that you'll combine it with sauces, dressings, and a rainbow of ingredients in the future.

how to select

I always recommend purchasing the best-quality meat, seafood, and eggs that your budget allows. I steer clear of anything factory farmed and opt instead for pastured, grass-fed, and hormone- and antibiotic-free options. Meat from grass-fed animals is not only leaner with a more robust nutrient profile (way more beneficial omega-3s), it also just tastes better! Similar health benefits can be found in wild-caught seafood, which is why I try to avoid farmed fish and shrimp. Most farmed seafood has been raised in high-density aquaculture tanks and is doused with antibiotics, pesticides, and other contaminants, which is not great for you or the environment.

how to store

In general, cooked meat and seafood will last 3 to 4 days in the fridge, and up to 3 months in the freezer, in an airtight container. If the protein is in a soup or stew, it may last an extra day or so in the fridge, but learn to trust your nose and taste buds. If something smells or tastes funky, throw it out.

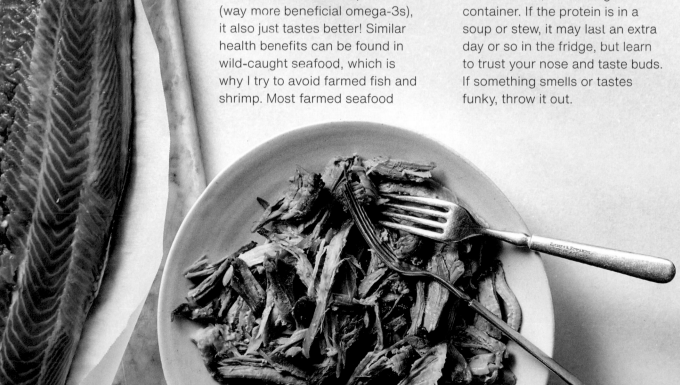

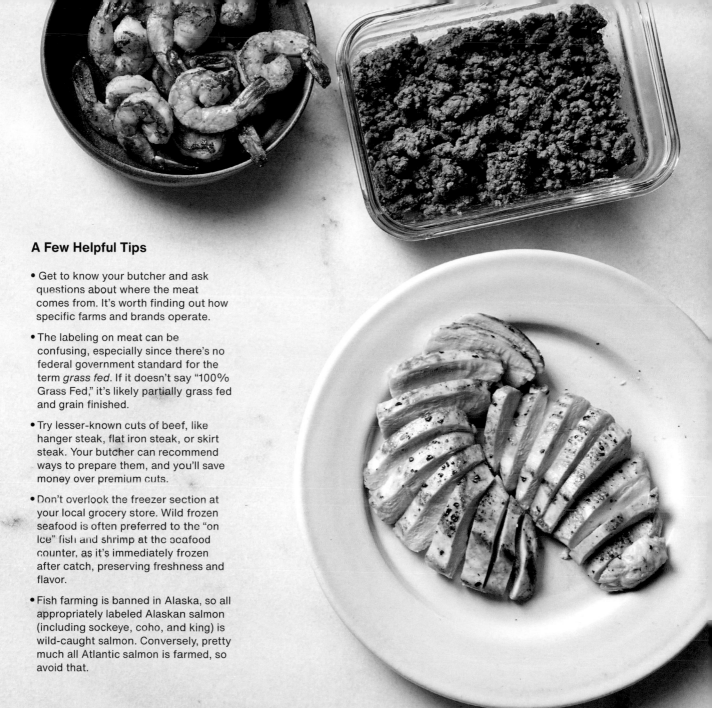

A Few Helpful Tips

- Get to know your butcher and ask questions about where the meat comes from. It's worth finding out how specific farms and brands operate.

- The labeling on meat can be confusing, especially since there's no federal government standard for the term *grass fed*. If it doesn't say "100% Grass Fed," it's likely partially grass fed and grain finished.

- Try lesser-known cuts of beef, like hanger steak, flat iron steak, or skirt steak. Your butcher can recommend ways to prepare them, and you'll save money over premium cuts.

- Don't overlook the freezer section at your local grocery store. Wild frozen seafood is often preferred to the "on ice" fish and shrimp at the seafood counter, as it's immediately frozen after catch, preserving freshness and flavor.

- Fish farming is banned in Alaska, so all appropriately labeled Alaskan salmon (including sockeye, coho, and king) is wild-caught salmon. Conversely, pretty much all Atlantic salmon is farmed, so avoid that.

CAN YOU *REALLY* FREEZE AND REHEAT COOKED SALMON (AND OTHER FISH)?

I get this question all the time, and my answer is yes, you can! When you reheat fish, the texture will be slightly different from when you first cooked it (you have to know that going in), but here's what you can do: thaw in the fridge overnight, then reheat covered (to retain moisture) in a 275°F (135°C) oven for 10 to 15 minutes. Reheating gently is key, so avoid the microwave if possible. A better option is flaking the fish cold on top of a salad. You can also turn leftover fish into patties, a dip, or toss into a soup or curry!

eggs

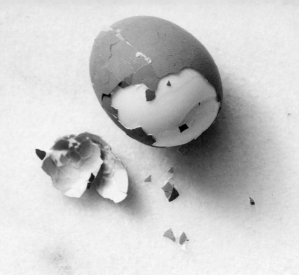

Put an egg on it! Just don't make me choose between soft-boiled, hard-boiled, and poached eggs—I love them all. Jammy soft-boiled eggs are great on avocado toast or in egg cups with a sprinkle of everything bagel seasoning; firm and perfectly cooked hard-boiled eggs are great in summertime's favorite potato salad or turned into deviled eggs; and poached eggs are just asking to be topped on skillet breakfast hashes and grilled vegetables (let that golden, oozy yolk coat everything). There's no denying eggs are the champs of meal prep. No matter how you cook them, they're endlessly adaptable for breakfast, lunch, and dinner. Frittatas can be served for brunch, bell peppers stuffed with eggs, like my Breakfast Stuffed Bell Peppers (page 97), can be served for breakfast *or* dinner, and hard-boiled eggs can be a midmorning snack or topped on just about anything for a protein boost.

how to select

The best eggs you can buy are pasture raised, ideally from your local farmers' market. If you're buying from the grocery store, just make sure to look for the "Certified Humane" or "Animal Welfare Approved" stamps (most of the other labels on egg cartons are simply marketing). Yes, pasture-raised eggs are pricier, but they're also richer in vitamins A, E, D, and omega-3s, so it's money well spent. Plus, when chickens roam in outdoor space, you'll notice a more vibrant yolk, a compact white, and a thicker shell.

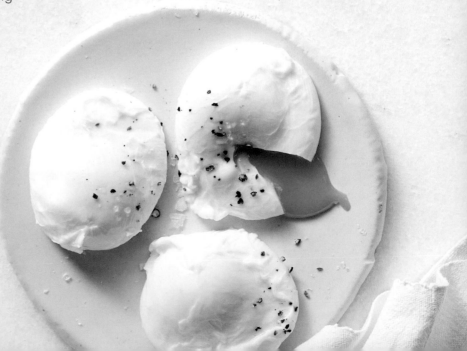

how to meal prep

Poach: Bring a medium pot of water to a boil, then reduce the heat to a simmer. While waiting for the water to boil, crack an egg into a small fine-mesh sieve over a bowl. Swirl the egg in the sieve until the liquidy egg whites have been removed, while the thick egg whites remain. Then place the egg in a ramekin or small bowl. Stir 1 to 2 tablespoons vinegar (optional but recommended) into the simmering water. Gently pour the egg from the ramekin into the pot. If adding multiple eggs, space them out in the pot. Cook for 3 to 4 minutes, depending on how soft you like your poached eggs. Use a slotted spoon to remove the egg. Place the eggs in an ice-water bath, then store them in an airtight container in the fridge for up to 2 days. To reheat, add some hot water to a small bowl or cup and add the poached egg until it's warmed through, about 20 to 30 seconds.

Helpful tip: For poached eggs, if you're just making one, you can gently swirl a vortex in the pot and drop the egg in the middle. This will help to ensure a tight white around the yolk.

Soft and Hard Boiled: Bring a medium pot of water to a boil. Ensure there's enough water in the pot to cover the eggs by about 1 inch (2.5 cm). While waiting for the water to boil, prepare an ice-water bath in a large bowl. Once the water is boiling, reduce the heat to low and use a skimmer or slotted spoon to gently add the eggs to the water. Turn up the heat to bring the water back to a boil. Cook for 6 to 8 minutes for soft-boiled eggs and 12 to 14 minutes for hard-boiled eggs. Remove the eggs and immediately submerge them in the ice-water bath to stop them from cooking (this also helps make it easier to remove the shell). If you'd like to serve them warm, remove from the ice-water bath after 15 seconds, then peel.

To store: Submerge them in the ice-water bath for 5 minutes, or until fully cooled, before placing them in an airtight container in the fridge for 3 to 4 days for soft-boiled eggs, and up to 7 days for hard-boiled eggs. For maximum freshness, keep the eggs in their shells.

quick-assembly meals

Now that you've learned how to meal prep individual ingredients, here comes the fun part—assembling them into tasty mix-and-match meals! This is the heart of the Downshiftology approach to meal prep, where a random assortment of food containers magically turns into mouthwatering meals. On the following pages, I've got a few ideas for you, but keep in mind that these are not a hard-and-fast formula but are simply meant to serve as inspiration!

There are five essential categories I consider prepping every week for balanced meals, each of which offers an array of possibilities:

1. Protein: Roasted chicken, shredded chicken, baked salmon, slow-cooker pulled pork, chickpea curry, turkey patties, and so on

2. Veggies: Sheet pan of roasted veggies, spiralized veggies, fresh veggies, or any combination of those

3. Starch: Sweet potato, quinoa, lentils, mashed root vegetables

4. Snacks: Hummus, tzatziki, roasted potato wedges, crisp vegetable sticks

5. Breakfast: Hard- or soft-boiled eggs, chia pudding, overnight oats, homemade granola, pancakes, frittatas

I tend to prep a couple of items from each category, depending on what I'm craving. Again, the goal is not to have all meals set and done but to have enough healthy ingredients prepped so that you can assemble most of your meals quickly.

After meal prepping this way for several years, I find that what I love most is how it's expanded my creativity in the kitchen. It leads me to combine ingredients in ways that I would have never thought previously. In fact, some of my most delicious meals are ones where I just toss a bunch of things together, thinking, "Well, let's see how this turns out?!"—and it ends up knock-your-socks-off amazing!

1

This warm-weather meal prep celebrates a bounty of fresh produce *and* bright flavor. It includes juicy strawberries, raw zucchini noodles, crisp celery, and soft-boiled eggs, along with simply made components such as chia pudding, a peas and prosciutto side dish, and flaked salmon. These come together to create just what your body craves in the spring and summer—light, fresh, and healthy meals. Just set aside a little time on Sunday morning to prep these items for tasty meals throughout the week!

item	method	time	storage
boiled eggs (see page 65)	Stovetop	6 to 14 minutes (depending on preference)	Store in the fridge for 3 to 4 days for soft boiled, and up to 1 week for hard boiled.
flaked salmon (page 199)	Oven	10 to 14 minutes	Store in the fridge for 3 to 4 days, or in the freezer for up to 3 months.
peas and prosciutto (page 231)	Stovetop	10 minutes	Store in the fridge for 4 to 5 days.
zucchini noodles (see page 56)	Spiralizer	5 minutes	Store in the fridge for 3 to 4 days.
celery (see page 42)	Knife	5 minutes	Store in a jar of water in the fridge for 1 week.
tzatziki (page 253)	Bowl	10 minutes	Store in the fridge for 4 to 5 days.
lemon vinaigrette (page 260)	Bowl	10 minutes	Store in the fridge for up to 1 week.
chia pudding (see page 117)	Bowl	4 hours or overnight	Store in the fridge for 4 to 5 days, or in the freezer for up to 3 months.
strawberries	Wash	5 minutes	Store in the fridge for 4 to 5 days.

additional fresh and pantry items needed:

- Red Onion
- Avocados
- Arugula
- Sliced Almonds
- Endive Leaves
- Mayonnaise
- Cucumber
- Parsley and Dill

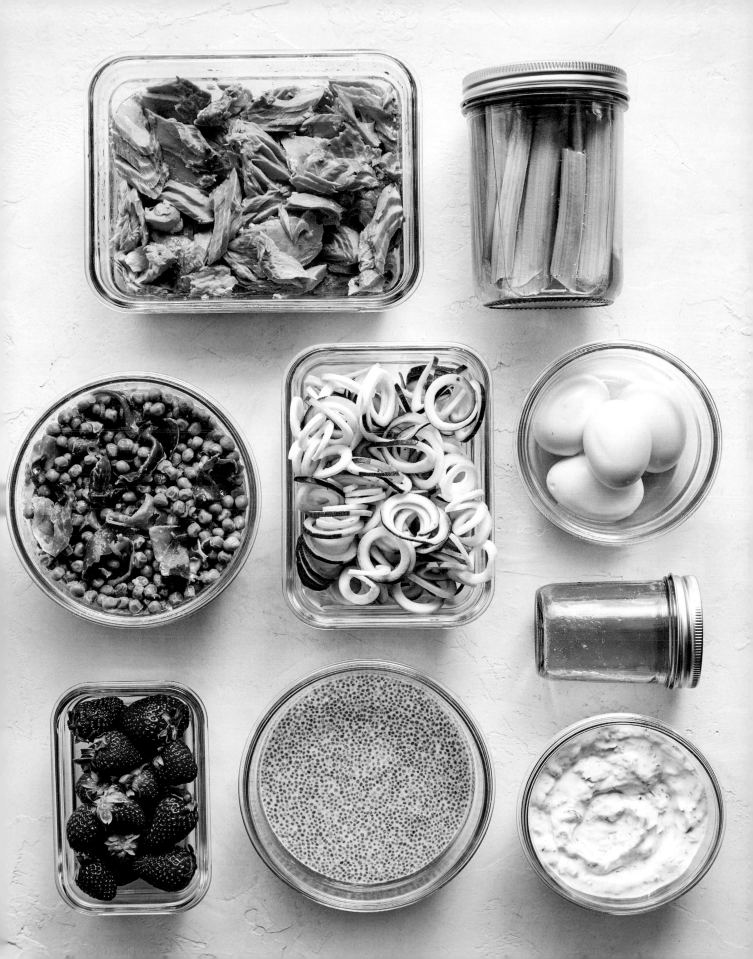

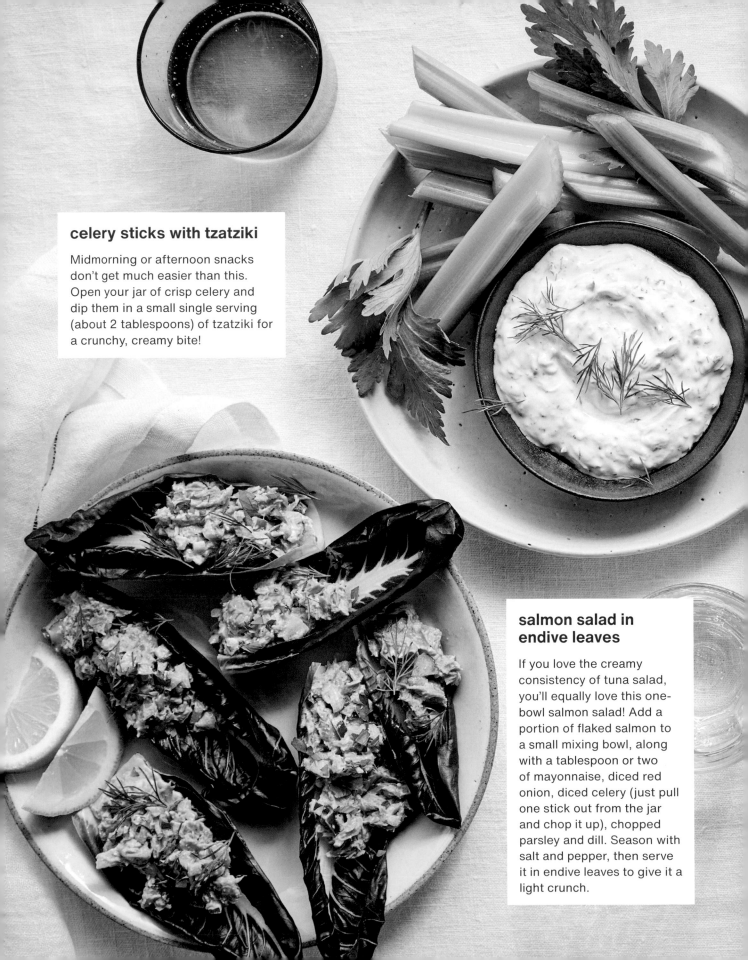

celery sticks with tzatziki

Midmorning or afternoon snacks don't get much easier than this. Open your jar of crisp celery and dip them in a small single serving (about 2 tablespoons) of tzatziki for a crunchy, creamy bite!

salmon salad in endive leaves

If you love the creamy consistency of tuna salad, you'll equally love this one-bowl salmon salad! Add a portion of flaked salmon to a small mixing bowl, along with a tablespoon or two of mayonnaise, diced red onion, diced celery (just pull one stick out from the jar and chop it up), chopped parsley and dill. Season with salt and pepper, then serve it in endive leaves to give it a light crunch.

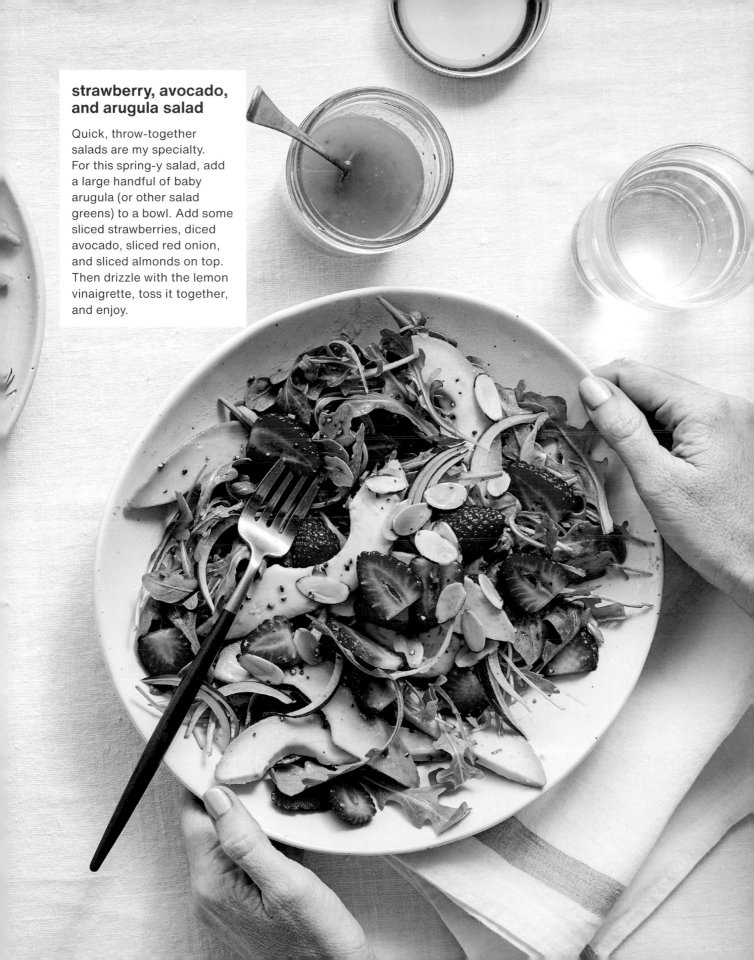

strawberry, avocado, and arugula salad

Quick, throw-together salads are my specialty. For this spring-y salad, add a large handful of baby arugula (or other salad greens) to a bowl. Add some sliced strawberries, diced avocado, sliced red onion, and sliced almonds on top. Then drizzle with the lemon vinaigrette, toss it together, and enjoy.

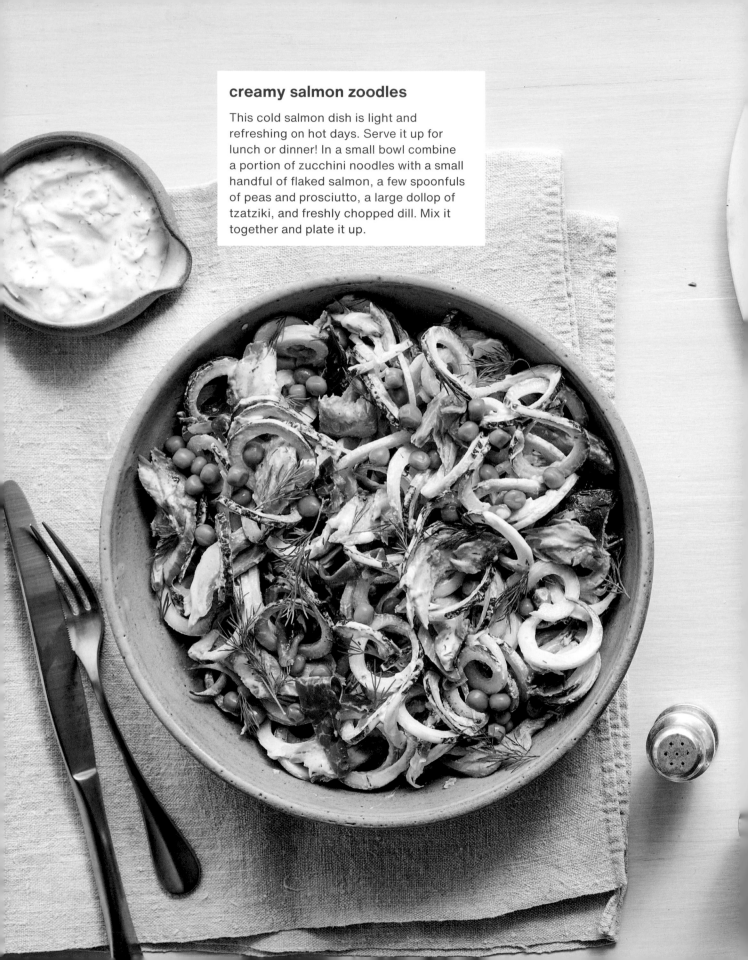

creamy salmon zoodles

This cold salmon dish is light and refreshing on hot days. Serve it up for lunch or dinner! In a small bowl combine a portion of zucchini noodles with a small handful of flaked salmon, a few spoonfuls of peas and prosciutto, a large dollop of tzatziki, and freshly chopped dill. Mix it together and plate it up.

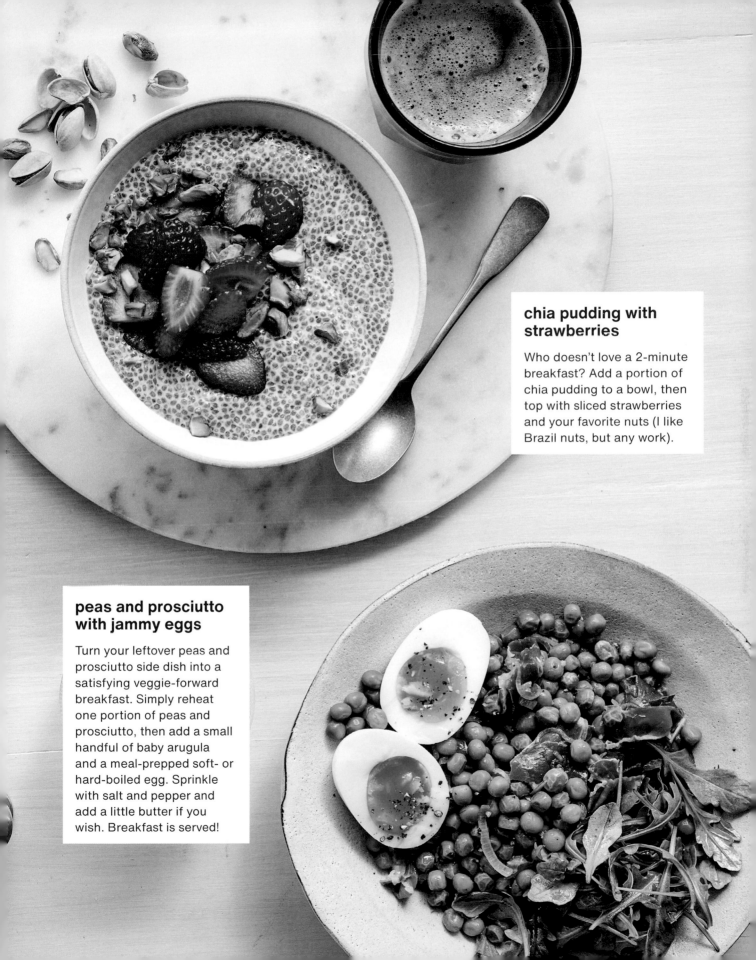

chia pudding with strawberries

Who doesn't love a 2-minute breakfast? Add a portion of chia pudding to a bowl, then top with sliced strawberries and your favorite nuts (I like Brazil nuts, but any work).

peas and prosciutto with jammy eggs

Turn your leftover peas and prosciutto side dish into a satisfying veggie-forward breakfast. Simply reheat one portion of peas and prosciutto, then add a small handful of baby arugula and a meal-prepped soft- or hard-boiled egg. Sprinkle with salt and pepper and add a little butter if you wish. Breakfast is served!

meal prep idea 2

Sunny, festive, and colorful meals are what this meal prep is all about! If you're anything like me, you'd rather spend time outdoors than in the kitchen with the oven blazing when it's hot outside, so I've kept cooking to a minimum in this meal prep. Featured flavors include juicy mango and blueberries, crisp cucumber, and zesty lime for a simple nine-item meal prep with Cali vibes.

item	method	time	storage
cilantro lime shrimp (page 187)	Stovetop	30 minutes	Store in the fridge for 3 to 4 days.
mango	Knife	15 minutes	Store in the fridge for 4 to 5 days.
coconut rice (page 240)	Stovetop	10 minutes	Store in the fridge for 4 to 5 days, or in the freezer for up to 3 months.
blueberry pancakes (page 122)	Stovetop	30 minutes	Store in the freezer for up to 3 months.
baby persian cucumbers (see page 44)	Wash	5 minutes	Store in the fridge for 3 to 4 days.
green onions (see page 50)	Knife	5 minutes	Store in the fridge for up to 1 week.
homemade granola (page 106)	Oven	40 minutes	Store at room temperature for several weeks, or in the freezer for up to 3 months.
key lime tartelettes (page 291)	Blender	4 hours and 15 minutes	Store in the fridge for 1 week, or in the freezer for up to 3 months.
lemon vinaigrette (page 260)	Bowl	10 minutes	Store in the fridge for up to 1 week.

additional fresh and pantry items needed:

- Limes
- Avocados
- Cilantro
- Tomatoes
- Sour Cream
- Butter Leaf Lettuce
- Blueberries and Blackberries
- Goat Cheese
- Banana
- Yogurt
- Maple Syrup
- Pecans
- Basil and Mint
- Unsweetened Coconut Flakes

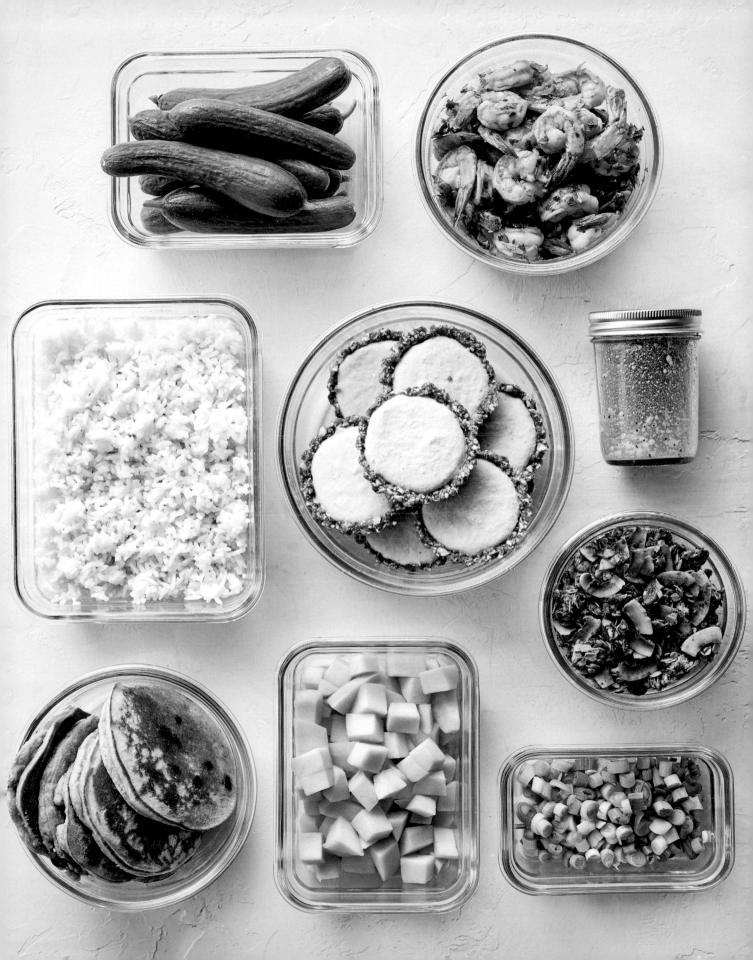

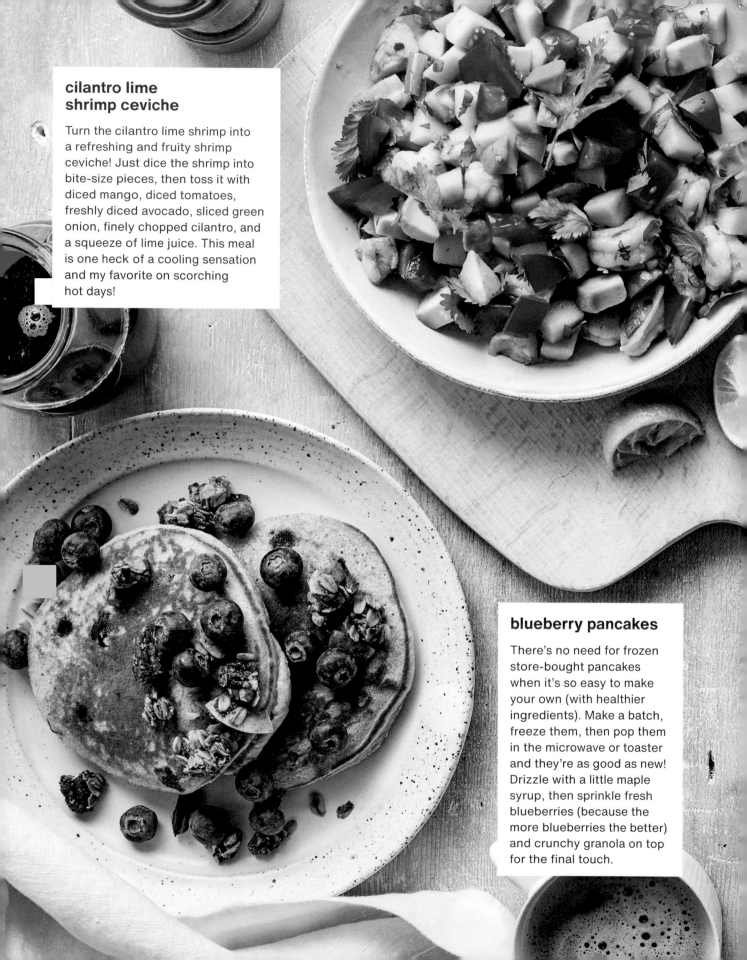

cilantro lime shrimp ceviche

Turn the cilantro lime shrimp into a refreshing and fruity shrimp ceviche! Just dice the shrimp into bite-size pieces, then toss it with diced mango, diced tomatoes, freshly diced avocado, sliced green onion, finely chopped cilantro, and a squeeze of lime juice. This meal is one heck of a cooling sensation and my favorite on scorching hot days!

blueberry pancakes

There's no need for frozen store-bought pancakes when it's so easy to make your own (with healthier ingredients). Make a batch, freeze them, then pop them in the microwave or toaster and they're as good as new! Drizzle with a little maple syrup, then sprinkle fresh blueberries (because the more blueberries the better) and crunchy granola on top for the final touch.

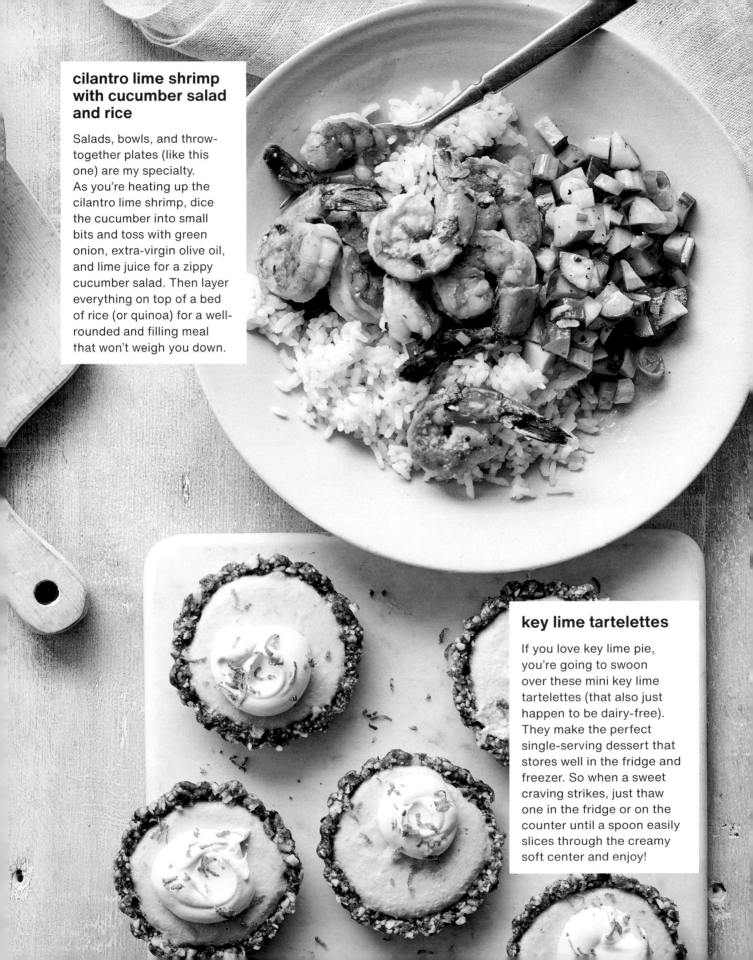

cilantro lime shrimp with cucumber salad and rice

Salads, bowls, and throw-together plates (like this one) are my specialty. As you're heating up the cilantro lime shrimp, dice the cucumber into small bits and toss with green onion, extra-virgin olive oil, and lime juice for a zippy cucumber salad. Then layer everything on top of a bed of rice (or quinoa) for a well-rounded and filling meal that won't weigh you down.

key lime tartelettes

If you love key lime pie, you're going to swoon over these mini key lime tartelettes (that also just happen to be dairy-free). They make the perfect single-serving dessert that stores well in the fridge and freezer. So when a sweet craving strikes, just thaw one in the fridge or on the counter until a spoon easily slices through the creamy soft center and enjoy!

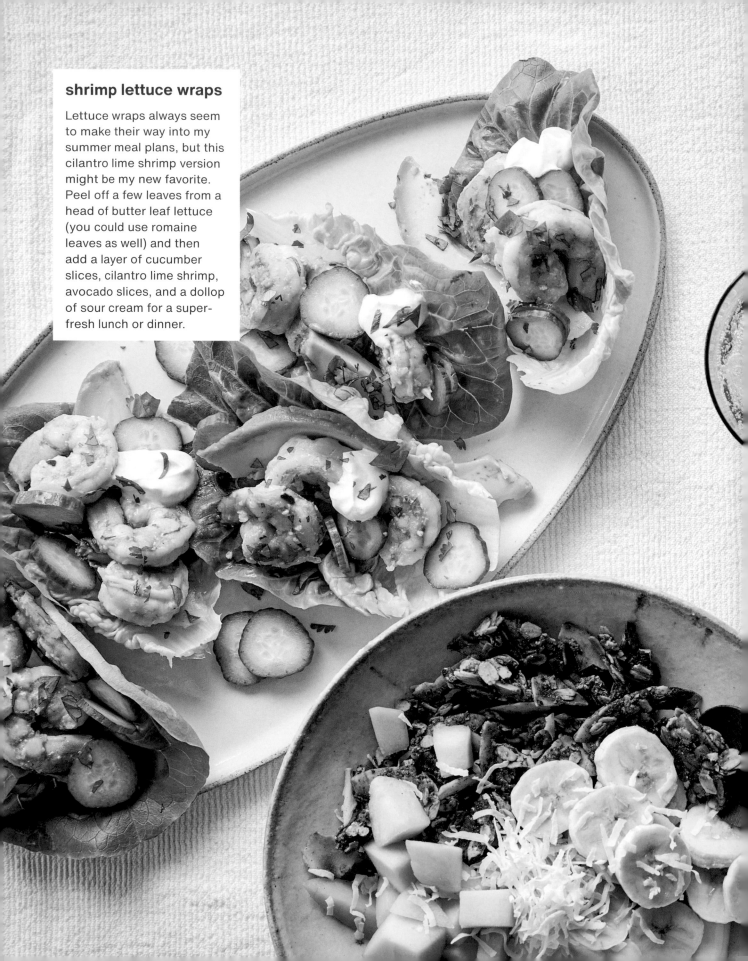

shrimp lettuce wraps

Lettuce wraps always seem to make their way into my summer meal plans, but this cilantro lime shrimp version might be my new favorite. Peel off a few leaves from a head of butter leaf lettuce (you could use romaine leaves as well) and then add a layer of cucumber slices, cilantro lime shrimp, avocado slices, and a dollop of sour cream for a super-fresh lunch or dinner.

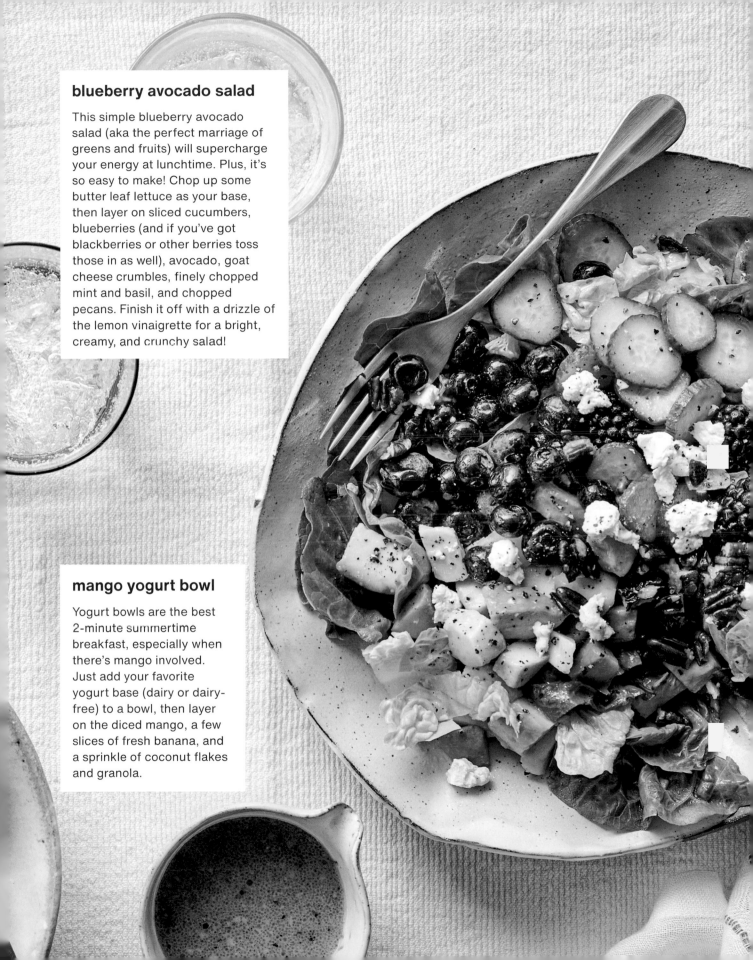

blueberry avocado salad

This simple blueberry avocado salad (aka the perfect marriage of greens and fruits) will supercharge your energy at lunchtime. Plus, it's so easy to make! Chop up some butter leaf lettuce as your base, then layer on sliced cucumbers, blueberries (and if you've got blackberries or other berries toss those in as well), avocado, goat cheese crumbles, finely chopped mint and basil, and chopped pecans. Finish it off with a drizzle of the lemon vinaigrette for a bright, creamy, and crunchy salad!

mango yogurt bowl

Yogurt bowls are the best 2-minute summertime breakfast, especially when there's mango involved. Just add your favorite yogurt base (dairy or dairy-free) to a bowl, then layer on the diced mango, a few slices of fresh banana, and a sprinkle of coconut flakes and granola.

meal prep idea 3

With how incredibly delicious and filling this cold-weather meal prep is, you won't even realize that it's vegetarian. It's the perfect antidote to overindulgent and holiday-heavy meals and is loaded with veggie superstar ingredients, including chickpeas, broccoli, cabbage, and carrot. Want to feel awesome when everyone else feels sluggish? Whip up this meal prep!

item	method	time	storage
coconut chickpea curry (page 210)	Stovetop	30 minutes	Store in the fridge for 4 to 5 days, or in the freezer for up to 3 months.
lemon herb rice (page 243)	Stovetop	30 minutes	Store in the fridge for 4 to 5 days, or in the freezer for up to 3 months.
cassava flour tortillas (page 265)	Stovetop	30 minutes	Store in the fridge for 4 to 5 days, or in the freezer for up to 3 months.
red cabbage (see page 36)	Knife	5 minutes	Store in the fridge for 4 to 5 days.
spiralized carrot (see page 40)	Spiralizer	5 minutes	Store in the fridge for 3 to 4 days.
apple cider vinaigrette (page 261)	Bowl	10 minutes	Store in the fridge for up to 1 week.
garlic sautéed beet greens (page 262)	Stovetop	10 minutes	Store in the fridge for 3 to 4 days.
broccoli (see page 30)	Knife	10 minutes	Store in the fridge for 4 to 5 days.
overnight oats (see page 101)	Bowl	8 hours or overnight	Store in the fridge for 3 to 4 days.

additional fresh and pantry items needed:

- Sour Cream
- Cilantro
- Apples

- Walnuts and Brazil Nuts
- Pumpkin Seeds (Pepitas)
- Tomatoes

- Green Onions
- Ginger
- Frozen Edamame
- Avocados

- Eggs
- Goat Cheese
- Kiwi
- Maple Syrup

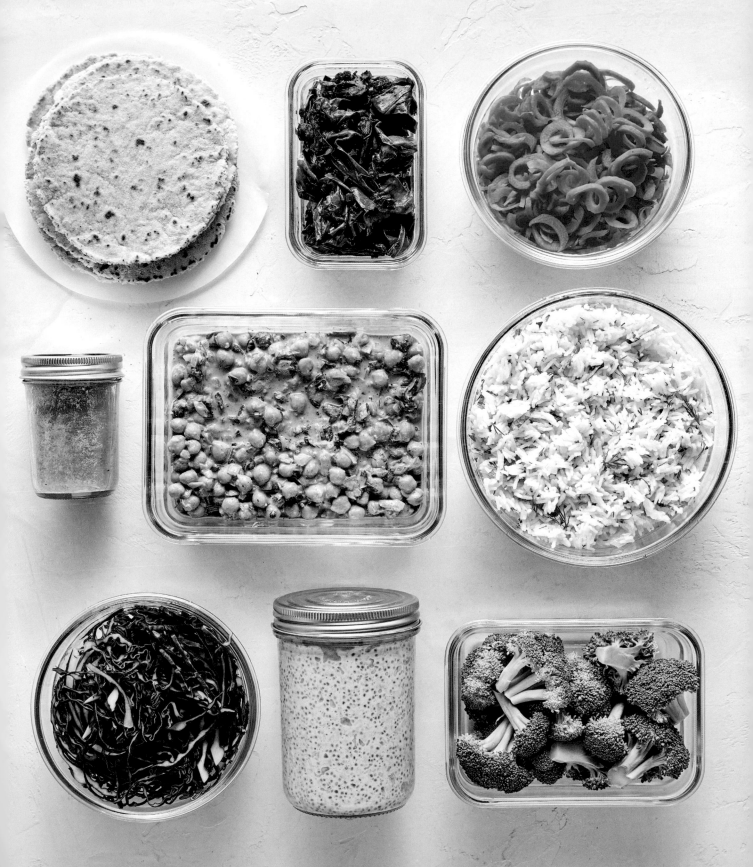

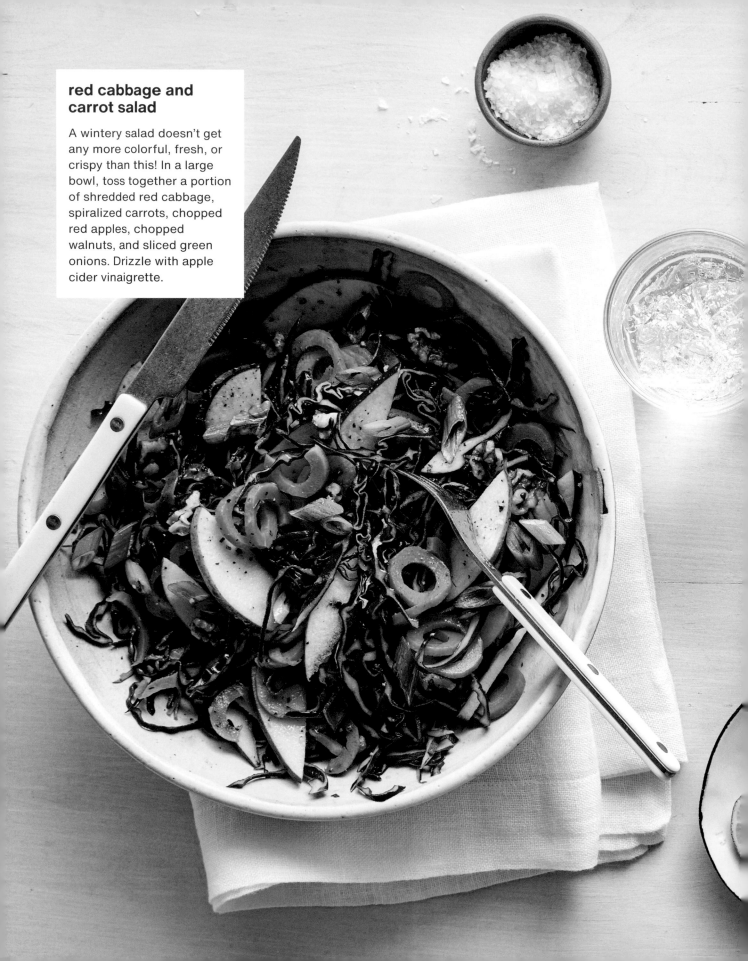

red cabbage and carrot salad

A wintery salad doesn't get any more colorful, fresh, or crispy than this! In a large bowl, toss together a portion of shredded red cabbage, spiralized carrots, chopped red apples, chopped walnuts, and sliced green onions. Drizzle with apple cider vinaigrette.

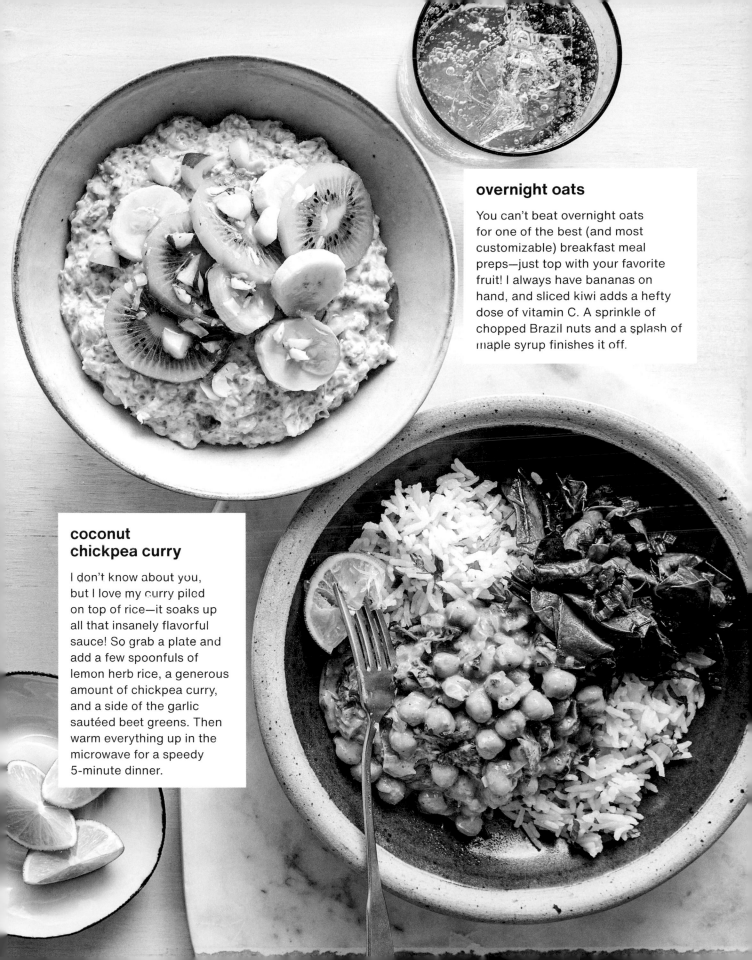

overnight oats

You can't beat overnight oats for one of the best (and most customizable) breakfast meal preps—just top with your favorite fruit! I always have bananas on hand, and sliced kiwi adds a hefty dose of vitamin C. A sprinkle of chopped Brazil nuts and a splash of maple syrup finishes it off.

coconut chickpea curry

I don't know about you, but I love my curry piled on top of rice—it soaks up all that insanely flavorful sauce! So grab a plate and add a few spoonfuls of lemon herb rice, a generous amount of chickpea curry, and a side of the garlic sautéed beet greens. Then warm everything up in the microwave for a speedy 5-minute dinner.

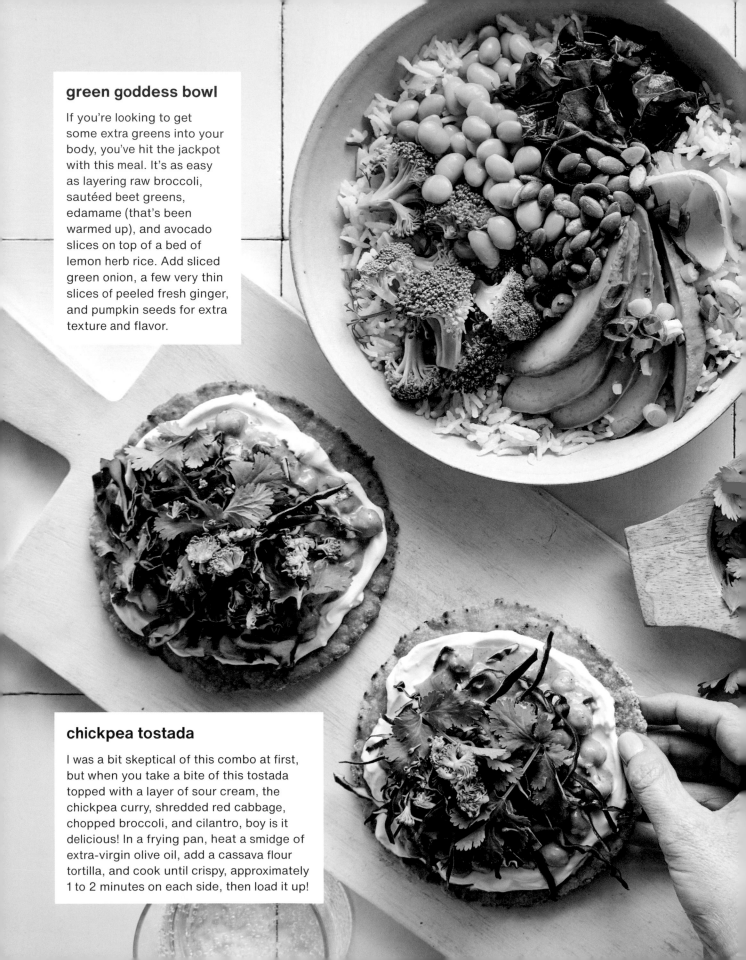

green goddess bowl

If you're looking to get some extra greens into your body, you've hit the jackpot with this meal. It's as easy as layering raw broccoli, sautéed beet greens, edamame (that's been warmed up), and avocado slices on top of a bed of lemon herb rice. Add sliced green onion, a few very thin slices of peeled fresh ginger, and pumpkin seeds for extra texture and flavor.

chickpea tostada

I was a bit skeptical of this combo at first, but when you take a bite of this tostada topped with a layer of sour cream, the chickpea curry, shredded red cabbage, chopped broccoli, and cilantro, boy is it delicious! In a frying pan, heat a smidge of extra-virgin olive oil, add a cassava flour tortilla, and cook until crispy, approximately 1 to 2 minutes on each side, then load it up!

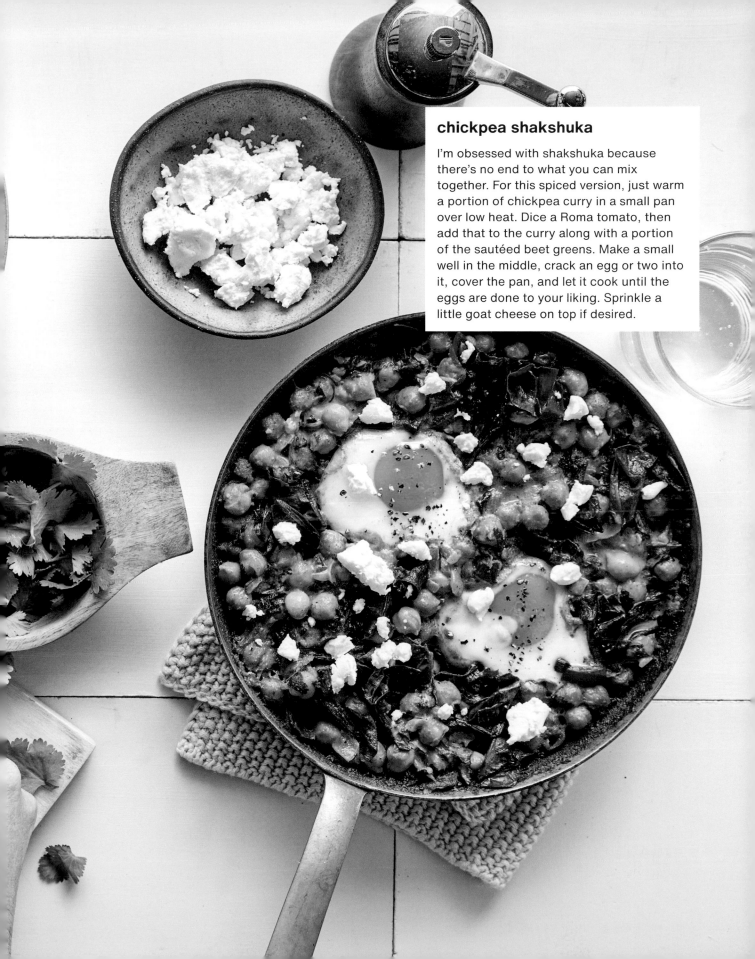

chickpea shakshuka

I'm obsessed with shakshuka because there's no end to what you can mix together. For this spiced version, just warm a portion of chickpea curry in a small pan over low heat. Dice a Roma tomato, then add that to the curry along with a portion of the sautéed beet greens. Make a small well in the middle, crack an egg or two into it, cover the pan, and let it cook until the eggs are done to your liking. Sprinkle a little goat cheese on top if desired.

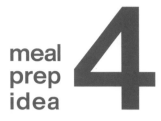

meal prep idea 4

You can always count on roasted chicken for a year-round meal-prep option. And with ingredients like roasted cauliflower steaks, black lentils, garlicky roasted tomatoes, and colorful bell peppers, this meal prep unintentionally (though maybe it was subconsciously) has a Mediterranean flair to it—you know that's my favorite. Some of these may look fancy-ish, but I promise you they're easy to assemble in just a few minutes.

item	method	time	storage
roasted chicken (see page 179)	Oven	2 hours and 25 minutes	Store in the fridge for 3 to 4 days, or in the freezer for up to 3 months.
spicy roasted cauliflower steaks (page 236)	Oven	30 minutes	Store in the fridge for 3 to 4 days, or in the freezer for up to 3 months.
hummus (page 254)	Blender	5 minutes	Store in the fridge for 1 week, or in the freezer for up to 3 months.
garlic herb roasted tomatoes (page 239)	Oven	25 minutes	Store in the fridge for 4 to 5 days.
mini bell peppers (see page 28)	Wash	5 minutes	Store in the fridge for 1 to 2 weeks.
black lentils (see page 60)	Stovetop	30 minutes	Store in the fridge for 4 to 5 days, or in the freezer for up to 3 months.
basil pesto (page 252)	Blender	15 minutes	Store in the fridge for 4 to 5 days, or in the freezer for up to 3 months.
red onion (see page 50)	Knife	5 minutes	Store in the fridge for up to 1 week.
balsamic vinaigrette (page 260)	Bowl	10 minutes	Store In the fridge for up to 1 week.

additional fresh and pantry items needed:

- Baby Spinach
- Pine Nuts
- Parsley and Chives
- Feta Cheese
- Avocados
- Mayonnaise
- Eggs

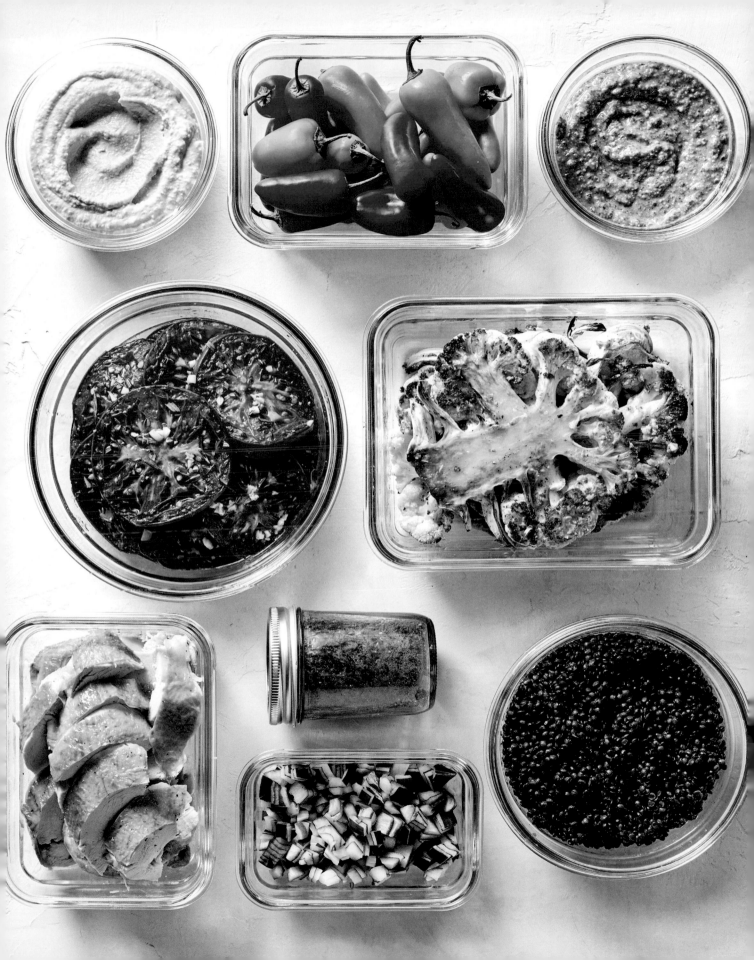

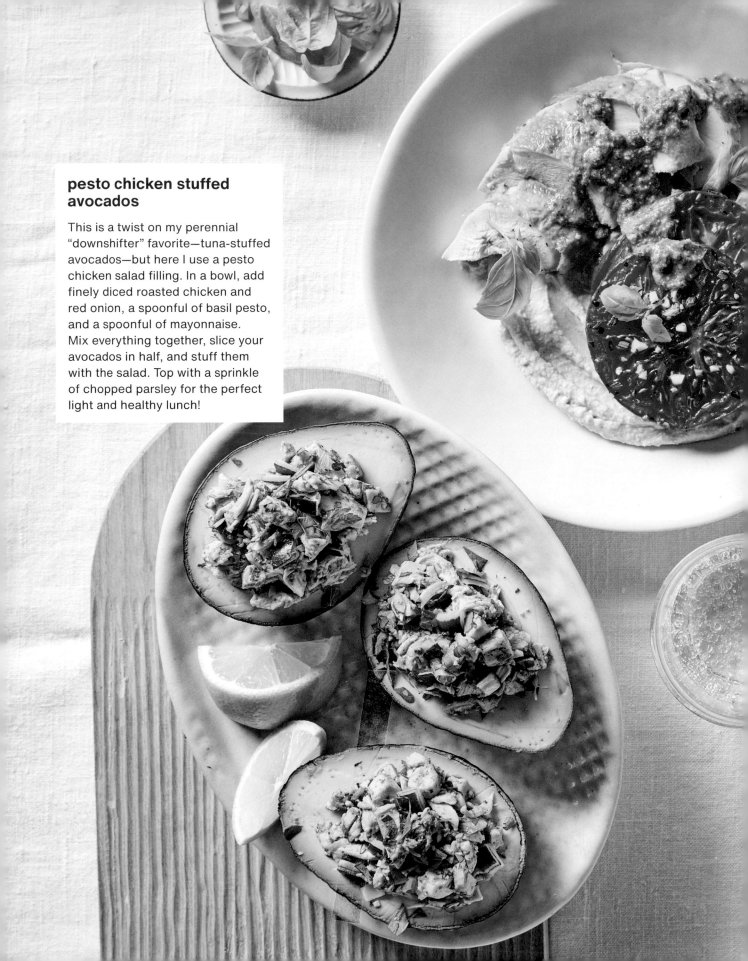

pesto chicken stuffed avocados

This is a twist on my perennial "downshifter" favorite—tuna-stuffed avocados—but here I use a pesto chicken salad filling. In a bowl, add finely diced roasted chicken and red onion, a spoonful of basil pesto, and a spoonful of mayonnaise. Mix everything together, slice your avocados in half, and stuff them with the salad. Top with a sprinkle of chopped parsley for the perfect light and healthy lunch!

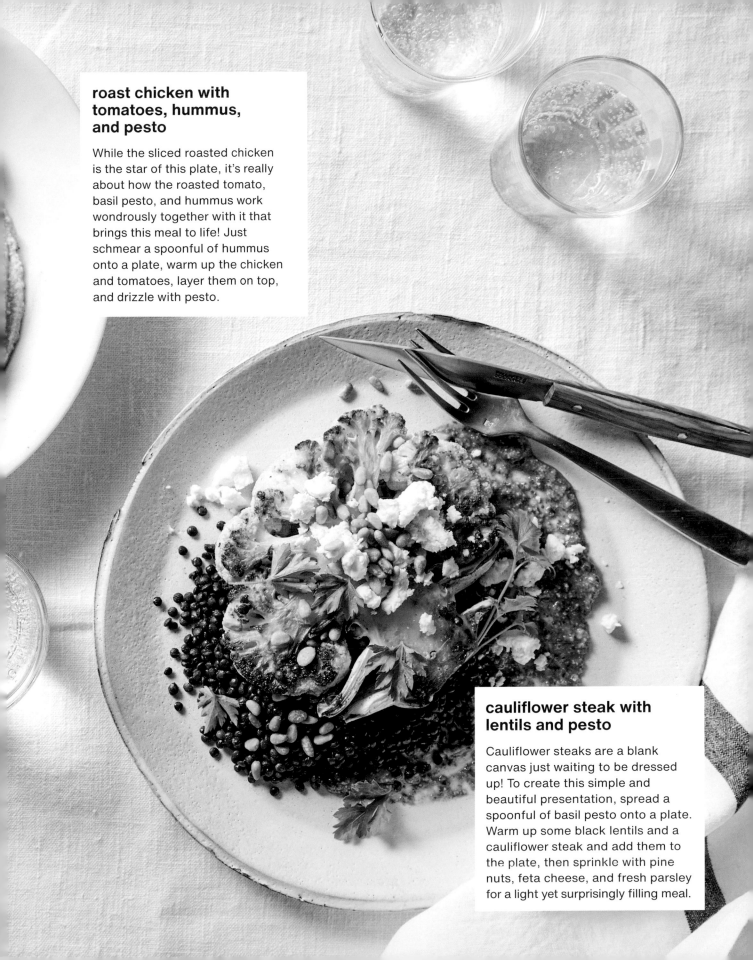

roast chicken with tomatoes, hummus, and pesto

While the sliced roasted chicken is the star of this plate, it's really about how the roasted tomato, basil pesto, and hummus work wondrously together with it that brings this meal to life! Just schmear a spoonful of hummus onto a plate, warm up the chicken and tomatoes, layer them on top, and drizzle with pesto.

cauliflower steak with lentils and pesto

Cauliflower steaks are a blank canvas just waiting to be dressed up! To create this simple and beautiful presentation, spread a spoonful of basil pesto onto a plate. Warm up some black lentils and a cauliflower steak and add them to the plate, then sprinkle with pine nuts, feta cheese, and fresh parsley for a light yet surprisingly filling meal.

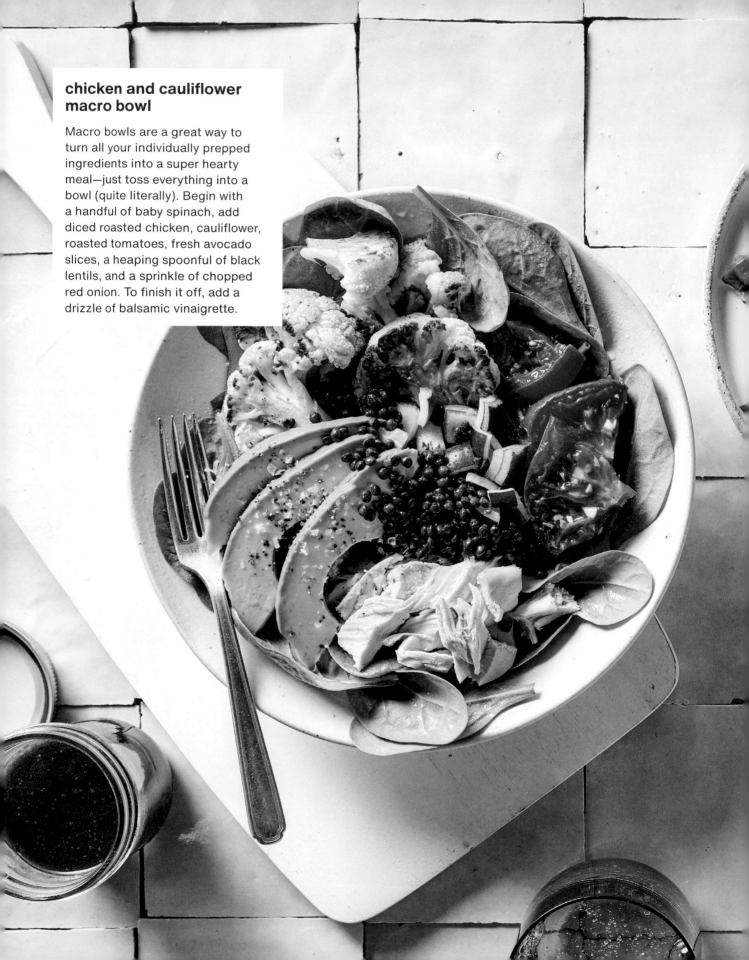

chicken and cauliflower macro bowl

Macro bowls are a great way to turn all your individually prepped ingredients into a super hearty meal—just toss everything into a bowl (quite literally). Begin with a handful of baby spinach, add diced roasted chicken, cauliflower, roasted tomatoes, fresh avocado slices, a heaping spoonful of black lentils, and a sprinkle of chopped red onion. To finish it off, add a drizzle of balsamic vinaigrette.

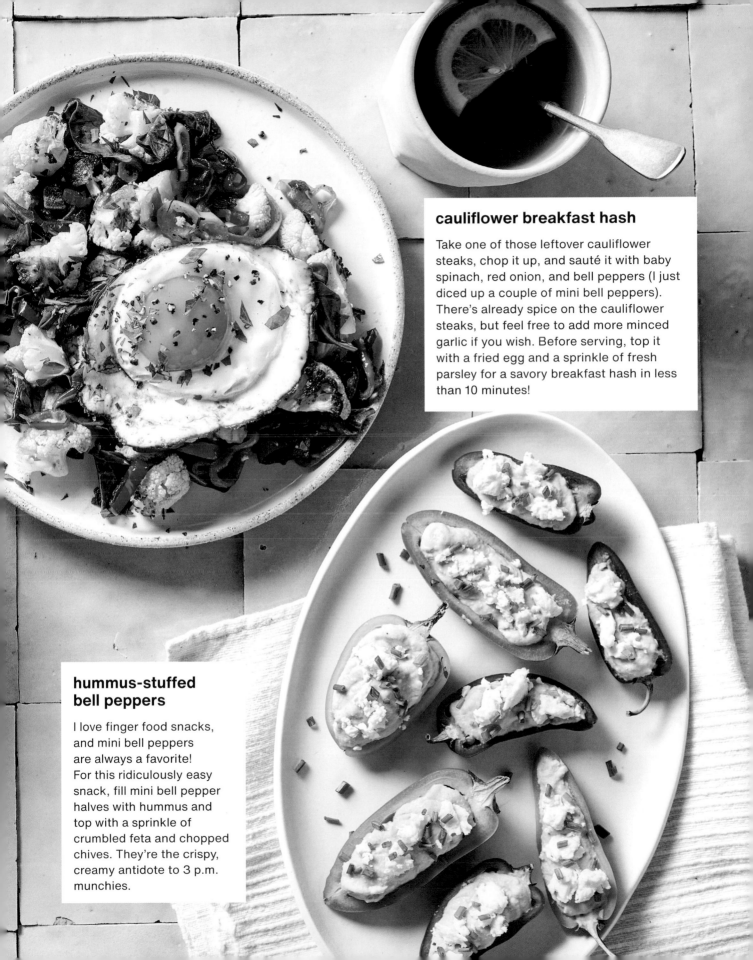

cauliflower breakfast hash

Take one of those leftover cauliflower steaks, chop it up, and sauté it with baby spinach, red onion, and bell peppers (I just diced up a couple of mini bell peppers). There's already spice on the cauliflower steaks, but feel free to add more minced garlic if you wish. Before serving, top it with a fried egg and a sprinkle of fresh parsley for a savory breakfast hash in less than 10 minutes!

hummus-stuffed bell peppers

I love finger food snacks, and mini bell peppers are always a favorite! For this ridiculously easy snack, fill mini bell pepper halves with hummus and top with a sprinkle of crumbled feta and chopped chives. They're the crispy, creamy antidote to 3 p.m. munchies.

nourishing breakfasts

I'm a breakfast girl through and through. I love my hearty fridge clean-out breakfast scrambles, tossing chopped veggies and whatever's left over in the fridge into my eggs. I also love colorful chia puddings with layers of fruit, nuts, and seeds. In fact, you could say it's a personal mission of mine to get you to eat more veggies and fresh fruit at breakfast. Because let's be honest, breakfast tends to be the most lackluster beige meal of the day (hello, cereal and toast).

Breakfast is the most important meal to kick-start our brains and nourish us until lunch, but it's also the meal people struggle with the most to make from scratch. For many of us, mornings are often frenzied as we juggle a bunch of to-dos before making a mad dash out the door. Translation: Breakfast is when we need meal prep the most!

In this chapter, you'll find a wide variety of healthy breakfast options from sweet to savory that you can prepare in advance, and in many cases, you'll be set for the week. I'm a big proponent of starting the day with veggies as often as possible, but I'm also human and crave something sweet or carb-y from time to time. So you'll find an assortment of options ranging from Peaches and Cream Baked Oatmeal (page 102) to Spiralized Beet Frittata (page 105), to Mediterranean Sheet Pan Eggs (page 94), to Breakfast Stuffed Bell Peppers (page 97). These are all healthy items you can make in advance, store, then assemble or reheat in a jiffy.

mediterranean sheet pan eggs

This might just be one of my favorite "cooking for a crowd" breakfast recipes. It looks fancy and impressive, but it's incredibly easy to make. You can easily customize the ingredients for seasonality or a brunch theme. If that weren't enough, the thin layer of baked eggs is perfect for topping on toast, rolling into a tortilla, or serving as the base of a breakfast salad. Endless options! **serves 12**

2 cups (250g) cherry tomatoes, halved

6 garlic cloves, minced

½ medium red onion, thinly sliced

2 tablespoons extra-virgin olive oil

14 large eggs

1 medium zucchini, thinly sliced

2 cups (40g) baby arugula, plus more for garnish

¼ cup (28g) crumbled feta cheese, plus more for garnish

½ teaspoon kosher salt

Pinch of freshly ground black pepper to taste

1. Preheat the oven to 400°F (200°C). In a medium bowl, drizzle the cherry tomatoes, garlic, and red onion with the oil and toss to coat. Arrange on a rimmed half sheet pan (18 × 13 inches / 46 x 33cm). Bake for 15 to 20 minutes, until the tomatoes start to blister.

2. While the tomatoes are roasting, whisk together the eggs in a large mixing bowl. Add the zucchini, arugula, feta cheese, salt, and pepper, then stir to combine.

3. Remove the sheet pan from the oven, give the tomatoes a toss with a spatula, then pour the egg mixture on top. Reduce the oven temperature to 350°F (180°C) and bake for approximately 20 minutes, or until the eggs are just cooked through. Garnish with feta cheese and arugula.

storage

Store in an airtight container in the fridge (with parchment paper between the slices) for 3 to 4 days, or in the freezer for up to 3 months.

to reheat

If frozen, thaw in the fridge overnight. Reheat in the oven at 350°F (180°C) for 10 minutes, or in the microwave for 1 minute, until warmed through.

helpful tip

If you plan to freeze, I suggest swapping out the tomatoes and zucchini for bell pepper and asparagus. Due to the amount of moisture in the tomatoes and zucchini, they're more likely to become watery when thawed and reheated.

Serving size: 1 piece

Calories: 130

Fat: 9g

Saturated fat: 3g

Carbs: 3g

Fiber: 1g

Sugar: 2g

Protein: 8g

Cholesterol: 219mg

Sodium: 134mg

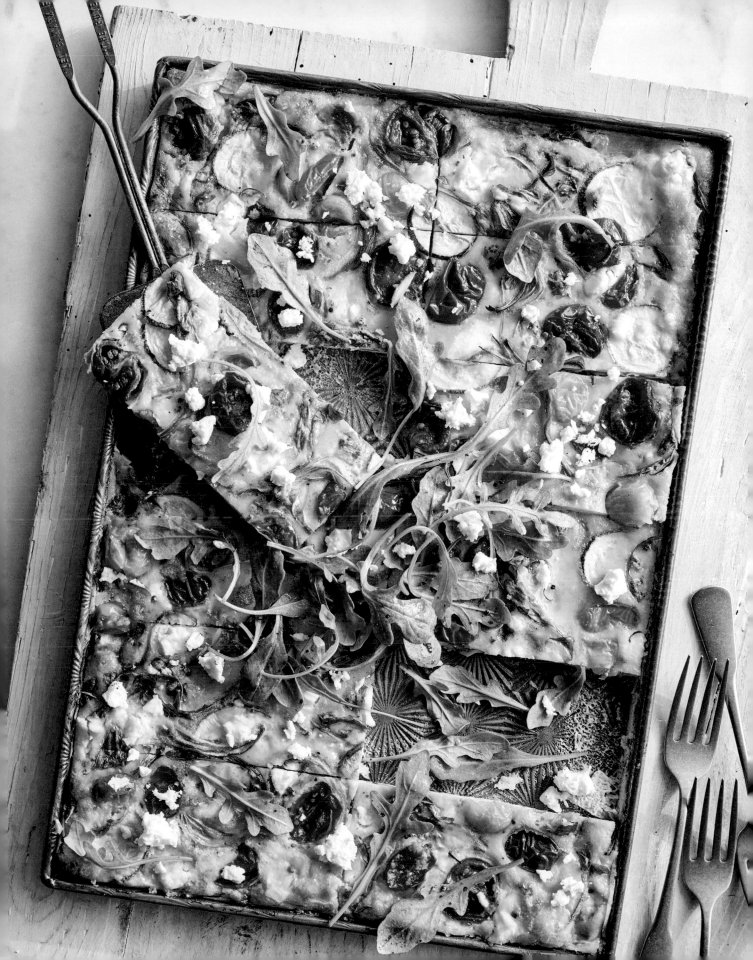

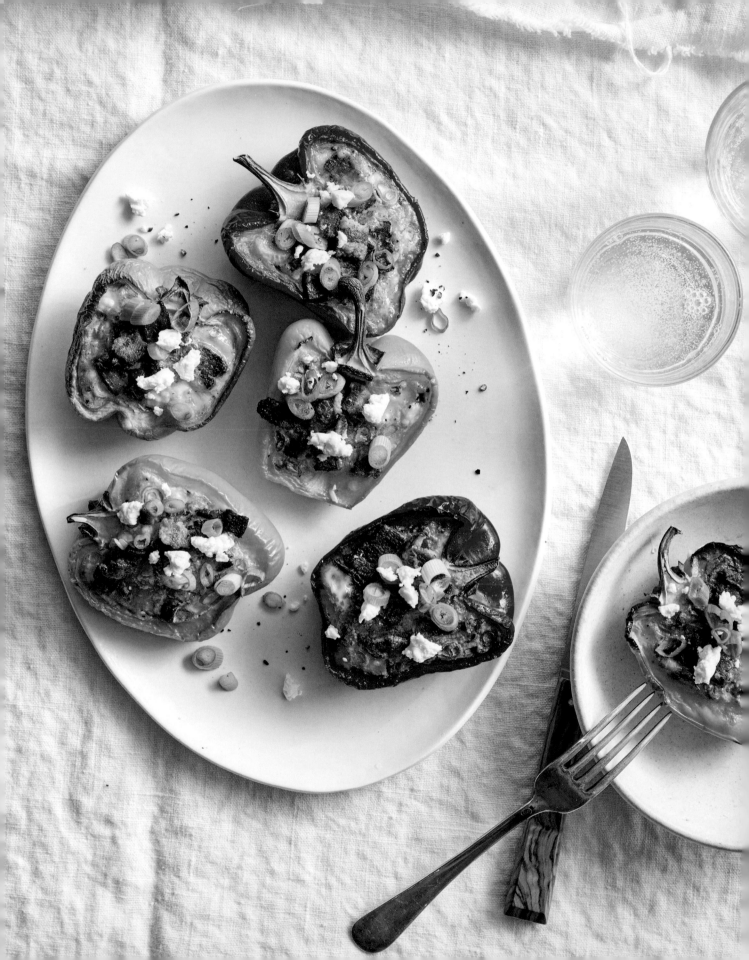

breakfast stuffed bell peppers

Stuffed bell peppers are regularly used in dinner meal prep, but they're equally great for breakfast! Think of them as egg "muffins" but with an added veggie boost. What I really love is how each stuffed pepper half is perfectly portioned with your breakfast favorites: eggs, bacon, goat cheese, and a sprinkle of green onions. Just place one on your plate with a few slices of avocado and breakfast is ready. **serves 4**

storage

Store in an airtight container in the fridge for 3 to 4 days, or in the freezer for up to 3 months (if you stack them, place parchment paper in between them).

to reheat

If frozen, thaw in the fridge overnight. Reheat in a covered casserole dish in the oven at 350°F (180°C) for 15 minutes, or in the microwave for 1 to 2 minutes, until warmed through.

helpful tip

If the bell peppers are a bit wobbly in the pan, you can slice a little bit off the bottom to help stabilize them. Just be careful not to slice all the way through. Stabilizing the bell pepper also prevents the egg mixture from leaking out.

8 slices bacon, cut into ½-inch (1.3cm) pieces

10 large eggs

3 green onions (white and green parts), thinly sliced

½ cup (56g) crumbled herbed goat cheese

½ teaspoon kosher salt

¼ teaspoon freshly ground black pepper

3 medium bell peppers, halved and seeded

1. Preheat the oven to 375°F (190°C).

2. In a large skillet, cook the bacon over medium heat until crispy, then use a slotted spoon to remove the pieces to a paper towel–lined plate.

3. In a medium bowl (preferably with a pour spout), whisk together the eggs, green onions, goat cheese, salt, and pepper. Stir in the crispy bacon.

4. In a 13 × 9-inch (33 × 23cm) baking dish, place the bell peppers cut side up. Fill the cavities with the egg mixture and bake for 35 to 40 minutes, until the egg filling is cooked through.

Serving size:
½ bell pepper

Calories: 222
Fat: 15g
Saturated fat: 5g
Carbs: 5g
Fiber: 2g
Sugar: 3g
Protein: 17g
Cholesterol: 326mg
Sodium: 423mg

apple cinnamon instant oatmeal (family size)

Who doesn't love those little store-bought packets of instant oatmeal? They're perfectly portioned, come in a variety of flavors that are so sweet they almost feel like dessert rather than breakfast, and are super easy to make—all you've got to do is add water or milk. This recipe is a family size or meal-prep size of everyone's favorite flavor: apple cinnamon. The best part is that it has less sugar than store-bought versions *plus* flaxseeds for extra nutrients. A win all around. **makes 10 individual servings**

4 cups (416g) gluten-free quick-cooking oats

1 cup (60g) finely diced dried apples

½ cup (56g) ground flaxseed

¼ cup (40g) maple sugar or coconut sugar

1 tablespoon ground cinnamon

1 teaspoon kosher salt

1. In a large bowl, stir together the oats, dried apples, flaxseed, maple sugar, cinnamon, and salt.

2. To make a single serving of oatmeal (microwave): Scoop ½ cup (52g) of the oat mixture into a bowl and add 1 cup (240ml) water or milk. Stir together until it's combined. Microwave the oats for 1½ to 2 minutes, or until they reach your desired consistency.

3. To make a single serving of oatmeal (stovetop): In a small saucepan, bring 1 cup (240ml) water or milk to a boil. Stir in ½ cup (52g) of the oat mixture to the saucepan, then reduce the heat to medium-low. Simmer the oats for 5 minutes, or until they reach your desired consistency.

storage

Store the dry oat mixture in an airtight container in your pantry for up to 3 months.

get creative

Feel free to swap in another dried fruit for the apples (raisins, dried blueberries, or dried cranberries are great), or even add your favorite chopped nuts to the mix.

helpful tip

You can omit the sugar and make this recipe entirely sugar-free or just add a splash of maple syrup on top before serving if you prefer.

Serving size:
½ cup (45g)

Calories: 226
Fat: 5g
Saturated fat: 1g
Carbs: 41g
Fiber: 6g
Sugar: 8g
Protein: 7g
Cholesterol: 0mg
Sodium: 121mg

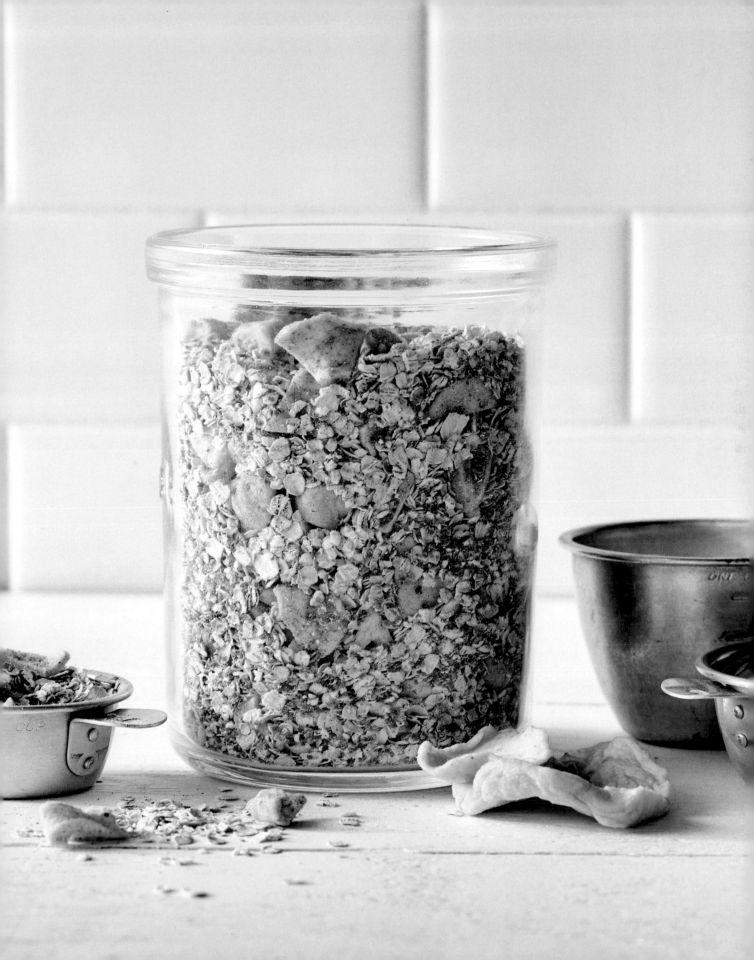

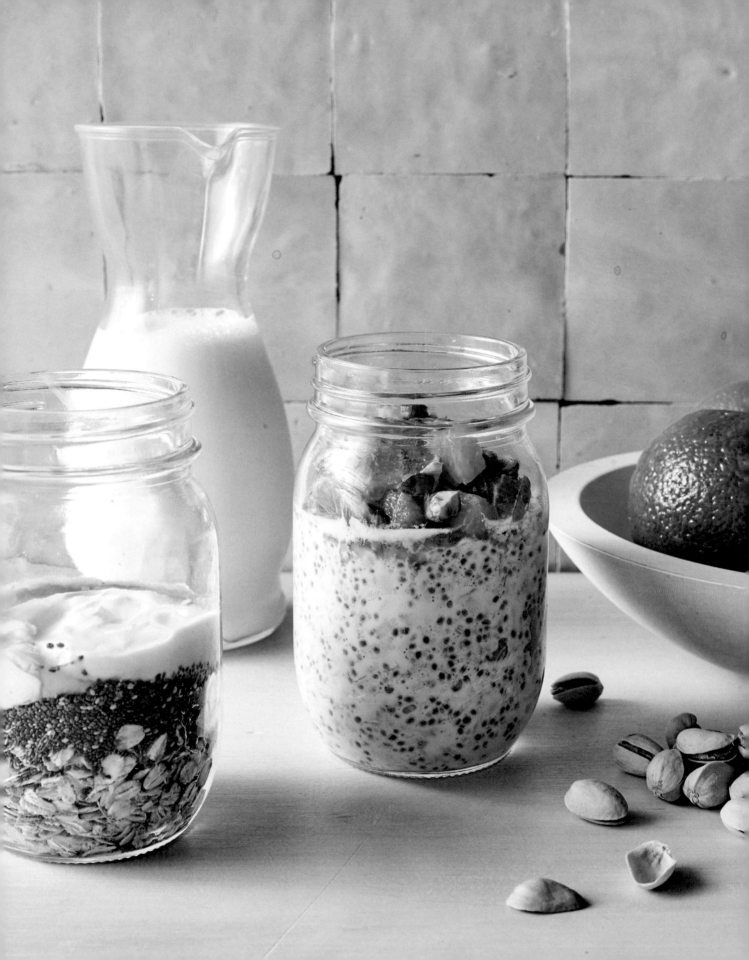

orange pistachio overnight oats

storage

Store in an airtight container in the fridge for 3 to 4 days, or in the freezer for up to 3 months. To thaw a frozen serving, just place it in the fridge the day before.

helpful tip

You can use quick-cooking oats rather than rolled oats in this recipe, but the texture will be more mushy and porridge-like.

If you want a healthy breakfast but don't have much time in the morning, overnight oats were made for you. Honestly, it's as easy as stirring together a couple of ingredients in a jar, placing it in the fridge overnight, and enjoying the next morning. On hot days you can enjoy overnight oats cool from the fridge (what I do most often), but on cold days you can warm them in a pot on the stove or in the microwave.

The beauty of overnight oats is that you can keep them simple or get as creative as you'd like. The base recipe is delicious and filling, but if you want to spruce it up, you can add a variety of toppings and mix-ins, including fresh fruit, nuts, seeds, spices, jams, and more. Lately, I'm loving this orange and pistachio combo. I tend to default to berries, so this switch-up keeps my breakfast interesting! **serves 1**

BASE OVERNIGHT OATS

½ cup (54g) gluten-free old-fashioned rolled oats

½ cup (120ml) milk (dairy or dairy-free)

¼ cup (57g) plain Greek yogurt (dairy or dairy-free)

1 tablespoon chia seeds

1 tablespoon pure maple syrup

FOR THE ORANGE PISTACHIO TOPPING

¼ cup (40g) diced orange

1 tablespoon roughly chopped pistachios

1 tablespoon pure maple syrup

Pinch of ground ginger or cinnamon

1. To make the base: Place the oats, milk, yogurt, chia seeds, and maple syrup in a pint-size mason jar or other storage container. Stir well to combine.

2. Let the oat mixture soak in the fridge for at least 2 hours, but it's best to soak overnight for 8 hours. This will yield a creamier consistency.

3. To top the base: Top with the orange, pistachios, maple syrup, and spice before serving.

Serving size: 1 recipe

Calories: 485
Fat: 13g
Saturated fat: 3g
Carbs: 78g
Fiber: 11g
Sugar: 31g
Protein: 17g
Cholesterol: 5mg
Sodium: 111mg

peaches and cream
baked oatmeal

While overnight oats are great for individual grab-and-go breakfasts or snacks, baked oatmeal is perfect for serving family and guests. It's essentially an oatmeal casserole made from oats, milk, eggs, fruit, and spices. When it bakes in the oven, the top gets golden and slightly crisp while the middle stays soft and moist, so it's got more texture and oomph to it than regular stovetop oatmeal. Like most things with oats, it's a blank canvas for flavor, though I'm quite partial to this peaches and cream version. And to make it *extra* creamy, I just add a dollop of yogurt on top before serving. **serves 6**

2 cups (216g) gluten-free old-fashioned rolled oats

½ cup (42g) sliced almonds

1 teaspoon ground cinnamon

½ teaspoon baking soda

½ teaspoon kosher salt

1 peach, pitted and pureed

1¾ cups (420ml) milk (dairy or dairy-free)

¼ cup (80ml) honey or pure maple syrup

2 large eggs

2 teaspoons vanilla extract

2 tablespoons melted unsalted butter or coconut oil

2 peaches, pitted and cut into chunks

1. Preheat the oven to 375°F (190°C). Grease a 9-inch (23cm) square baking dish.

2. In a large bowl, stir together the oats, almonds, cinnamon, baking soda, and salt.

3. In a medium bowl, whisk together the pureed peach, milk, honey, eggs, vanilla, and butter. Pour the wet mixture into the dry mixture, add the diced peaches, stir it all together, and then transfer the mixture to the prepared baking dish. Bake for 40 to 45 minutes, until set.

storage

Store in an airtight container in the fridge for 4 to 5 days, or in the freezer for up to 3 months. Just cut the oatmeal into portions before freezing so it's easy to reheat a single serving.

to reheat

Thaw any frozen portions in the fridge overnight. Bake covered with aluminum foil in a 350°F (180°C) oven for 15 to 20 minutes. You can also reheat in the microwave for 1 to 2 minutes, until warmed though.

helpful tip

I puree the peach in a mini food processor. If you don't have a food processor, chop it up, add it to a mason jar, and puree with an immersion blender.

Serving size: ⅙th of recipe (about 1¼ cups/ 230g)

Calories: 315

Fat: 12g

Saturated fat: 4g

Carbs: 43g

Fiber: 6g

Sugar: 19g

Protein: 9g

Cholesterol: 72mg

Sodium: 274mg

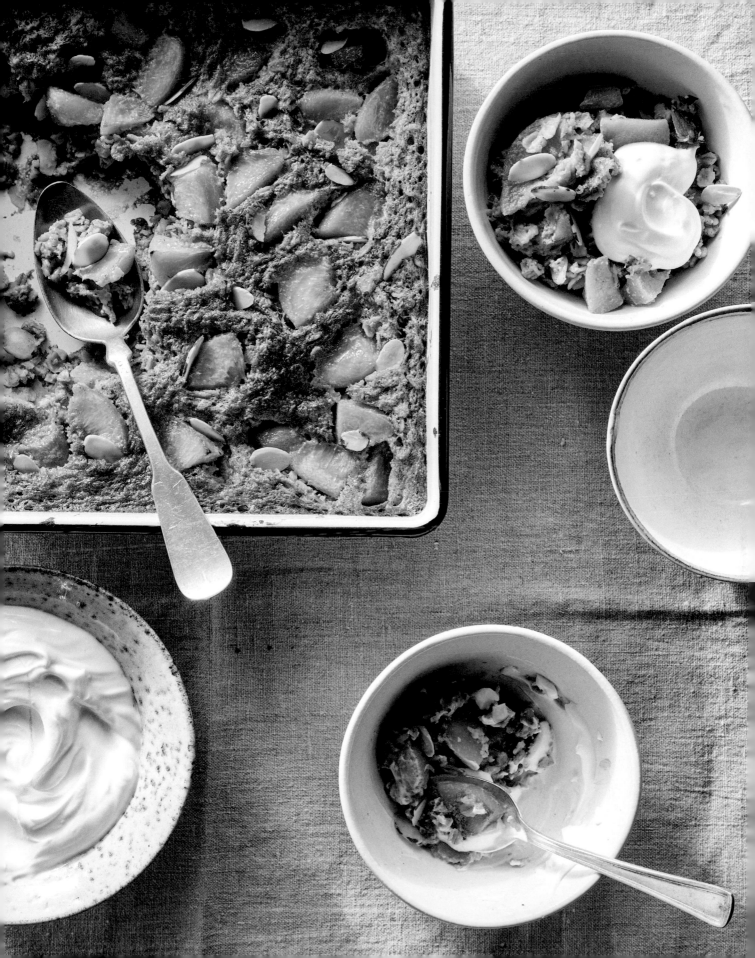

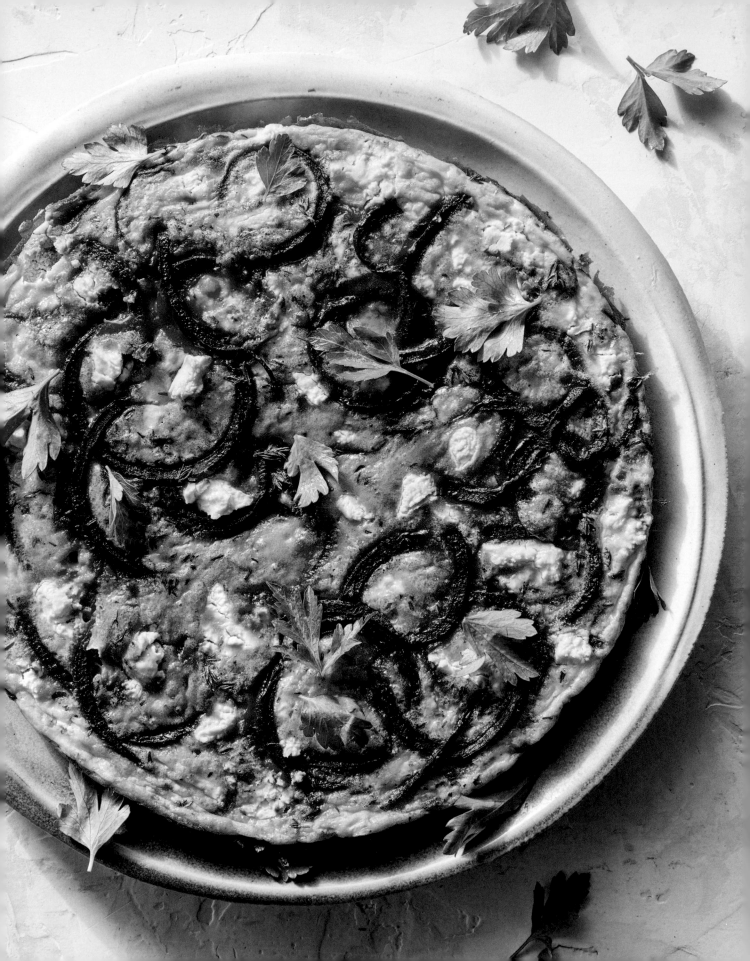

spiralized beet frittata

A frittata sounds fancy and sometimes it even looks fancy, but it's really just an incredibly easy, crustless quiche. All you need are some eggs, a little yogurt or cream, and whatever vegetables and herbs you'd like to toss in. They're the ultimate fridge clean-out recipe (along with egg scrambles) and can be served up for any meal of the day. You could make a frittata every week and never get bored! But there's one reason why I especially love this frittata—it sneaks a super healthy big red beet into your breakfast routine. And when was the last time you had beets for breakfast? Exactly. Time to change that! **serves 6**

1 large red beet, peeled and spiralized into noodles

2 tablespoons extra-virgin olive oil

½ medium yellow onion, diced

2 garlic cloves, minced

10 large eggs

½ cup plain Greek yogurt (dairy or dairy-free)

1 tablespoon chopped fresh thyme

½ teaspoon kosher salt

Pinch of freshly ground black pepper, to taste

1 cup (112g) crumbled goat cheese

1. Preheat the oven to 400°F (200°C). Use kitchen shears to snip the beet noodles into smaller pieces.

2. In a 10-inch (25cm) oven-safe skillet, heat the oil over medium heat. Add the onion and beet and sauté for 7 to 10 minutes, until tender. Add the garlic and sauté for another minute.

3. Meanwhile, in a large bowl, whisk together the eggs, yogurt, thyme, salt, and pepper until creamy.

4. Pour the egg mixture into the skillet and cook for 2 to 3 minutes, until the edge of the frittata just starts to firm up. Sprinkle the goat cheese on top and transfer the skillet to the oven. Bake for 15 to 20 minutes, until the eggs are set.

Serving size:
⅙ of frittata

Calories: 246
Fat: 18g
Saturated fat: 6g
Carbs: 6g
Fiber: 1g
Sugar: 4g
Protein: 16g
Cholesterol: 321mg
Sodium: 313mg

homemade granola (two ways)

When I was first diagnosed with celiac disease, I quickly learned by reading packaging labels that most store-bought granolas weren't gluten-free. Bummed that I couldn't enjoy those chunky, crunchy, clusters of oats, nuts, and other goodies, I began making my own with what I had in my pantry. These granolas are both naturally sweetened with either honey or maple syrup, perfectly spiced, have loads of texture to help form the best little clusters and—bonus—the maple almond granola is also grain-free. Making a batch of homemade granola is seriously easy, and when you're done, you've got something sweet, nutty, and crunchy to sprinkle on yogurt, chia pudding, or fresh fruit. **makes about 6 cups**

storage

Store in an airtight container at room temperature for several weeks, or in the freezer for up to 3 months.

get creative

Once your granola has baked, dried, and cooled, you can add a variety of mix-ins, including raisins, dried cherries, dried apricots, and yes, even chocolate chips.

honey oat granola

2½ cups (270g) gluten-free old-fashioned rolled oats

1 cup (120g) raw pecans, roughly chopped

½ cup (40g) unsweetened coconut flakes

¼ cup (28g) ground flaxseed

½ cup (160ml) honey

¼ cup (57ml) melted coconut oil

2 teaspoons vanilla extract

1 tablespoon ground cinnamon

½ teaspoon kosher salt

maple almond granola

2½ cups (210g) sliced almonds

½ cup (70g) raw cashews, roughly chopped

½ cup (62g) shelled raw sunflower seeds

½ cup (65g) raw pumpkin seeds (pepitas)

¼ cup (80ml) pure maple syrup

2 tablespoons blackstrap molasses

2 teaspoons vanilla extract

1 tablespoon ground cinnamon

½ teaspoon kosher salt

1. Preheat the oven to 300°F (150°C). Line a rimmed baking sheet with parchment paper.

2. In a large bowl, stir together the ingredients, then spread in an even layer on the prepared baking sheet.

3. Bake the granola for 25 to 30 minutes, stirring halfway through. The granola is done when it's lightly golden, though do keep an eye

Serving size (honey oat): ⅓ cup (30g)

Calories: 275
Fat: 17g
Saturated fat: 7g
Carbs: 30g
Fiber: 5g
Sugar: 12g
Protein: 5g
Cholesterol: 0mg
Sodium: 49mg

Serving size (maple almond): ⅓ cup (30g)

Calories: 183
Fat: 13g
Saturated fat: 1g
Carbs: 11g
Fiber: 3g
Sugar: 5g
Protein: 6g
Cholesterol: 0mg
Sodium: 44mg

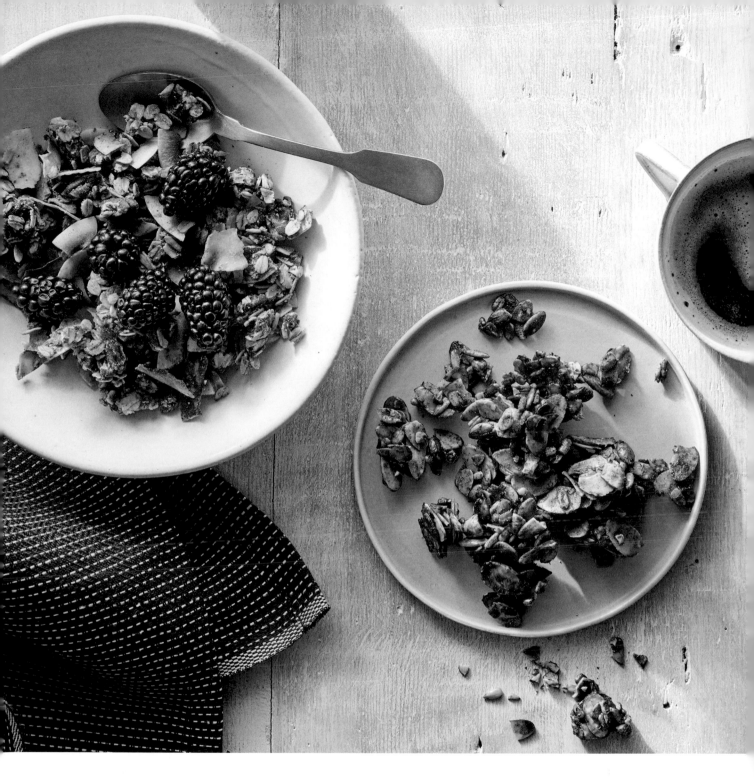

on it as it can burn quickly toward the end. When you remove it from the oven, it will still feel wet and sticky but will harden up as it cools.

4. Let the granola cool completely, then use your fingers to crumble it into pieces. If you'd like, you can toss with any optional add-ins before storing away (see Get Creative).

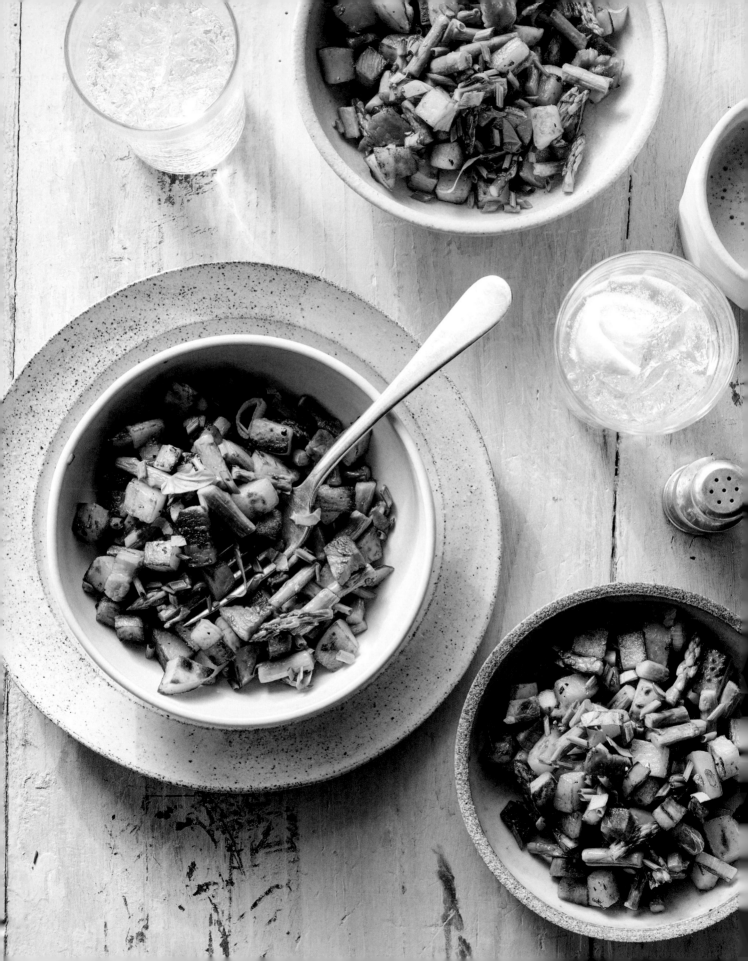

asparagus pancetta breakfast hash

When spring has sprung and I've got bundles of fresh greens from the farmers' market, this one-pan breakfast hash is first on my to-do list. Skinny asparagus, lively green onions, and aromatic herbs give it that energetic spring vibe, but the crispy pancetta and creamy potatoes are what make it so addictively delicious. Top it with jammy, soft-boiled eggs or poached eggs, and trust me, you will be in breakfast heaven. Yes, it's *that* darn good. **serves 4**

¼ **pound (112g) pancetta, diced**

1 **pound (454g) Yukon Gold potatoes, peeled and diced into small cubes**

½ **teaspoon kosher salt, plus more as needed**

¼ **teaspoon freshly ground black pepper, plus more as needed**

½ **pound (227g) skinny asparagus, woody ends trimmed, cut into ½-inch (1.3cm) pieces**

3 **green onions, sliced and separated into white and green parts**

1 **tablespoon roughly chopped fresh basil**

1 **tablespoon roughly chopped fresh chives**

1. In a large sauté pan over medium heat, cook the pancetta until crispy on all sides, about 10 minutes. Remove it with a slotted spoon to a paper towel–lined plate.

2. Add the potatoes in a single flat layer in the pan. Season with salt and pepper and let them crisp up, without stirring, for several minutes. Then flip them and repeat, until all sides are evenly browned, 10 to 12 minutes total. If the pan starts to look dry, you can add 1 to 2 tablespoons of additional oil as needed.

3. Add the asparagus and the white parts of the onion to the pan and stir. Cover the pan and let this cook for 5 to 7 minutes, stirring occasionally, until the asparagus is crisp-tender.

4. Remove the lid and add the green parts of the onion and the crispy pancetta to the pan. Stir for another minute to warm through. Turn off the heat and stir in the basil and chives. Taste and season with more salt and pepper if desired.

Serving size:
1 cup (126g)

Calories: 225
Fat: 13g
Saturated fat: 2g
Carbs: 22g
Fiber: 3g
Sugar: 2g
Protein: 8g
Cholesterol: 20mg
Sodium: 540mg

raspberry crumble bars

If granola bars and a dessert crisp came together in one recipe, they would be these raspberry crumble bars. Are they breakfast? Dessert? An on-the-go snack? Well, probably all the above, so use your best judgment (and maybe even a little restraint . . . if possible). Almond flour and rolled oats make up the base, and the filling is a generous amount of raspberry and chia seed jam. The top crumble is the oat base plus chopped pecans, with no added sugar, so it's not overly sweet. Hmm, I think I just convinced myself this is breakfast.

serves 9

storage

Store in an airtight container in the fridge for 4 to 5 days.

helpful tip

Let the bars cool completely before slicing into them—otherwise, they'll fall apart. But if they do, they'll make a tasty, messy topping on yogurt or ice cream!

FOR THE BASE

2½ cups (300g) almond flour

1 cup (108g) gluten-free old-fashioned rolled oats

½ teaspoon ground cinnamon

⅓ cup (80ml) melted butter or coconut oil

¼ cup (80ml) pure maple syrup

1 teaspoon vanilla extract

FOR THE FILLING

12 ounces (340g) fresh raspberries

2 tablespoons pure maple syrup

1 teaspoon fresh lemon juice

1 tablespoon chia seeds

1 tablespoon tapioca flour

FOR THE TOPPING

¼ cup (30g) raw pecans, roughly chopped

1. Preheat the oven to 350°F (180°C).

2. To make the base: In a medium bowl, stir together the flour, oats, cinnamon, butter, maple syrup, and vanilla extract until combined. Place a quarter of the crumble base in a small bowl and set aside.

3. Line an 8-inch (20cm) square pan with parchment paper going over the sides by about an inch. Add the crumble base and press it down firmly and evenly. Bake for 13 to 15 minutes, until lightly golden.

4. To make the filling: In a small pot over medium heat, combine the raspberries, maple syrup, and lemon juice. Simmer for 5 to 7 minutes, stirring occasionally and using the back of the spoon to help break down the raspberries. Once they have a puree-like texture, turn off the heat and stir in the chia seeds and tapioca flour.

5. Remove the base from the oven and spread the raspberry filling on top.

Serving size: 1 bar

Calories: 370

Fat: 23g

Saturated fat: 6g

Carbs: 35g

Fiber: 8g

Sugar: 11g

Protein: 11g

Cholesterol: 18mg

Sodium: 3mg

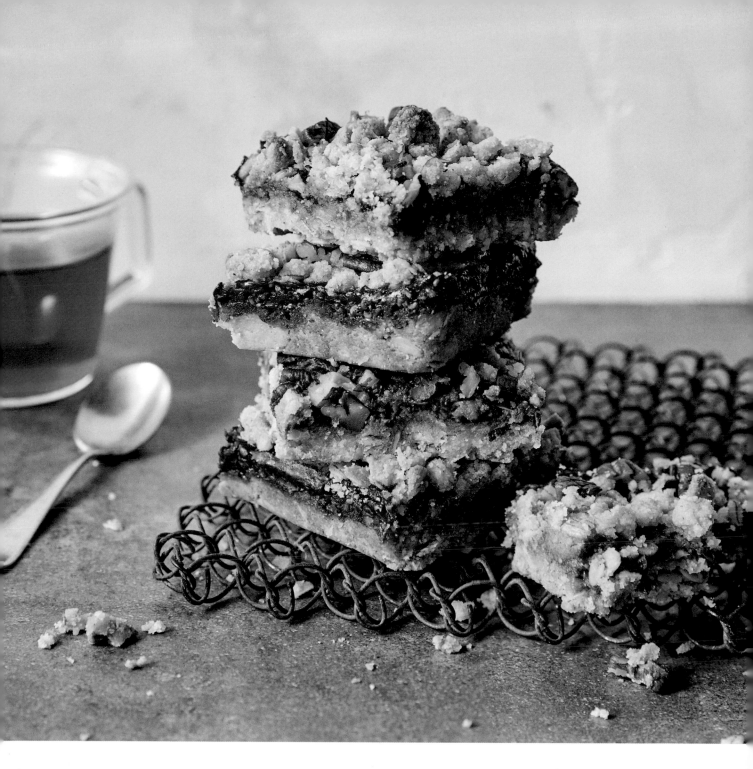

6. To make the topping: Add the chopped pecans to the reserved crumble and stir together. Sprinkle on top of the raspberry layer, and lightly press it into the raspberries, just so it sticks a bit to the middle layer. Bake for 25 to 30 minutes, until the top is golden.

7. Remove the crumble from the oven and let it cool completely in the pan. Once cooled, remove it from the pan and slice it into bars.

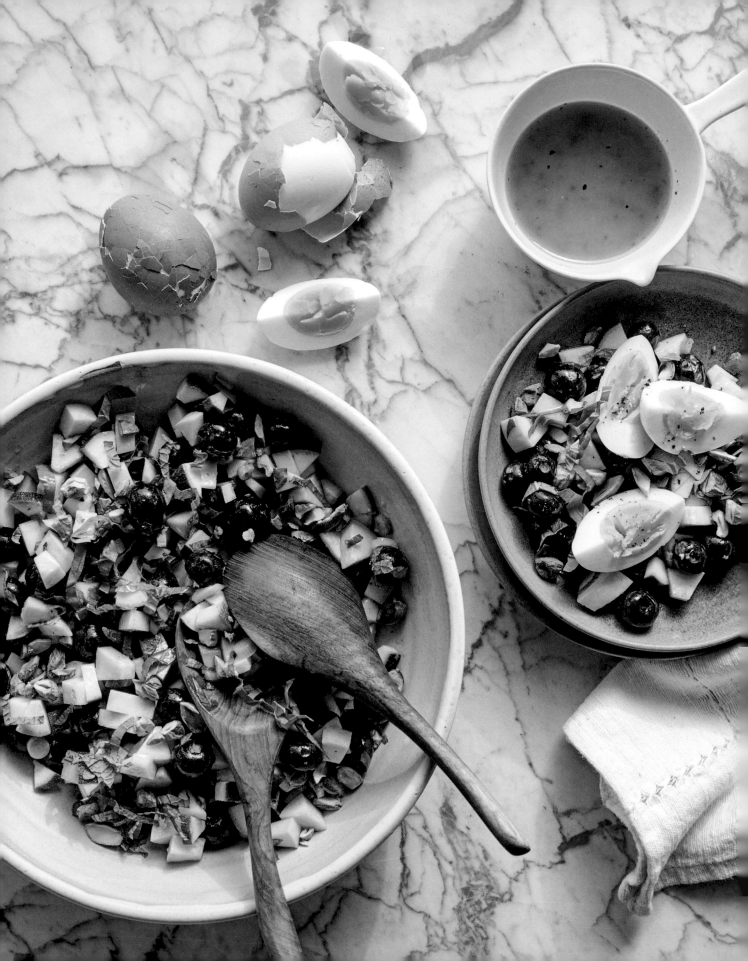

zucchini and blueberry breakfast salad

Salad for breakfast? Count me in! Especially when it's loaded with juicy anti-inflammatory blueberries and refreshing zucchini, then brightened with lemony flavor. The addition of hard-boiled eggs make it breakfast ready and protein packed, but it's the fresh basil and mint that gives it that garden-fresh salad spin. I feel like I'm always on a quest to remind people of two things: first, that you can eat any food any time of day, and second, to eat more veggies for breakfast. This recipe—a salad recipe—is a good-for-you way to start the day. **serves 4**

3 tablespoons extra-virgin olive oil

1½ tablespoons fresh lemon juice (from about ½ lemon)

1 small garlic clove, minced

1 teaspoon honey

½ teaspoon kosher salt

Freshly ground black pepper

1 medium zucchini

1 medium yellow summer squash

6 ounces (170g) blueberries

1 green onion (white and green parts), thinly sliced

¼ cup (30g) roughly chopped pistachios

3 tablespoons thinly sliced fresh basil

2 tablespoons thinly sliced fresh mint

4 hard-boiled eggs (see page 65), peeled and quartered

1. In a small bowl, whisk together the oil, lemon juice, garlic, honey, salt, and pinch of pepper and set aside.

2. Trim the ends off the zucchini and summer squash, then slice them into quarters lengthwise. Slice each of those quarters in half lengthwise once again, then slice across for a small dice and place in a large bowl.

3. Add the blueberries, green onion, chopped pistachios, basil, and mint. Drizzle with the dressing and give it a gentle toss.

4. Top with the hard-boiled eggs and season with a little extra sprinkle of salt and pepper before serving.

green goddess scrambled eggs

There might just be more greens than eggs in this recipe. And I'm okay with that! I adore fridge clean-out scrambles—they're the throw-together recipe I show most often on Instagram. And while you can use a variety of vegetables, I often find myself with frozen peas in the freezer and baby spinach and broccoli in the fridge just waiting to be used up. A quick sauté with a little onion and garlic turns a handful of simple ingredients into an easy, nutrient-packed green goddess scramble. It's a great way to sneak in greens at breakfast (add another layer of green with a side of avocado!), and leftovers are just as delicious the next day. **serves 4**

8 large eggs

¼ teaspoon kosher salt

Pinch of freshly ground black pepper

1 tablespoon extra-virgin olive oil

¼ cup (32g) diced yellow onion

½ cup (60g) broccoli rice or finely chopped broccoli

½ cup (85g) frozen peas

2 garlic cloves, minced

2 cups (70g) loosely packed baby spinach

Avocado slices, for garnish

1. In a large bowl, whisk together the eggs, salt, and pepper until light and foamy. Set aside.

2. In a large pan, heat the oil over medium heat and sauté the onion for 2 to 3 minutes, until softened. Add the broccoli and peas and sauté another minute, then add the garlic and spinach and sauté for 1 to 2 minutes more, until the spinach has wilted.

3. Pour the eggs on top of the vegetables and use a silicone spatula to push the edges of the eggs toward the middle, gently flipping them, then let them resettle. Continue this process until the eggs are just set.

4. Remove the eggs to a plate and serve with a few slices of avocado.

storage
Let the eggs cool slightly, then store in an airtight container in the fridge for 3 to 4 days, or in the freezer for up to 3 months.

to reheat
Thaw in the fridge overnight. Reheat in a lightly buttered or greased pan on the stove. You can also microwave in 15-second increments, stirring in between, until warmed through. Be careful not to over-reheat as the eggs can turn spongy and dry.

get creative
Turn the scrambled eggs into a breakfast burrito or quesadilla with a little cheese and a tortilla, or a collard green breakfast wrap (yes, more greens!).

helpful tip
If you plan to store and reheat all the scrambled eggs, it's best to slightly undercook them on the stove. That way, they'll stay moist and fluffy when reheated.

Serving size:
1 cup (150g)

Calories: 216

Fat: 14g

Saturated fat: 4g

Carbs: 7g

Fiber: 2g

Sugar: 3g

Protein: 15g

Cholesterol: 373mg

Sodium: 226mg

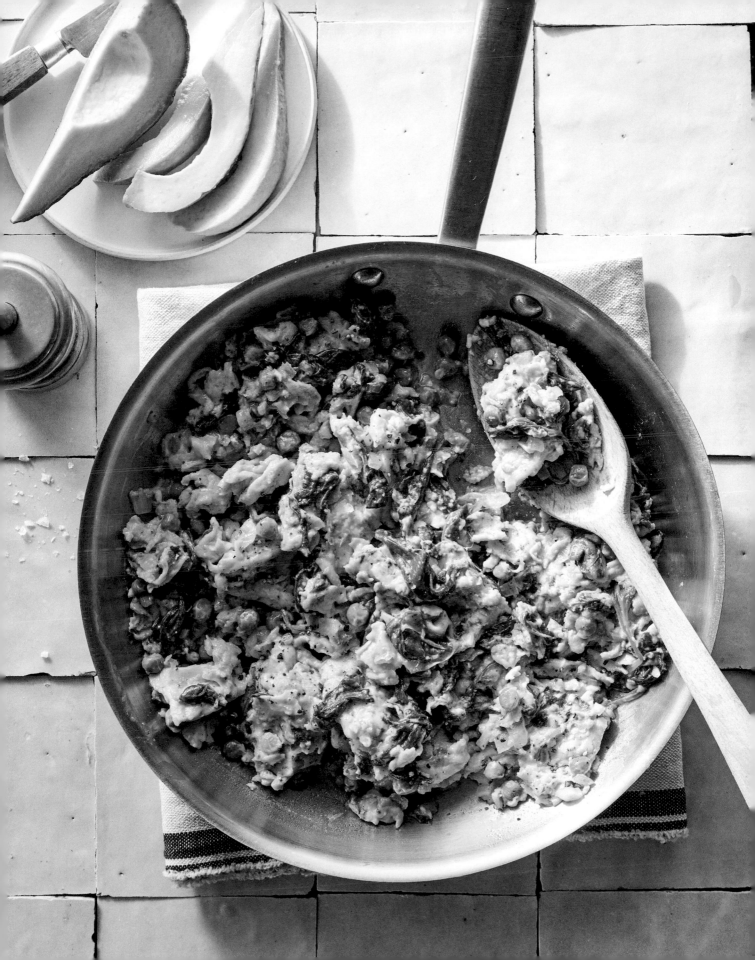

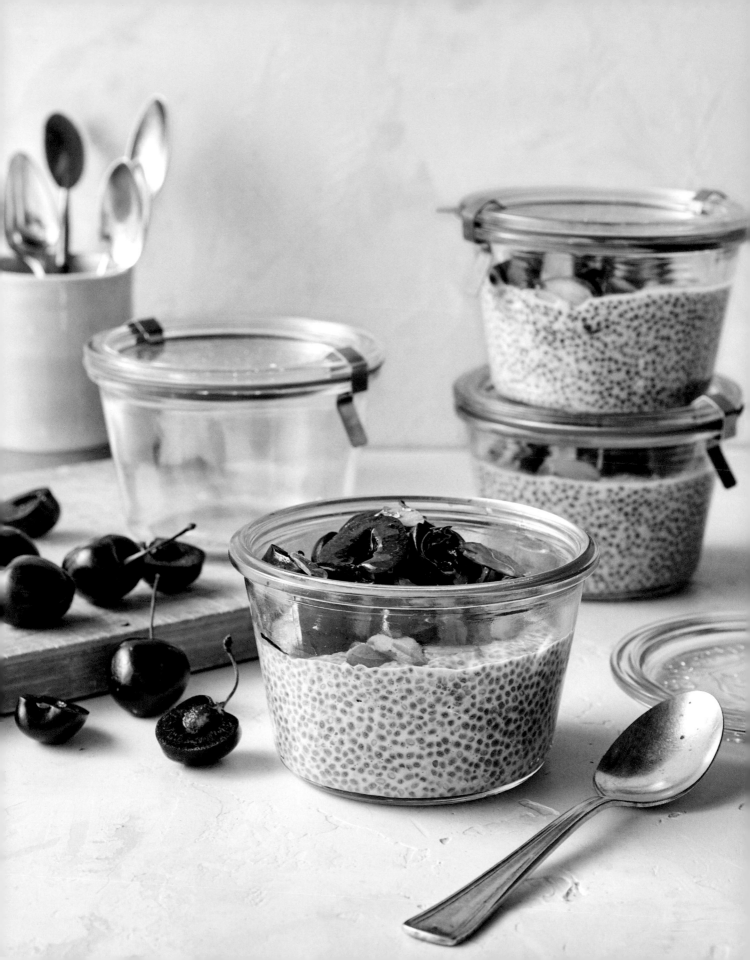

cherry almond chia pudding

Chia pudding might just be the easiest healthy breakfast you can make. All you have to do is stir chia seeds and milk together along with any sweetener of your choice, and a couple of hours later you've got the most delicious pudding. I've got a single serving for you below, but you can also make a large batch (just double, triple, or quadruple the base), then freeze individual portions for several weeks or months. Topping combinations are virtually endless, but this cherry almond chia pudding is divine and tastes like cherry clafouti!

serves 1

storage

Store in an airtight container the fridge for 4 to 5 days, or in the freezer for up to 3 months. To thaw a frozen serving, just place it in the fridge the day before.

get creative

Other toppings for chia pudding include fresh fruit (strawberries, blueberries, blackberries, raspberries, kiwi, mango, and pineapple are great additions), fruit purees, nut butters, dried fruit, and spices.

BASE CHIA PUDDING

½ cup (120ml) dairy or dairy-free milk

2 tablespoons chia seeds

1 teaspoon pure maple syrup

½ teaspoon vanilla extract

FOR THE CHERRY ALMOND TOPPING

10 cherries, pitted and halved

¼ teaspoon pure maple syrup

¼ teaspoon almond extract

Sprinkle of sliced almonds

1. To make the pudding: In a small bowl, stir together the milk, chia seeds, maple syrup, and vanilla. Let it sit for 10 to 15 minutes, then stir again once the seeds have started to gel.

2. To make the topping: In a separate small bowl, stir together the cherries, maple syrup, and almond extract. Pour on top of the chia pudding, then cover the bowl and place in the refrigerator for at least 1 hour. Top with sliced almonds before serving. Chia pudding can also be made overnight for breakfast the next morning (my preferred method).

Serving size: 1 recipe

Calories: 243

Fat: 11g

Saturated fat: 1g

Carbs: 30g

Fiber: 10g

Sugar: 17g

Protein: 6g

Cholesterol: 0mg

Sodium: 91mg

frozen yogurt bark

During those summer months of sweltering heat (it can get mighty hot in Southern California), I make a batch of this cooling and refreshing yogurt bark. Think of it as a frozen yogurt Popsicle in bark form. It's incredibly easy to make—you don't have to fiddle with any sticks or Popsicle molds, and you can endlessly switch up the toppings. The combo I seem to make most often is strawberries and granola. It's sweet, crunchy, packed with protein, and perfect for those 11 a.m. munchies. **serves 8**

3 cups (680g) plain Greek yogurt (dairy or dairy-free)

¼ cup (80ml) pure maple syrup or honey

½ teaspoon vanilla extract

1 cup (120g) sliced strawberries

⅓ cup (30g) Homemade Granola (page 106)

1. Line a sheet pan with parchment paper.

2. In a medium bowl, stir together the yogurt, maple syrup, and vanilla. Spread the yogurt mix on the parchment paper to an even ½-inch (1.3cm) thickness.

3. Top the yogurt mix with the sliced strawberries and granola. Freeze for 2 to 3 hours, or until firm. Break into pieces and serve.

storage
Store in the freezer in an airtight container for up to 3 months.

get creative
Feel free to swap in blueberries, kiwi fruit, peaches, or your favorite fruit, along with chopped nuts for the granola. While I love full-fat Greek yogurt for its ultra-creamy texture, you can also use low-fat or nonfat yogurt.

Serving size:
About 3 pieces (90g)

Calories: 138

Fat: 5g

Saturated fat: 3g

Carbs: 16g

Fiber: 1g

Sugar: 14g

Protein: 9g

Cholesterol: 14mg

Sodium: 40mg

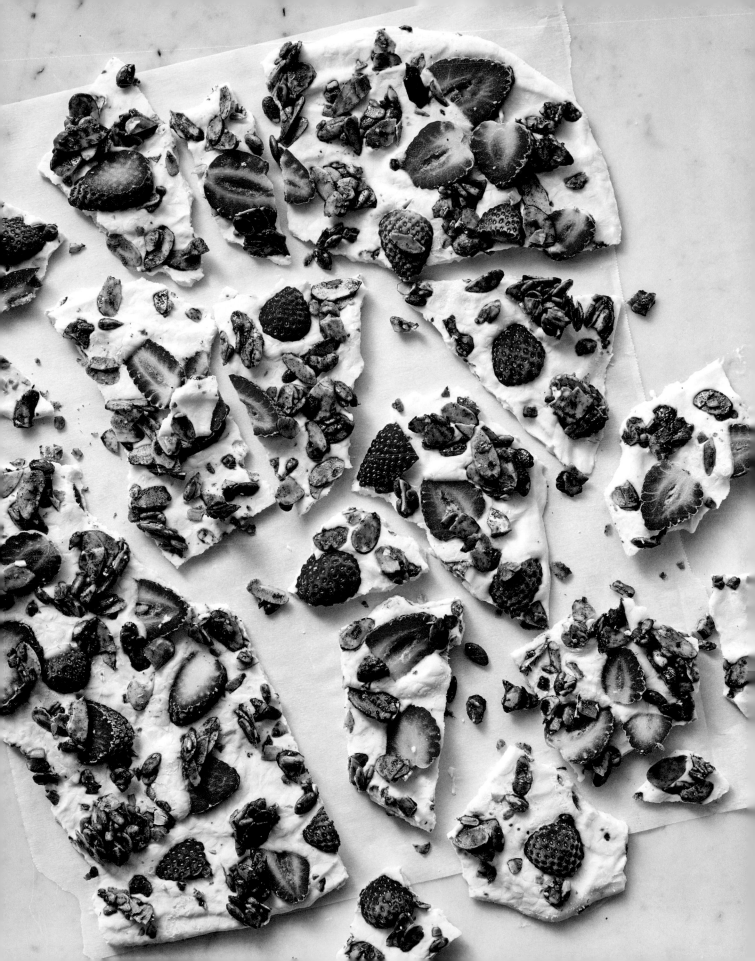

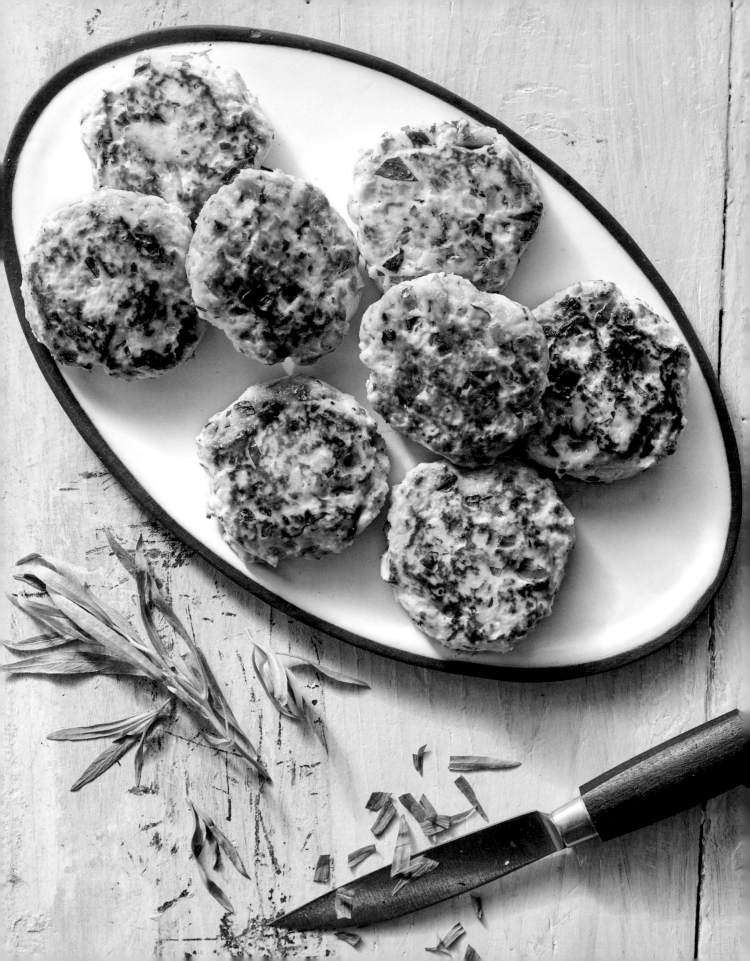

chicken, maple, and tarragon breakfast patties

Breakfast patties, when served alongside eggs and sautéed veggies or hash browns, are reminiscent of your favorite diner or cafe breakfast (but with no line or wait!). And while pork may be the go-to meat for breakfast sausages, these chicken-based patties are equally hearty and distinctly delicious with their touch of maple sweetness. The best part is that you can easily double (or even triple) this batch and freeze them. serves 8

1 pound (454g) ground chicken

⅓ cup (43g) finely diced yellow onion

2 garlic cloves, minced

2 tablespoons pure maple syrup

1 teaspoon kosher salt

½ teaspoon freshly ground black pepper

2 tablespoons finely chopped fresh tarragon

2 tablespoons avocado oil or extra-virgin olive oil

1. In a large bowl, use your hands to mix together the ground chicken, onion, garlic, maple syrup, salt, pepper, and tarragon until well combined.

2. Evenly divide the mixture into 8 portions. Use your hands to form 8 small patties and place them on a plate.

3. In a large skillet, heat the oil on medium-high heat. Cook the patties for 3 to 4 minutes on each side, until golden. Use a spatula to remove the patties to a paper towel–lined plate.

Serving size: 1 patty

Calories: 149

Fat: 9g

Saturated fat: 2g

Carbs: 5g

Fiber: 0g

Sugar: 3g

Protein: 14g

Cholesterol: 61mg

Sodium: 184mg

blueberry pancakes

You can't go wrong with Sunday morning pancakes that are thick, fluffy, and dotted with juicy blueberries. Several years ago, I tried every possible gluten-free, grain-free, dairy-free pancake recipe I could find. But most came out too dense, too gritty, too almond-y or too coconut-y. So I created my own recipe, using a triumvirate of flours for the perfect texture! A drizzle of maple syrup is a must, as is a side of crispy bacon or Chicken, Maple, and Tarragon Breakfast Patties (page 121). And if you don't mention that they're free of gluten, grain, and dairy, they could easily be mistaken for traditional pancakes (so best keep that to yourself). **serves 4**

½ cup (60g) almond flour

⅓ cup (40g) tapioca flour

¼ cup (30g) coconut flour

½ teaspoon baking soda

¼ teaspoon kosher salt

4 large eggs

½ cup (120ml) milk (dairy or dairy-free)

1 tablespoon pure maple syrup, plus more to drizzle

1 teaspoon apple cider vinegar

1 teaspoon vanilla extract

1 cup (148g) blueberries, plus more to garnish

Butter or oil, such as coconut oil or avocado oil, to coat skillet

1. In a large bowl, whisk together the almond flour, tapioca flour, coconut flour, baking soda, and salt.

2. In a medium bowl, whisk together the eggs, milk, maple syrup, vinegar, and vanilla. Pour the wet ingredients into the dry and stir until well combined, then fold in the blueberries. If needed, let the batter sit for 3 to 5 minutes to thicken up.

3. Heat a large skillet or griddle and melt the butter on medium-high heat.

4. Spoon small heaps of the batter into the skillet. Keeping your pancakes 3 to 4 inches (7.6 to 10.2cm) in diameter will make them much easier to flip. Let them cook for 2 to 3 minutes on one side, then flip and cook for an additional 1 to 2 minutes.

storage

Store in an airtight container in the fridge for 4 to 5 days, or in the freezer for up to 3 months. To freeze, place them in a single layer on a piece of parchment paper in the freezer for 1 to 2 hours, until frozen. Then transfer them to a storage container and stack the frozen pancakes.

to reheat

Pop the pancakes in your toaster or reheat in the microwave for 1 minute if thawed, or 2 to 3 minutes, if frozen.

helpful tip

I use baking soda plus vinegar to create fluffy pancakes (it's a lovely chemical reaction of bubbles), but you could swap both of those items for 1 teaspoon of baking powder.

Serving size: 2 pancakes

Calories: 271

Fat: 14g

Saturated fat: 3g

Carbs: 26g

Fiber: 5g

Sugar: 10g

Protein: 11g

Cholesterol: 187mg

Sodium: 390mg

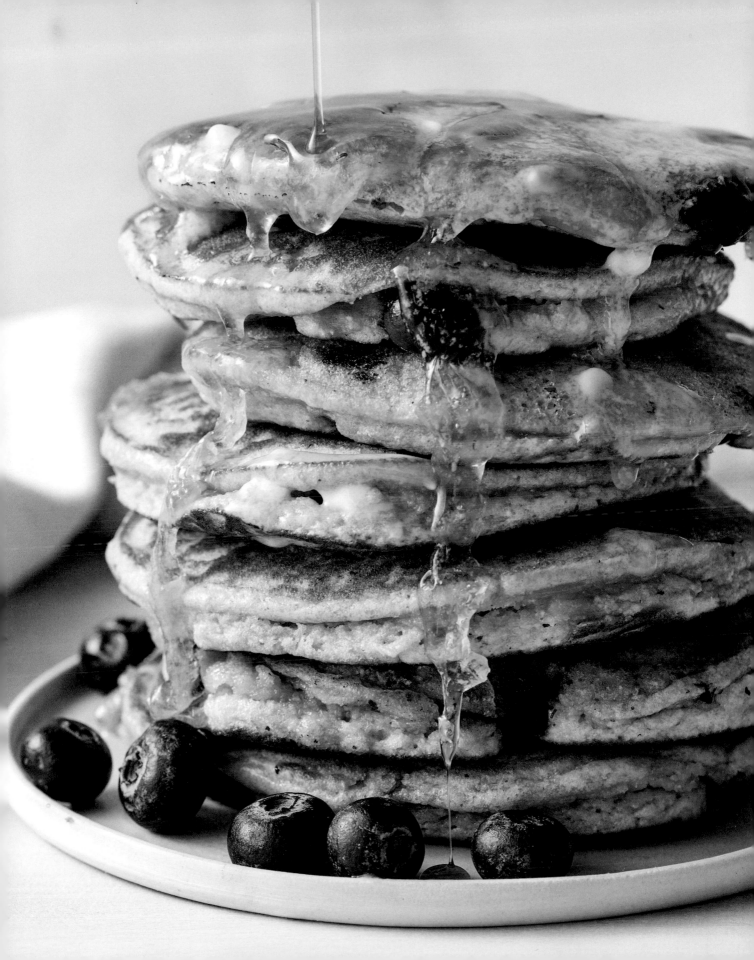

durable salads

Salads reign supreme for getting a hefty amount of vegetables in your diet. That's why I always encourage you to eat at least one salad a day, whether it's as a main meal, light lunch, or side salad to accompany another recipe.

When it comes to meal prep, I find that people often skip salads because they're afraid the salads will wilt and go mushy or that ingredients may brown. And that can definitely happen if you don't choose the *right* ingredients. My dad always joked that salads were "rabbit food" because of all the leafy greens, and let's be honest, leafy greens are somewhat synonymous with salads. However, you won't find any leafy green salads in this chapter! Nor will you find any avocado (shocker, I know), apples, or other ingredients that will discolor when stored in the fridge.

Instead, you'll find salads that are durable enough to last several days and tasty enough that you'll want to eat them for several days (the most important part). Some of them, like the Mango Curried Chicken Salad (page 127) are hearty enough to be a stand-alone main meal, while others like my Grilled Corn and Zucchini Salad (page 139) are the perfect light, fresh, summertime side dish—you could also add shredded meat from a roasted chicken (see page 179) to turn it into a main dish. In other words, there are lots of options to help you easily meet your daily salad goals!

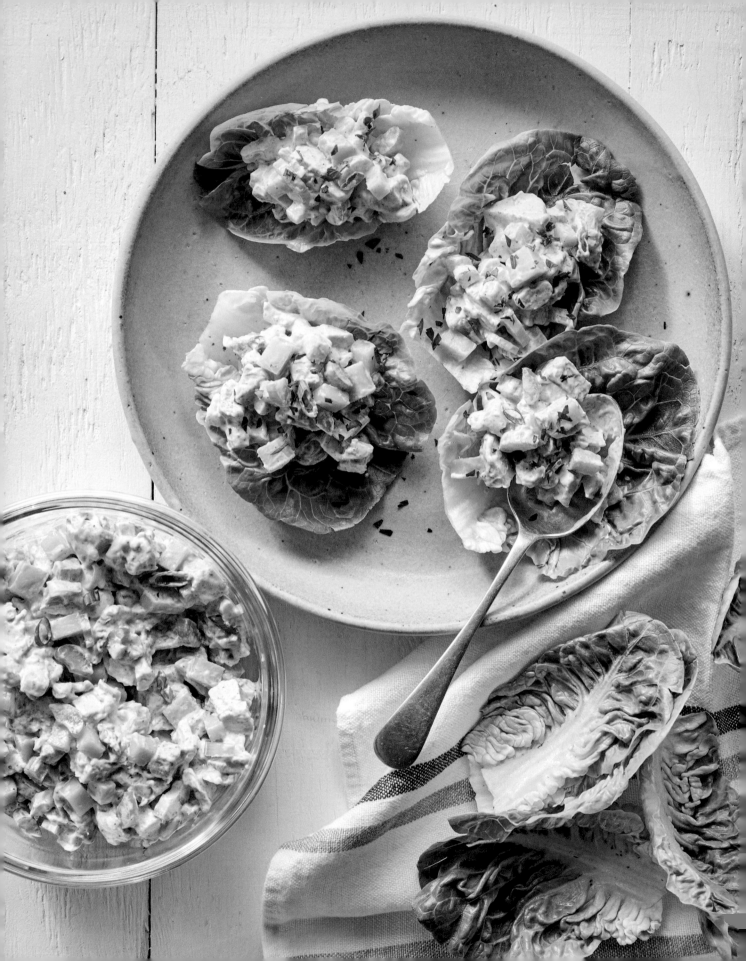

mango curry chicken salad

storage

Store in an airtight container in the fridge for 4 to 5 days.

ways to serve

In addition to enjoying this salad by itself (which is what I usually do), you can pile it on gluten-free bread to make a sandwich, or roll it up in lettuce leaves or a grain-free tortilla to make a wrap.

helpful tip

When shopping for a ripe mango at the market, look for a slightly soft texture (similar to a ripe avocado). If your mango is a bit hard or completely green, you can speed up the ripening process by placing it in a paper bag at room temperature for a couple of days.

Serving size:
1½ cups (262g)

Calories: 650
Fat: 40g
Saturated fat: 7g
Carbs: 23g
Fiber: 3g
Sugar: 17g
Protein: 51g
Cholesterol: 144mg
Sodium: 466mg

This sweet and spicy twist on chicken salad is the perfect blend of juicy sweet mango, spicy curry, vibrant herbs, and crunchy cashew bits in a lusciously creamy base. Chicken salad is a much-loved classic and for good reason—it's delicious! But this version is entirely next level. Not only is it fresh and exciting, it's durable enough to last up to five days in the fridge, well theoretically anyway—if you can keep it in your fridge that long, you've certainly got more willpower than I do! **serves 6**

2 pounds (907g) boneless, skinless chicken breasts

2 mangoes, peeled, pitted, and diced

2 celery ribs, diced

4 green onions (white and green parts), thinly sliced

½ cup (70g) raw cashews, roughly chopped

2 tablespoons roughly chopped fresh parsley

2 tablespoons roughly chopped fresh cilantro

½ teaspoon kosher salt

½ teaspoon freshly ground black pepper

1 cup (220g) mayonnaise

3 tablespoons fresh lemon juice (from about 1 lemon)

1 tablespoon curry powder

1. Place the chicken in a wide pot and cover by about 1 inch of cold water. Set over medium heat, add a generous pinch of salt, and bring the water to a gentle boil. Reduce the heat to a low simmer and cover.

2. Let the chicken simmer for 8 to 12 minutes, or until an instant-read thermometer reads 160°F (71°C). Use tongs to transfer the chicken to a plate and let it rest for a couple of minutes, then place it in the fridge until it's completely cooled, about 15 minutes.

3. Set the cooled chicken on a cutting board and dice into ½-inch (1.3cm) pieces. Place it in a large mixing bowl and add the diced mango, celery, green onions, cashews, parsley, cilantro, salt, and pepper.

4. In a separate small bowl, whisk together the mayonnaise, lemon juice, and curry powder. Stir this mixture into the chicken until combined. Cover the bowl with plastic wrap and refrigerate until chilled, about 30 minutes, then serve as you like (see Ways to Serve).

shaved brussels sprouts, fennel, and mandarin salad with lemon vinaigrette

I love this salad for two reasons. First, shaved Brussels sprouts are a great way to bulk up a salad with healthy greens that won't wilt. And second, both Brussels sprouts and mandarin oranges are seasonal winter ingredients. I'm hoping this recipe nudges you toward a salad during what is typically the overindulgent holiday period (wink wink). This salad is great for a light, restorative lunch, but if you want to turn it into a full meal, just add some shredded roasted chicken (see page 179) or even flaked cod (see page 191). **serves 6**

storage

Store in an airtight container in the fridge for 3 to 4 days.

helpful tip

You can use a knife or a mandoline to shave the Brussels sprouts. The mandoline is quick and easy, but please do use a cut-proof glove—those suckers are sharp!

FOR THE LEMON VINAIGRETTE

⅓ cup (80ml) extra-virgin olive oil

¼ cup (60ml) fresh lemon juice

1 teaspoon Dijon mustard

½ teaspoon honey

1 garlic clove, minced

½ teaspoon kosher salt

Freshly ground black pepper

FOR THE SALAD

1 pound (454g) Brussels sprouts, ends trimmed, and shaved or thinly sliced

6 mandarin oranges, peeled and segmented

2 green onions (white and green parts), thinly sliced

¾ cup (63g) sliced almonds

1 medium fennel bulb, fronds removed, cored and very thinly sliced

¼ cup (22g) grated pecorino Romano cheese

1. To make the dressing: In a small bowl, whisk together vigorously the oil, lemon juice, mustard, honey, garlic, salt, and pepper until blended and emulsified.

2. To make the salad: In a large mixing bowl, combine the shaved Brussels sprouts, mandarin oranges, green onions, sliced almonds, fennel, and pecorino Romano cheese. Drizzle the dressing on top and toss the salad to combine.

Serving size:
2 cups (226g)

Calories: 295

Fat: 21g

Saturated fat: 3g

Carbs: 23g

Fiber: 7g

Sugar: 12g

Protein: 8g

Cholesterol: 3mg

Sodium: 225mg

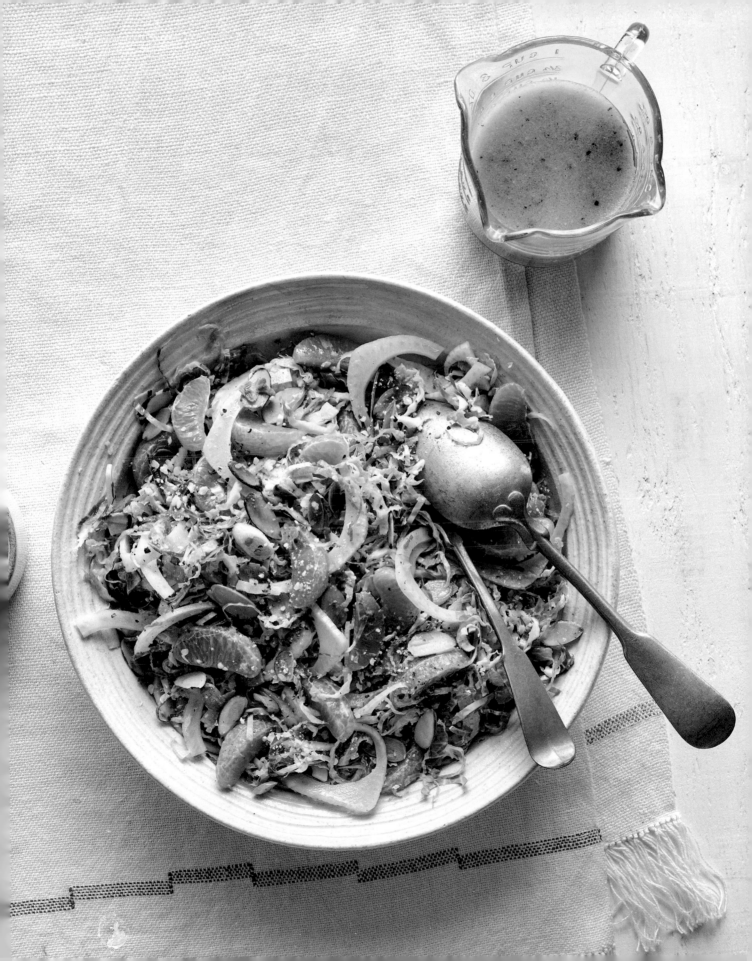

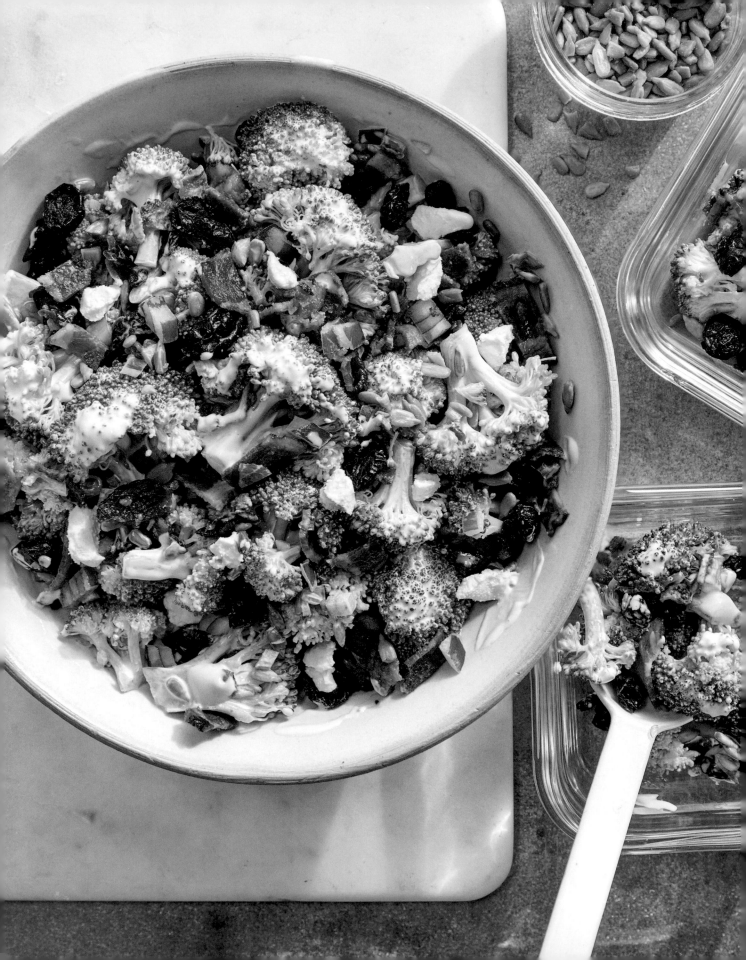

broccoli salad with crispy bacon, sunflower seeds, and cranberries

storage

Store in an airtight container in the fridge for 4 to 5 days.

dietary swaps

The beauty of a broccoli salad is that it's easy to customize. Bacon, dried fruit, cheese, and seeds are usually involved, and you can tweak each of these to your dietary preference. Feel free to use raisins instead of dried cranberries or slivered almonds instead of sunflower seeds. You could also make this salad dairy-free by eliminating the goat cheese and using a nondairy yogurt.

helpful tip

If you're wondering what to do with the broccoli stem, spiralize it! You can spiralize it just as you would a zucchini. It's delicious!

For a salad that can consistently surprise and delight you, look no further than this simple, unassuming broccoli salad. It may be easy to make, but this salad recipe is loaded with flavor. It's simultaneously crispy, creamy, sweet, and savory. And did I mention bacon is involved? The mayonnaise-based dressing ties everything together, and I "up" the creaminess factor by adding a little yogurt. It adds just the right sweetness and tang. **serves 6**

8 slices bacon

1 large head of broccoli, florets sliced into bite-size pieces

⅓ cup (43g) diced red onion

½ cup (60g) dried unsweetened cranberries

½ cup (62g) shelled raw sunflower seeds

¼ cup (28g) crumbled goat cheese

½ cup (110g) mayonnaise

¼ cup (57g) plain Greek yogurt (dairy or dairy-free)

1. Preheat the oven to 400°F (200°C). Arrange the bacon slices on a rimmed baking sheet lined with parchment paper and cook for 15 to 20 minutes, until crispy. Transfer the bacon to a paper towel–lined plate to drain and cool.

2. While the bacon is cooking, in a large mixing bowl, combine the broccoli florets, red onion, dried cranberries, sunflower seeds, and goat cheese.

3. In a small bowl, stir together the mayonnaise and yogurt. Add the bacon and dressing to the mixing bowl and toss to combine.

Serving size:
2 cups (203g)

Calories: 352
Fat: 27g
Saturated fat: 6g
Carbs: 18g
Fiber: 6g
Sugar: 5g
Protein: 11g
Cholesterol: 27mg
Sodium: 299mg

roasted butternut squash, kale, and lentil salad with maple balsamic vinaigrette

This warm and comforting salad is my antidote to cold-weather blues (yes, even in Southern California it gets cold!). The butternut squash gets slightly caramelized after a stop in the oven, the kale gives you a good dose of nutrients during those months you need it most, and the French lentils are sturdy enough to hold their shape after lots of tossing (and won't become soggy after storing in the fridge). Heads up: There's a good number of portions in this salad, so it'll last you and a significant other for the week, or you can serve it during the holidays as the perfect side dish. **serves 8**

storage

Store in an airtight container in the fridge for 4 to 5 days. Serve chilled, at room temperature, or warmed up in the microwave.

helpful tip

Lentil salads get even better after they have a chance to soak up the flavor in the dressing, so feel free to make this a day (or more) in advance of serving.

FOR THE MAPLE BALSAMIC VINAIGRETTE

¼ cup (60ml) extra-virgin olive oil

3 tablespoons balsamic vinegar

1 teaspoon Dijon mustard

1 small garlic clove, minced

1 tablespoon pure maple syrup

½ teaspoon kosher salt

Pinch of freshly ground black pepper

FOR THE SALAD

1 butternut squash (about 2½ pounds/1.1kg), peeled, seeded, and diced into ½-inch (1.3cm) cubes

2 tablespoons extra-virgin olive oil

1 teaspoon kosher salt

½ teaspoon freshly ground black pepper

1½ cups (250g) French lentils, picked over and rinsed

1 bunch of kale, stemmed, leaves roughly chopped

1 shallot, finely diced

½ cup (60g) raw pumpkin seeds (pepitas)

½ cup (60g) dried unsweetened cranberries

¼ cup (28g) crumbled feta cheese

Roughly chopped fresh parsley, for garnish

Serving size:
1¼ cups (175g)

Calories: 346

Fat: 15g

Saturated fat: 3g

Carbs: 45g

Fiber: 10g

Sugar: 8g

Protein: 12g

Cholesterol: 3mg

Sodium: 144mg

1. Preheat the oven to 400°F (200°C).

2. To make the dressing: In a small bowl, whisk together the oil, vinegar, mustard, garlic, maple syrup, salt, and pepper.

3. To make the salad: On a rimmed baking sheet, toss the butternut squash with oil, salt, and pepper, then spread it out in an even layer. Roast for 40 to 45 minutes, tossing the cubes halfway through,

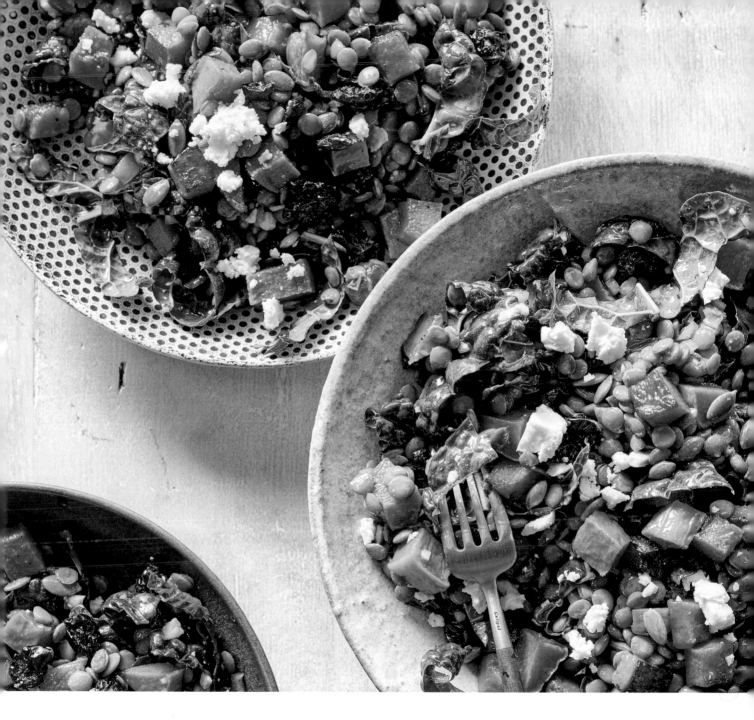

until tender and caramelized. Remove from the oven and set aside to cool slightly.

4. While the squash is roasting, in a small pot, bring 5 cups water and the lentils to a boil over high heat. Reduce the heat to low, cover the pot, and simmer the lentils for 15 to 20 minutes, until they are al dente, not mushy. Drain the lentils through a fine-mesh sieve.

5. In a large bowl, combine the butternut squash, kale, lentils, shallot, pepitas, cranberries, and feta cheese. Drizzle the dressing over the salad and toss to combine. Top with the parsley.

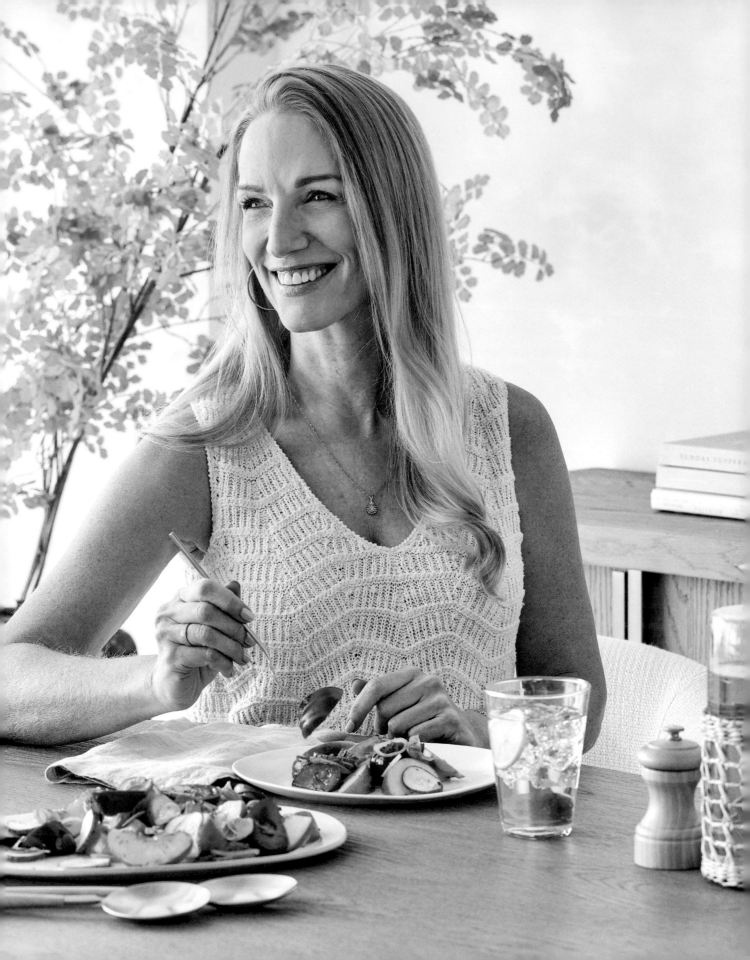

peach and tomato salad

storage

Store in an airtight container in the fridge for 3 to 4 days.

helpful tips

If you don't have peaches, you can swap in other stone fruits like nectarines, apricots, or plums (or just double the tomatoes). You can also swap sherry vinegar for the white balsamic vinegar. And if you're okay with dairy, this salad is extra scrumptious with a little creamy goat cheese or burrata.

This salad is summertime in a bowl. Fresh, juicy tomatoes, succulent peaches, and itty-bitty, crunchy Persian cucumbers are paired with garden fresh herbs and a thinly sliced shallot, then gently tossed with a sweet and mildly tangy white balsamic vinaigrette. It's simplicity at its finest, so seek out the best-of-the-best in-season peaches and tomatoes picked right at their prime—even if you have to jump the fence and snag them from your neighbors' garden. Just kidding (kind of). **serves 6**

FOR THE DRESSING

2 tablespoons extra-virgin olive oil

1 tablespoon white balsamic vinegar

1 teaspoon honey

Kosher salt and freshly ground black pepper to taste

FOR THE SALAD

4 large ripe tomatoes, cored and sliced into wedges

4 peaches, halved, pitted, and sliced into thick wedges

2 baby Persian cucumbers, thinly sliced

1 small shallot, very thinly sliced

2 tablespoons torn or roughly chopped fresh mint

2 tablespoons torn or roughly chopped fresh basil

1. To make the dressing: In a small bowl, whisk together the oil, vinegar, honey, and salt and pepper.

2. To make the salad: In a large mixing bowl, add the tomatoes, peaches, cucumbers, and shallot. Pour the dressing over the salad, add the mint and basil, and toss everything together to combine.

Serving size:
1½ cups (218g)

Calories: 120
Fat: 5g
Saturated fat: 1g
Carbs: 19g
Fiber: 3g
Sugar: 15g
Protein: 2g
Cholesterol: 0g
Sodium: 7g

potato, green bean, and egg salad with red wine vinaigrette

This French-inspired potato salad puts a decidedly elegant spin on classic potato salad with the addition of crisp-tender green beans, soft-boiled eggs with just a hint of a jammy yolk (8-minute eggs for the win in this recipe), and loads of fresh herbs. While many potato salads are tossed with a mayo-based dressing, this one has a tangy, garlicky vinaigrette that's light and fresh, complementing the springtime herbs perfectly. Just make sure to toss everything together before adding the eggs, otherwise the yolks will spill out, and not be *quite* as elegantly French (though still wonderfully delicious). serves 6

FOR THE RED WINE VINAIGRETTE

¼ cup (60ml) extra-virgin olive oil

2 tablespoons red wine vinegar

2 teaspoons Dijon mustard

2 garlic cloves, minced

½ teaspoon kosher salt

Freshly ground black pepper

FOR THE SALAD

1½ pounds (680g) small white potatoes

4 large eggs

1 pound (454g) green beans (preferably French haricots verts), trimmed

3 tablespoons roughly chopped fresh herbs, such as parsley, dill, and chives

Kosher salt and freshly ground black pepper

1. To make the vinaigrette: In a small bowl, whisk together the oil, vinegar, mustard, garlic, salt, and some pepper.

2. To make the salad: Bring a large pot of salted water (with a heaping tablespoon of salt added) to a boil. Add the potatoes to the pot, reduce the heat to a simmer, and cook until tender, about 20 minutes. Use a slotted spoon to remove the potatoes, transfer to a cutting board, and let cool.

3. While the potatoes are boiling, cook the eggs. Bring a medium pot of water to a boil, then reduce the heat to low, gently add in the eggs, and cook for 8 minutes, depending on how firm you like your yolk. Use a slotted spoon to transfer the eggs to an ice-water bath for a few minutes. Then crack, peel, and halve each one.

storage

Store in an airtight container in the fridge for 3 to 4 days.

helpful tip

Grab the smallest white potatoes that you can find for this recipe. If using new potatoes, I try to find ones that are about the same size as the eggs. If you'd like something even smaller, feel free to swap in fingerling or marble potatoes—but note that you may need to reduce the boiling time by up to 10 minutes.

Serving size: 1½ cups (235g)

Calories: 232

Fat: 13g

Saturated fat: 2g

Carbs: 23g

Fiber: 5g

Sugar: 3g

Protein: 8g

Cholesterol: 123g

Sodium: 153g

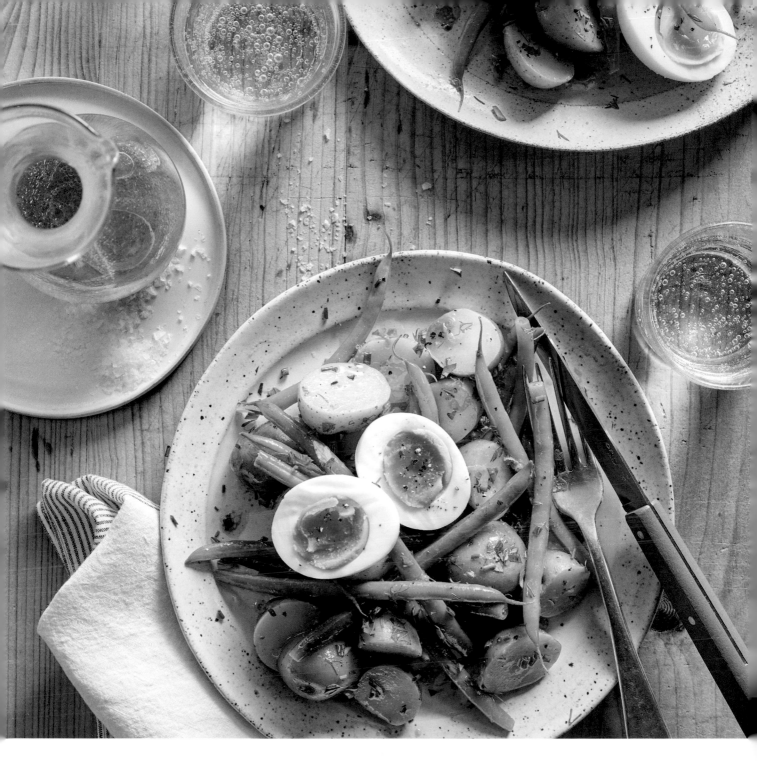

4. Return the medium pot of water to a boil and add the green beans. Cook until just tender, 4 to 5 minutes, then transfer to the ice-water bath. Drain and pat dry.

5. Cut the potatoes into halves, or in quarters if they're large, and place in a large bowl. Add green beans and herbs, then toss with the dressing. Before serving, arrange the eggs on top, and season with additional salt and pepper if desired.

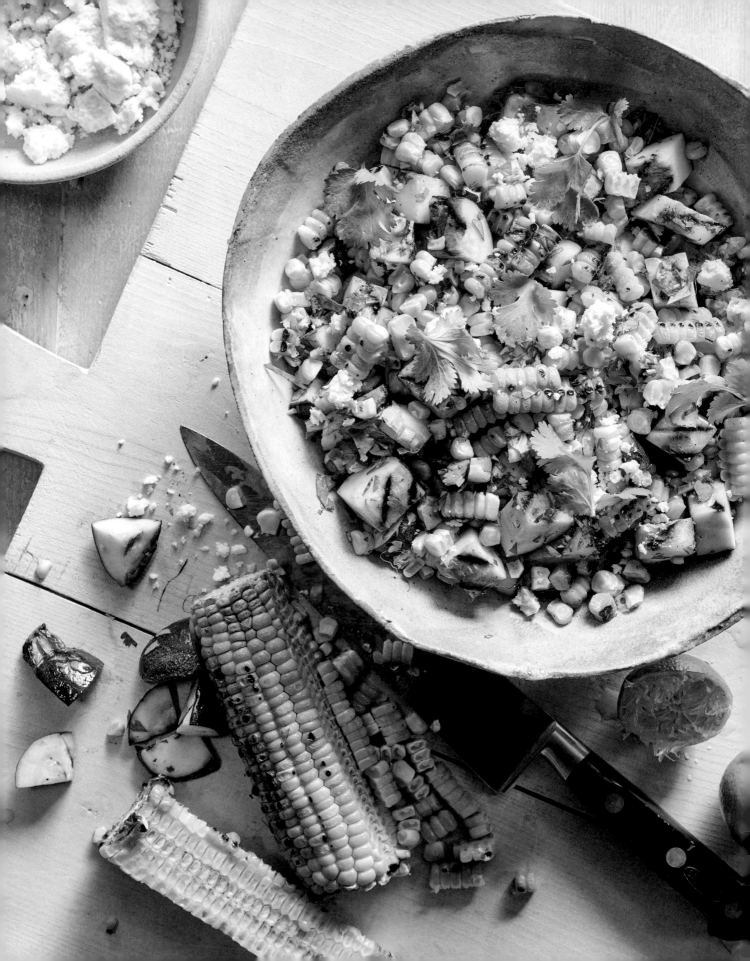

grilled corn and zucchini salad

storage

Store in an airtight container in the fridge for 4 to 5 days.

helpful tip

There's always a debate over whether you should grill corn with or without the husk. Leaving the husks on the corn protects it from the direct heat of the grill and gently steams it as it cooks. Removing the husks, as I've done in this recipe, gives it a more charred flavor, with a crisp-tender texture. Give it a try both ways and see which you prefer!

When I was developing and testing recipes for this cookbook, I took one bite of this salad and immediately said, "OMG yes, this is going on the must-include list!" Grilled zucchini and corn are slightly charred and deliciously smoky from the grill, and they get tossed with some jalapeño, cilantro, onion, garlic, and lime juice. It's light, fresh, and layered with flavor, and I guarantee it will get devoured fast! Sprinkle a little cotija or queso fresco cheese on top and serve this up at your next outdoor barbecue. **serves 6**

5 ears of corn, shucked

2 medium zucchini, halved lengthwise

5 tablespoons extra-virgin olive oil

1 jalapeño, seeded and finely diced

2 green onions (white and green parts), sliced

1 garlic clove, minced

1 bunch of fresh cilantro, roughly chopped

¼ cup (60ml) fresh lime juice (from about 2 limes)

½ teaspoon kosher salt

¼ teaspoon freshly ground black pepper

2 tablespoons cotija cheese or queso fresco

1. Preheat an outdoor grill or grill pan on the stove to medium-high heat.

2. Lightly brush the corn and zucchini with 3 tablespoons of the oil and grill for 8 to 10 minutes, flipping the zucchini halfway through and rotating the corn every couple of minutes, until all sides are slightly charred. Transfer to a plate and let cool enough to handle.

3. In a large mixing bowl, hold the corn upright by the cob and use a sharp knife to shave the kernels from the cob, top to bottom.

4. Slice the zucchini into quarters lengthwise, then cut across for a small dice, and add to the bowl with the corn. Add the jalapeño, green onions, garlic, cilantro, the remaining 2 tablespoons oil, the lime juice, salt, pepper, and cotija cheese to the bowl, then toss to combine.

Serving size:
1 cup (150g)

Calories: 200

Fat: 14g

Saturated fat: 2g

Carbs: 20g

Fiber: 3g

Sugar: 7g

Protein: 4g

Cholesterol: 3mg

Sodium: 156mg

shaved asparagus and smoked salmon salad

Want to make raw asparagus look fancy? Give it a shave with a vegetable peeler! This spring-green medley of asparagus, cucumber, dill, and chives is paired with smoked salmon for a protein boost, then drizzled with a bright lemon vinaigrette for a simple, yet vibrant salad. I'm using store-bought smoked salmon that requires no cooking, but you could also use cooked and flaked salmon in this recipe if you prefer. If all you can find is thin and lanky asparagus, make the Asparagus Pancetta Breakfast Hash (page 109), and save this recipe for when you can get thick spears (they're much easier to shave).

serves 4

storage

Store in an airtight container in the fridge for 2 to 3 days.

helpful tip

If you can't find small Persian cucumbers, use an English cucumber and cut the bigger rounds in half or quarters for bite-size pieces.

FOR THE DRESSING

3 tablespoons olive oil

½ teaspoon lemon zest

1 tablespoon fresh lemon juice

½ teaspoon Dijon mustard

¼ teaspoon kosher salt

Pinch of freshly ground black pepper

FOR THE SALAD

1 pound (454g) thick asparagus, woody ends trimmed

6 ounces (170g) smoked salmon, torn into small pieces

2 small Persian cucumbers, sliced into thin rounds

2 tablespoons roughly chopped fresh dill

2 tablespoons finely chopped fresh chives

1. To make the dressing: In a small bowl, whisk together the oil, lemon zest, lemon juice, mustard, salt, and pepper.

2. To make the salad: Use a vegetable peeler to shave the asparagus lengthwise into long, thin ribbons.

3. In a large bowl, combine the shaved asparagus, smoked salmon, cucumbers, dill, and chives. Pour the dressing over the salad and toss everything together to combine.

Serving size: 1½ cups (172g)

Calories: 172

Fat: 12g

Saturated fat: 2g

Carbs: 7g

Fiber: 3g

Sugar: 3g

Protein: 11g

Cholesterol: 10mg

Sodium: 374mg

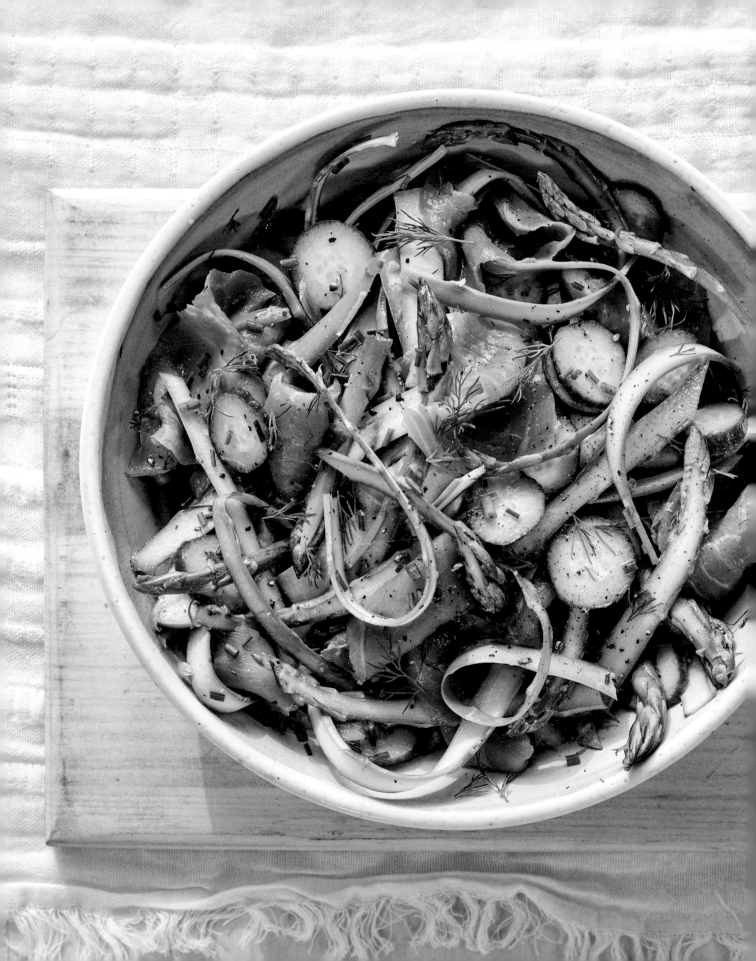

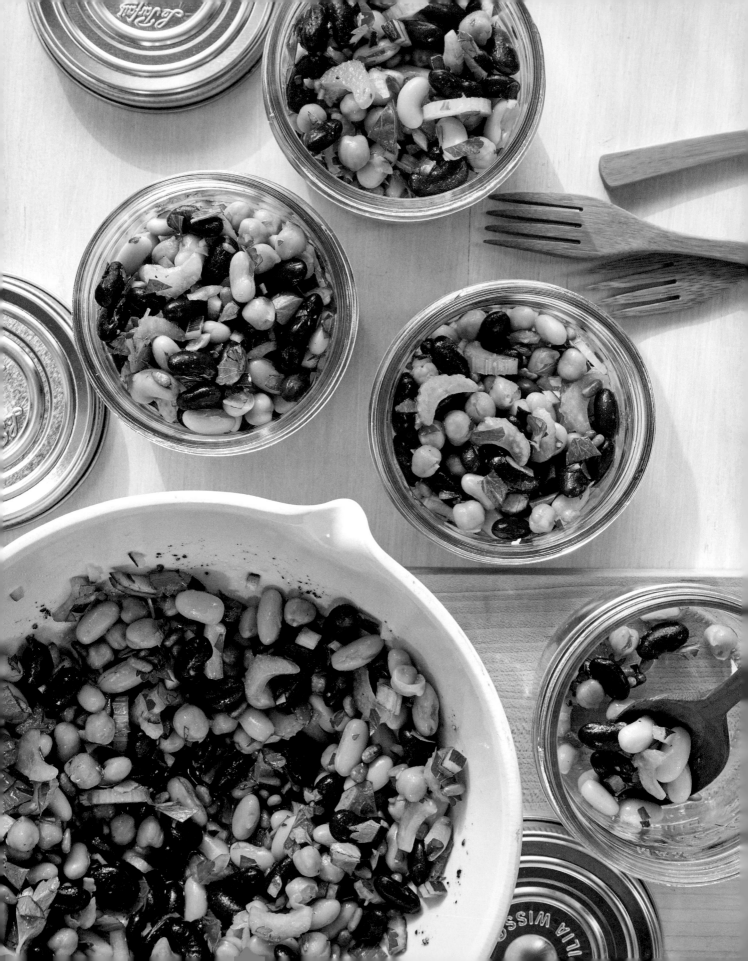

three-bean salad with pine nuts

This is quite possibly the easiest 15-minute salad you'll ever make, and the most durable too (it gets better and better as the beans marinate in the dressing). All you've got to do is open a few cans of beans, chop a few veggies, and toss everything together with a simple homemade dressing. Besides being economical, sturdy enough to hold up outdoors, and able to feed a crowd (double or triple the recipe), part of the beauty of three-bean salads is you can swap in your favorite beans. I'm using cannellini beans, kidney beans, and chickpeas, but if you prefer navy beans, pinto beans, black beans, or any other beans, by all means, use them! **serves 6**

FOR THE DRESSING

¼ cup (60ml) olive oil

¼ cup (60ml) apple cider vinegar

1 garlic clove, minced

1 tablespoon honey

½ teaspoon kosher salt

¼ teaspoon freshly ground black pepper

FOR THE SALAD

⅓ cup (46g) raw pine nuts

1 (15.5-ounce/439g) can cannellini beans, drained and rinsed

1 (15.5-ounce/439g) can kidney beans, drained and rinsed

1 (15.5-ounce/439g) can chickpeas, drained and rinsed

2 celery ribs, finely chopped

½ medium red onion, finely chopped

1 cup (20g) loosely packed fresh parsley, finely chopped

1. To make the dressing: In a small bowl, whisk together the oil, vinegar, garlic, honey, salt, and pepper.

2. To make the salad: Heat a small pan over medium-low heat and add the pine nuts. Toast for 3 to 4 minutes, stirring frequently, until lightly golden.

3. In a large bowl, combine the cannellini beans, kidney beans, chickpeas, celery, red onion, pine nuts, and parsley. Add the dressing and toss all the ingredients together until well combined.

Serving size:
1 cup (176g)

Calories: 361
Fat: 17g
Saturated fat: 2g
Carbs: 42g
Fiber: 11g
Sugar: 7g
Protein: 14g
Cholesterol: 0g
Sodium: 328g

roasted carrot and parsnip salad with lemon tahini dressing

When I visited Tel Aviv a few years back on a wellness trip I noticed two things on the table at virtually every meal: roasted veggies every which way and some form of tahini dressing. Plates and bowls of all shapes and sizes were filled to the brim with smoky, caramelized veggies in various rainbow assortments, and I'd often fill up on those veggies before the main meal ever arrived. Roasting vegetables coaxes out their natural sweetness and makes them universally more appealing, and tahini dressing adds a lemony, nutty, creaminess with a touch of richness. Traveling gives me such fabulous inspiration in the kitchen, and hopefully I've captured a small snippet of that pleasurable foodie trip for you with this roasted carrot and parsnip salad. **serves 4**

storage

Store in an airtight container in the fridge for 3 to 4 days.

FOR THE LEMON TAHINI DRESSING

2 tablespoons tahini

1 to 2 tablespoons water

1½ tablespoons fresh lemon juice, or more to taste

1 small garlic clove, minced

½ tablespoon pure maple syrup

¼ teaspoon kosher salt

Pinch of freshly ground black pepper

FOR THE SALAD

1 pound (454g) small carrots, halved lengthwise or quartered if thicker and cut into 2-inch pieces

1 pound (454g) parsnips, peeled, halved lengthwise or quartered if thicker, and cut into 2-inch pieces

2 tablespoons extra-virgin olive oil

½ teaspoon kosher salt

¼ teaspoon freshly ground black pepper

2 red onions, cut into ½-inch (1.3cm) wedges

2 tablespoons raw pine nuts

1 tablespoon raw sesame seeds, for garnish

1 tablespoon roughly chopped fresh parsley, for garnish

Serving size:
1¼ cups (137g)

Calories: 310

Fat: 16g

Saturated fat: 2g

Carbs: 41g

Fiber: 11g

Sugar: 15g

Protein: 5g

Cholesterol: 0mg

Sodium: 312mg

1. Preheat the oven to 425°F (220°C).

2. To make the dressing: In a small bowl, whisk together the tahini, water (to thin it out), lemon juice, garlic, maple syrup, salt, and pepper.

3. On a sheet pan, toss the carrots and parsnips with 1 tablespoon of the oil, ¼ teaspoon of the salt, and ⅛ teaspoon of the pepper.

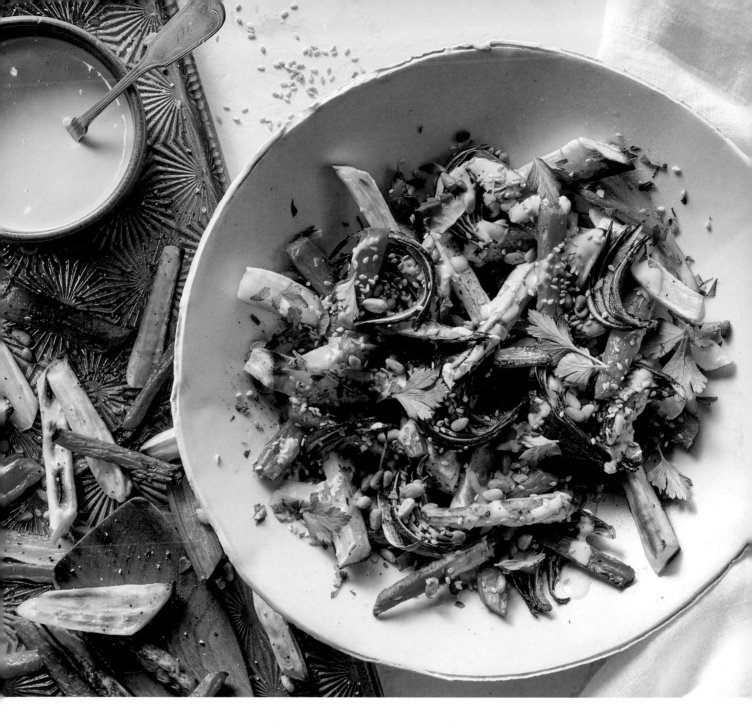

On a second sheet pan, toss the red onions with the remaining 1 tablespoon oil, ¼ teaspoon salt, and ⅛ teaspoon pepper. Roast both sheet pans for 20 to 25 minutes. The onions may need to roast a few minutes longer to allow them to fully soften and deeply caramelize. In the last 3 to 4 minutes of roasting, add the pine nuts to one of the pans to gently toast them.

4. Remove the vegetables and pine nuts from the oven and place them in a serving bowl. Drizzle the dressing over the vegetables and sprinkle with sesame seeds and parsley. Serve warm, chilled, or at room temperature.

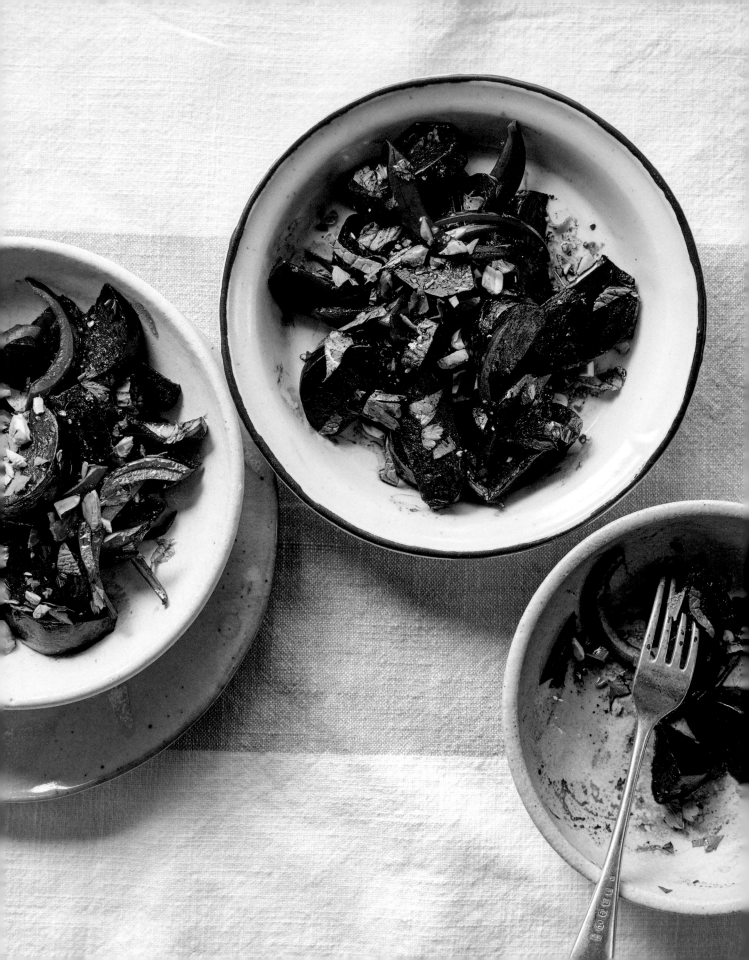

roasted beet salad
with pistachios

storage

Store in an airtight container in the fridge for 4 to 5 days.

get creative

A little sprinkle of feta or goat cheese pairs beautifully with the roasted beets.

I adore beets—did you see my breakfast Spiralized Beet Frittata (page 105)? Beets boast an impressive nutritional profile, they're packed with fiber, and they're great for heart health. Fun fact: Red veggies in general are great for the heart! This simple salad combines roasted beets with thinly sliced onion, fresh mint, parsley, and crunchy pistachios. It's great as a side, and it will last for days on end in the fridge (set aside the pistachios and sprinkle them over the salad before serving). You might even get an energy boost, which is a welcome side effect! **serves 4**

4 or 5 small red beets, ends trimmed

3 tablespoons extra-virgin olive oil

½ small red onion, thinly sliced

2 tablespoons roughly chopped fresh parsley

2 tablespoons roughly chopped fresh mint

2 tablespoons balsamic vinegar

½ teaspoon kosher salt

Pinch of freshly ground black pepper

1 tablespoon roughly chopped raw pistachios, for garnish

1. Preheat the oven to 425°F (220°C). Place the beets in a baking dish or Dutch oven. Drizzle with 1 tablespoon of the oil, toss to coat, cover the baking dish with aluminum foil (or with a lid if using a Dutch oven), and roast for 50 to 60 minutes, until the beets are fork-tender. Remove the baking dish from the oven and set the beets aside to cool. Once cool enough to handle, peel them and then cut into thin wedges.

2. In a large mixing bowl, toss the beets with the remaining 2 tablespoons oil, the red onion, parsley, mint, vinegar, salt, and pepper until combined. Sprinkle with the pistachios just before serving.

Serving size:
1 cup (125g)

Calories: 160
Fat: 11g
Saturated fat: 2g
Carbs: 14g
Fiber: 3g
Sugar: 9g
Protein: 2g
Cholesterol: 0mg
Sodium: 224mg

melon and shrimp salad

This shrimp, cantaloupe, and honeydew salad is quintessential
SoCal: cool, refreshing, and zingy, thanks to a lime and honey
dressing spiked with shallot and cilantro. It's light, bright, and
perfect for days when you're lounging at the pool or beach
(or sitting in front of your computer wishing you were at the
pool or beach!). Just pop the salad into your cooler and break
it out when you want a little respite from the sun (or screen).
serves 4

storage

Store in an airtight
container in the fridge
for 3 to 4 days.

FOR THE DRESSING

**2 tablespoons fresh lime juice
(from 1 to 2 limes)**

**1 tablespoon extra-virgin
olive oil**

**2 teaspoons finely chopped
shallot**

½ teaspoon honey

**2 tablespoons roughly chopped
fresh cilantro**

½ teaspoon kosher salt

FOR THE SALAD

1 tablespoon olive oil

**1 pound (454g) extra-large
shrimp, peeled and deveined**

**½ cantaloupe, seeded and flesh
scooped into balls**

**½ honeydew melon, seeded
and flesh scooped into balls**

1. To make the dressing: In a small bowl, whisk together the lime
juice, oil, shallot, honey, cilantro, and salt.

2. To make the salad: Heat the oil in a medium sauté pan over
medium heat. Add the shrimp and cook for 2 to 3 minutes on each
side, or until the shrimp is pink and opaque. Remove the shrimp to
plate and place in the fridge to cool.

3. Place the shrimp in a large bowl with the cantaloupe and
honeydew and toss with the dressing.

Serving size:
1¾ cups (260g)

Calories: 228

Fat: 8g

Saturated fat: 1g

Carbs: 23g

Fiber: 2g

Sugar: 19g

Protein: 17g

Cholesterol: 143mg

Sodium: 717mg

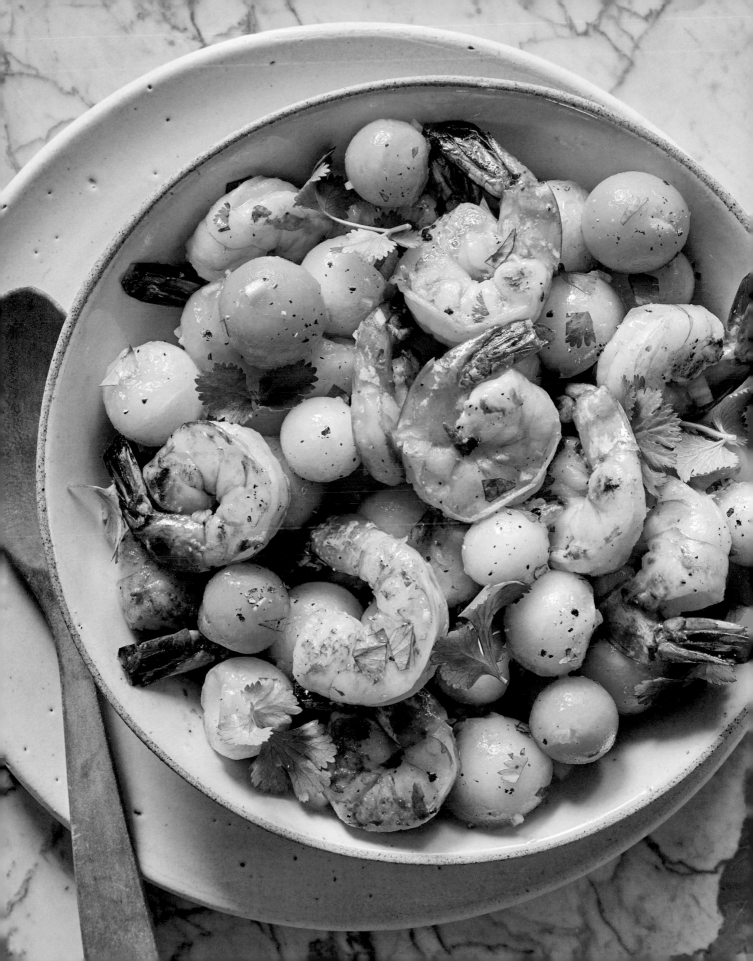

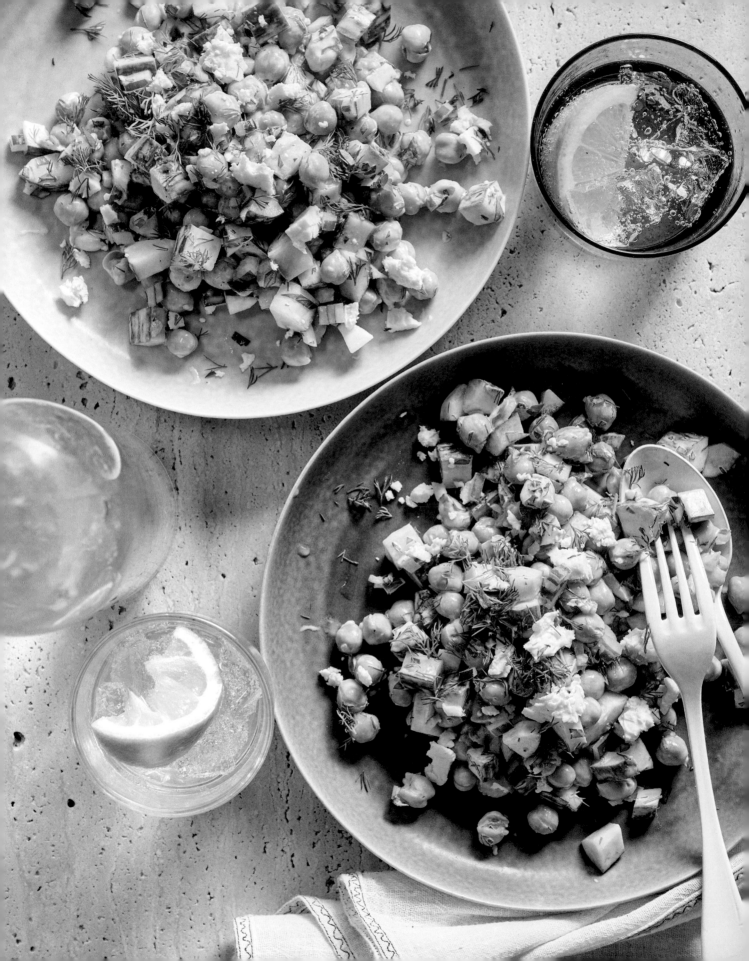

chickpea and cucumber salad with creamy yogurt dressing

storage

Store in an airtight container in the fridge for 4 to 5 days.

conversions

If you're using dried chickpeas, you'll need 1 cup. After soaking and cooking, they should expand to 3 cups, which is approximately the same quantity in 2 (15.5-ounce/439g) cans of chickpeas.

helpful tip

English cucumbers (also called hothouse cucumbers) are the ones you'll usually find individually wrapped in plastic at the grocery store. Their skin is thin and delicate, meaning there's no need to peel them for salads. You can use regular cucumbers as well, but I'd recommend peeling them first as they have a thicker skin that's often coated in wax.

Serving size:
1¼ cups (184g)

Calories: 201
Fat: 6g
Saturated fat: 1g
Carbs: 28g
Fiber: 8g
Sugar: 3g
Protein: 11g
Cholesterol: 4mg
Sodium: 253mg

This vegetarian salad can 100 percent hold its own against other creamy and crunchy lunchtime salads, like your classic tuna salad or chicken salad. It's light and fresh thanks to crisp cucumber and red onion, and it's also packed with plenty of plant-based protein to satisfy your hunger. If you're dairy-free, feel free to swap in nondairy yogurt, and if you'd like to make it even creamier naturally, just mash half of the chickpeas with a fork before mixing. If I were still in the corporate world, this would be a "take it to work" lunch on repeat. **serves 6**

FOR THE YOGURT DRESSING

½ cup (114g) plain Greek yogurt (dairy or dairy-free)

2 tablespoons mayonnaise

1 tablespoon fresh lemon juice

1 teaspoon Dijon mustard

½ teaspoon kosher salt

¼ teaspoon freshly ground black pepper

FOR THE SALAD

2 (15.5-ounce/439g) cans chickpeas, drained and rinsed

2 large English cucumbers, diced

⅓ cup finely diced red onion, or more to taste

2 tablespoons finely chopped fresh dill

2 tablespoons finely chopped fresh parsley

¼ cup (28g) crumbled feta cheese (optional)

1. To make the yogurt dressing: In a small bowl, stir together the yogurt, mayonnaise, lemon juice, mustard, salt, and pepper until creamy.

2. To make the salad: In a large bowl, combine the chickpeas, cucumber, red onion, dill, and parsley. Pour the dressing over the salad and toss well. If you'd like, sprinkle on the crumbled feta cheese. Refrigerate until ready to serve.

meaty mains

Often when people think of meal prep, the first thing that comes to mind is baking a few chicken breasts (which can be diced or sliced up), or slow-cooking some pork shoulder (which can be shredded into meals). And they're not wrong! It's the heart of big-batch cooking, where you cook more meat than you need for leftovers to enjoy throughout the week. That's exactly what meal prep is. But where I find most people go wrong is that they cook the *same* meat over and over, and over again, until they develop palate fatigue and get absolutely bored with the meal they've prepped.

Well, in this chapter, you'll have plenty of meaty mains to choose from—chicken, turkey, beef, pork, and lamb—and all with that necessary oomph in taste! Some, like the Garlic Rosemary Turkey Breast (page 176), are cooked simply with herbs and spices so that they can be eaten along with your favorite sides, diced into salads, or stuffed into wraps. I call that versatility at its finest! Others, like the Pepper Steak Stir-Fry (page 159) or Apple Cider Beef Stew (page 175) are your classic freezer-friendly big-batch meals that can be frozen and reheated on demand. In my meal prep world, back-to-back, same-same dinners are optional but never required (though you might just love these dishes so much you'll welcome it!).

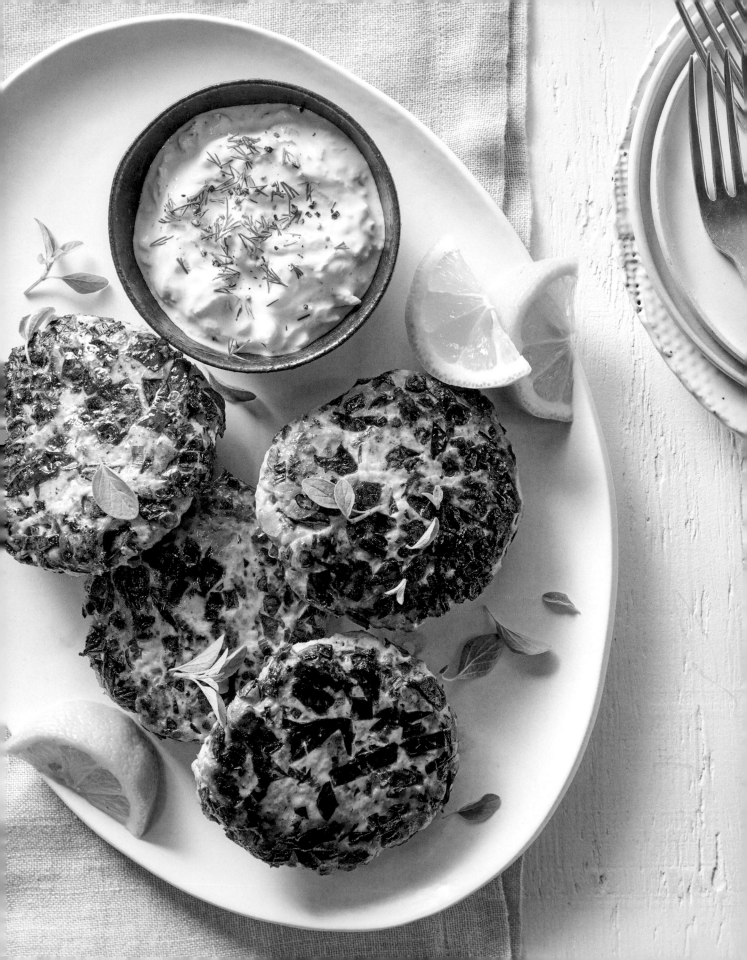

turkey spinach patties

Ground turkey is a healthy protein and easy to work with, but unfortunately, it's often used in bland and uninspired ways. Let's change that! These turkey patties are loaded with greens, and thanks to the spinach, green onions, garlic, and oregano, they've got heaps of Mediterranean-inspired flavor, especially when served with a dollop of creamy Tzatziki (page 253). I'm quite confident you'll love these, so plan ahead and make a double batch now, then freeze the extras to reheat later for an easy weeknight meal. **serves 4**

(page 253)

storage

Store in an airtight container in the fridge for 3 to 4 days, or in the freezer for up to 3 months.

to reheat

Preheat the oven to 350°F (180°C) and reheat for 4 to 5 minutes, until warmed through. You can also reheat the patties in the microwave for 1 to 2 minutes.

helpful tip

If you don't have fresh oregano, use dill or thyme. If you want to substitute with dried herbs, use just 1 teaspoon.

1 pound (454g) ground turkey

2 cups (70g) loosely packed baby spinach, roughly chopped

3 green onions (white and green parts), thinly sliced

3 garlic cloves, minced

1 tablespoon finely chopped fresh oregano

1 teaspoon kosher salt

½ teaspoon freshly ground black pepper

3 tablespoons olive oil

1. In a medium bowl, combine the turkey, spinach, green onions, garlic, oregano, salt, and pepper. Use your hands to mix everything together. Divide the mixture evenly and form 4 large patties.

2. In a large skillet over medium heat, heat the oil. Cook the patties for approximately 5 minutes per side, or until golden brown and cooked through.

Serving size: 1 patty

Calories: 181
Fat: 13g
Saturated fat: 3g
Carbs: 1g
Fiber: 0g
Sugar: 0g
Protein: 15g
Cholesterol: 60mg
Sodium: 195mg

lemon oregano roasted chicken legs and potatoes

Have you ever roasted whole chicken legs before? They're perfect for when you want a substantial portion of chicken on your plate (it's the chicken thigh plus the drumstick), and they're usually cheaper than smaller, individual cuts because there's less butchering involved. Hearty appetites love this cut! In this recipe, I place the chicken legs on top of diced potatoes, then drizzle everything with a bright, sun-drenched blend of lemon, garlic, and oregano. The chicken gets crispy on top, the potatoes get buttery soft, and together they make for one winner of a meal.   **serves 4**

4 whole chicken legs (thighs plus drumsticks)

2 lemons

¼ cup (60ml) extra-virgin olive oil

5 garlic cloves, minced

2 teaspoons dried oregano

1 teaspoon kosher salt

½ teaspoon freshly ground black pepper

2 pounds (907g) new potatoes, diced into 1-inch (2.5cm) pieces

1. Preheat the oven to 400°F (200°C). Pat the chicken dry with a paper towel and set aside.

2. In a small bowl, zest and juice 1 of the lemons. You should have about 1 tablespoon of zest and 3 tablespoons of juice. Add the oil, garlic, oregano, salt, and pepper and stir together.

3. Place the diced potatoes in a 13 × 9-inch (33 × 23cm) casserole dish and drizzle with half the lemon oil mixture, then toss to combine.

4. Arrange the chicken on top, drizzle with the remaining lemon oil mixture, and use your fingers or a brush to make sure the chicken is well coated. Thinly slice the remaining lemon and place the slices on top. Roast the chicken for 50 to 60 minutes, basting every 15 minutes with the pan drippings, until golden brown and an instant-read thermometer inserted into the thigh reads 170°F to 175°F (76°C to 80°C) and the potatoes are tender. If the top of the chicken is browning too quickly, cover the pan loosely with aluminum foil.

storage

Store both the chicken and potatoes together in an airtight container in the fridge for 3 to 4 days, or in the freezer for up to 3 months.

to reheat

If frozen, thaw in the fridge overnight. Reheat in a 350°F (180°C) oven for about 10 minutes, or in the microwave for 2 to 3 minutes, until warmed through.

helpful tip

While chicken is safe to eat at 165°F (74°C), chicken legs (which contain more connective tissue) are most tender when they're cooked to a slightly higher internal temperature. But that's perfect as it gives the potatoes enough time to cook!

Serving size:
1 chicken leg + 1⅓ cups (216g) potatoes

Calories: 982
Fat: 59g
Saturated fat: 14g
Carbs: 39g
Fiber: 6g
Sugar: 3g
Protein: 70g
Cholesterol: 301mg
Sodium: 603mg

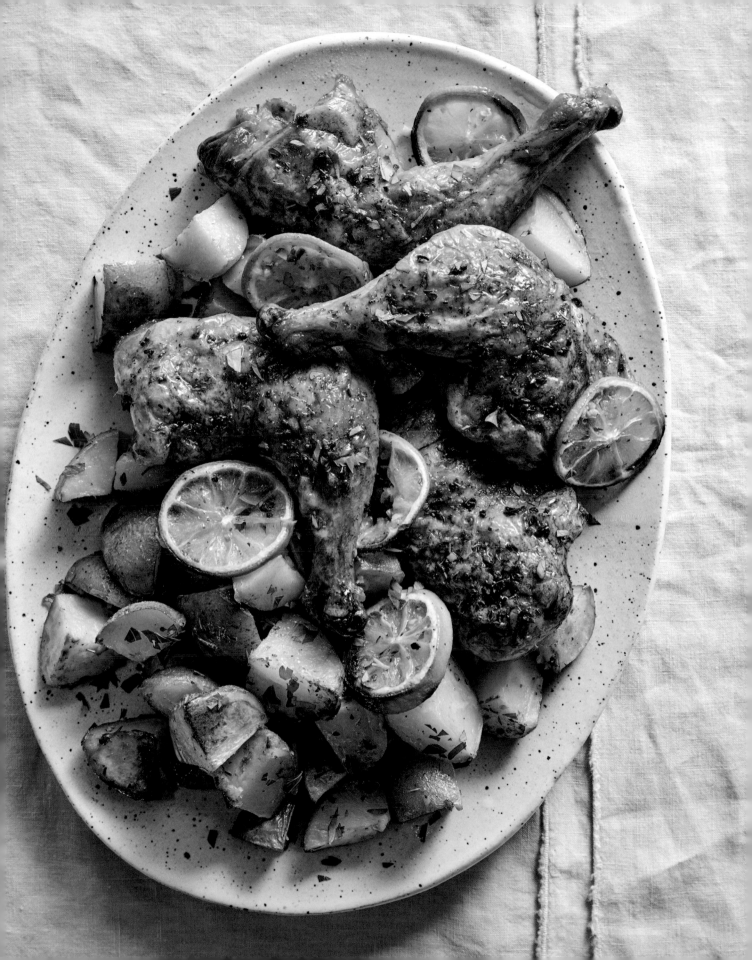

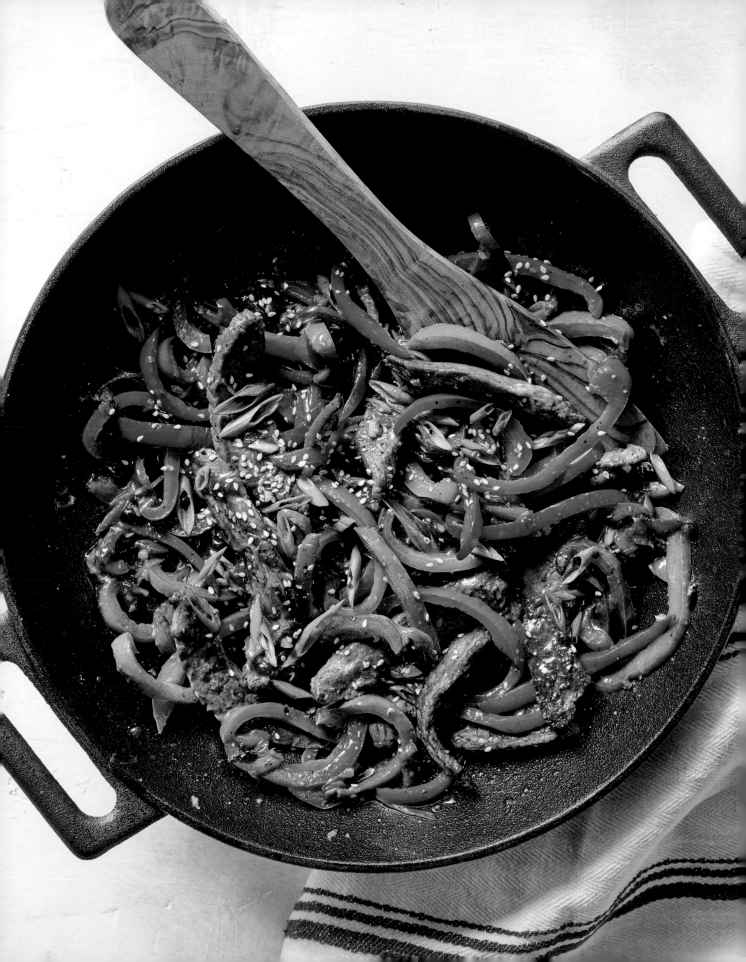

pepper steak stir-fry

storage

Store in an airtight container in the fridge for 4 to 5 days, or in the freezer for up to 3 months.

to reheat

Once thawed, reheat in a pan on the stove or in the microwave for 1 to 2 minutes, until warmed through.

helpful tip

You can also use skirt steak or top sirloin steak in this recipe. Just make sure to cut against the grain (the opposite direction of the fibers or striations) for the most tender pieces of meat.

This flavorful, quick Southeast Asian–inspired stir-fry combines melt-in-your-mouth steak and tender-crisp bell peppers in a savory-sweet sauce that's perfect for topping a pile of rice. I've always loved Asian takeout, but as a gluten-free gal it can be a bit tricky sometimes to navigate which sauces to avoid. This homemade version is naturally gluten-free, has a few more veggies in it, and can be served up in less than 20 minutes. **serves 6**

FOR THE SAUCE

⅓ cup (80ml) low-sodium tamari soy sauce or coconut aminos

2 teaspoons sesame oil

1 tablespoon coconut sugar

1 tablespoon arrowroot powder

FOR THE STEAK STIR-FRY

1 pound (454g) flank steak, thinly sliced against the grain

1 teaspoon freshly ground black pepper

¼ teaspoon kosher salt

2 tablespoons avocado oil or extra-virgin olive oil

2 large green bell peppers, seeded and thinly sliced

1 large red bell pepper, seeded and thinly sliced

1 medium yellow onion, thinly sliced

4 garlic cloves, minced

1 tablespoon minced peeled fresh ginger

Cooked rice, for serving (optional)

1 green onion (white and green parts), thinly sliced on a diagonal, for garnish

1. To make the sauce: In a small bowl, whisk together the tamari, sesame oil, coconut sugar, and arrowroot powder. Set aside.

2. To make the stir-fry: In a medium bowl, toss the sliced steak with the pepper and salt until coated. Heat a medium skillet or wok on medium-high heat and add 1 tablespoon of the avocado oil. Add the flank steak and sear for 1 to 2 minutes, until mostly browned but with a little bit of pink inside. Remove to a plate.

3. Leave any juices in the pan and add the remaining 1 tablespoon avocado oil along with the bell peppers and onion and sauté 2 to 3 minutes, until tender. Add the garlic and ginger to the skillet, stir for 30 seconds, then add the steak back to the skillet along with the sauce. Stir-fry for 1 to 2 minutes, until the sauce thickens. Serve over rice if you'd like and sprinkle the green onion on top.

Serving size:
1 cup (185g)

Calories: 346
Fat: 19g
Saturated fat: 5g
Carbs: 17g
Fiber: 3g
Sugar: 8g
Protein: 28g
Cholesterol: 77mg
Sodium: 967mg

gingered cashew chicken and sugar snap peas

I think I've become that person who now adds ginger to everything. It's good for the gut, it's good for the brain, and it's certainly good for the taste buds. I've added a heaping amount to this stir-fry cashew chicken along with a bunch of greens, in the form of sugar snaps and green onions. It's a lighter cashew chicken recipe with a bit more zing, and I love to serve it over rice, cauliflower rice, or even zucchini noodles. **serves 4**

FOR THE SAUCE

¼ cup (60ml) low-sodium chicken broth

¼ cup (60ml) low-sodium tamari soy sauce or coconut aminos

1 tablespoon dry sherry

1 tablespoon honey

1 teaspoon sesame oil

1 teaspoon rice vinegar or apple cider vinegar

1 tablespoon arrowroot powder

FOR THE CHICKEN STIR-FRY

¾ cup (105g) raw cashews

2 tablespoons avocado oil or extra-virgin olive oil

1 pound (454g) boneless, skinless chicken breast, cut into 1-inch pieces

½ teaspoon kosher salt

¼ teaspoon freshly ground black pepper

8 ounces (227g) sugar snap peas, trimmed

1 yellow bell pepper, seeded and chopped

4 green onions, thinly sliced and separated into white and green parts

4 garlic cloves, minced

1½ tablespoons finely grated peeled fresh ginger

Raw sesame seeds, for garnish

1. To make the sauce: In a small bowl, whisk together the broth, tamari, sherry, honey, sesame oil, vinegar, and arrowroot powder. Set aside.

2. To make the stir fry: In a small pan on medium-low heat, toast the cashews for 4 to 5 minutes, until lightly golden, flipping and tossing a few times. Set aside.

3. In a large skillet or wok on medium-high heat, add 1 tablespoon of the avocado oil and swirl the pan to coat the bottom. Add the chicken in a single flat layer. Season the chicken with the salt and pepper and cook until lightly browned, 4 to 5 minutes, stirring as needed. Remove the chicken to a plate.

storage

Store in an airtight container in the fridge for 4 to 5 days, or in the freezer for up to 3 months.

to reheat

Once thawed, reheat in a pan on the stove or in the microwave for 1 to 2 minutes, until warmed through.

get creative

If you can't find sugar snap peas at the market, swap in broccoli florets or chopped baby bok choy—both work great!

helpful tip

I love sugar snap peas, but they have a little string that runs on the concave side of the legume that can be annoying to chew on. Trim the peas by using a paring knife to slice off one end almost all the way through, then pull the string down the length of the pea. Trust me, it's worth the effort.

Serving size:
1½ cups (246g)

Calories: 495

Fat: 25g

Saturated fat: 5g

Carbs: 23g

Fiber: 2g

Sugar: 11g

Protein: 45g

Cholesterol: 97mg

Sodium: 940mg

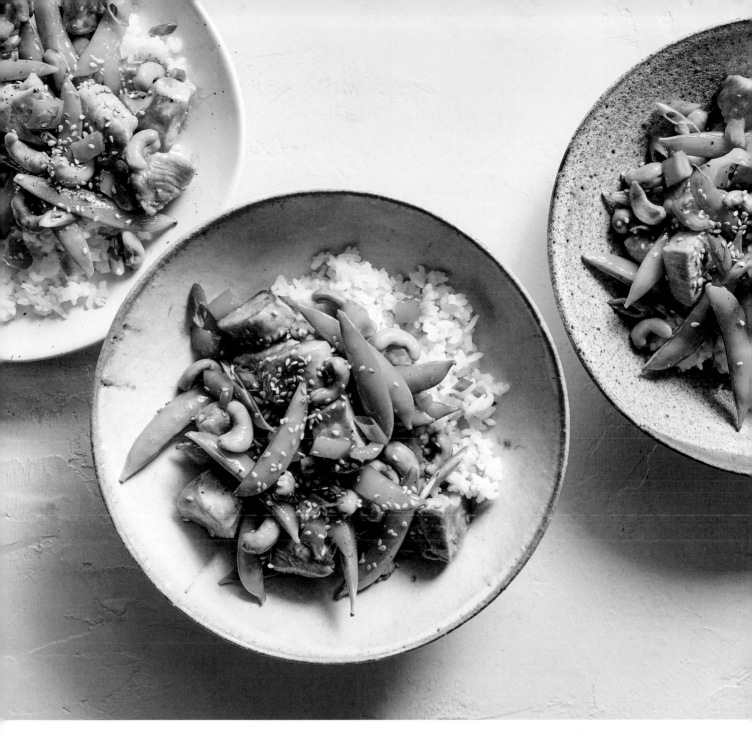

4. Leave any juices in the pan, then add the remaining 1 tablespoon avocado oil along with the sugar snap peas, bell pepper, and white parts of the green onion. Cook the vegetables until tender, 3 to 4 minutes.

5. Add the chicken back to the pan with the minced garlic and grated ginger. Stir for 30 seconds. Pour in the sauce (it may need to be quickly stirred again first) and stir-fry for another 1 to 2 minutes, until the sauce thickens. Remove from the heat, stir in the cashews and green parts of the green onion, garnish with sesame seeds, and serve.

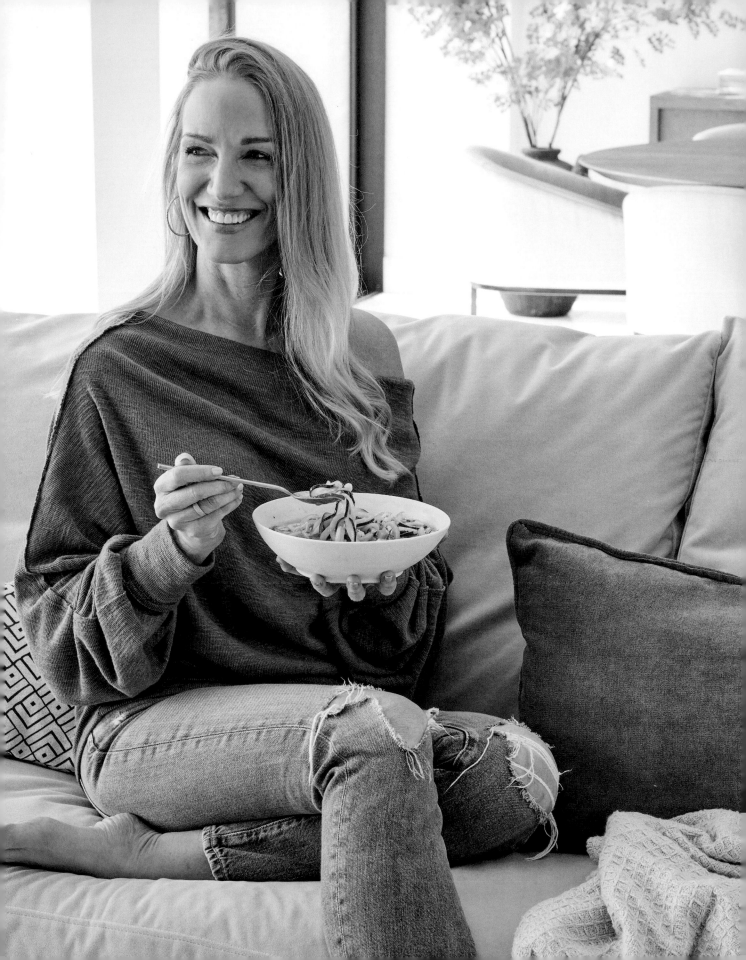

golden chicken zoodle soup

storage

Store in an airtight container in the fridge for 4 to 5 days, or in the freezer for up to 3 months.

to reheat

Reheat from frozen or chilled. Reheat a portion in a bowl in the microwave for 1 to 2 minutes if thawed, or 3 to 4 minutes if frozen, or in a pot on the stove until warmed through.

Chicken noodle soup has historically been the antidote for whatever ails you, yet I think it's possible to make it *even* healthier. Swap pasta noodles with zucchini "noodles" and then give the broth a massive boost with warming ginger and earthy turmeric. You've still got wholesome shredded chicken to fill you up, along with your mirepoix mix of onion, celery and carrots, but now each bowl has even more good-for-you vegetables and immune-boosting ingredients to bolster your wellness. If ever there was a flu-season soup to have ready-to-go from your freezer, it's this one! **serves 6**

2 tablespoons extra-virgin olive oil

½ medium yellow onion, diced

4 celery ribs, diced

3 medium carrots, sliced

4 garlic cloves, minced

6 cups (1.4L) low-sodium chicken broth

2 large boneless, skinless chicken breasts (8 ounces/227g each)

2 tablespoons grated peeled fresh ginger, or 2 teaspoons dried

2 tablespoons grated fresh turmeric, or 2 teaspoons dried

1 teaspoon ground coriander

1 teaspoon kosher salt

¼ teaspoon freshly ground black pepper

1 large zucchini, spiralized

2 tablespoons finely chopped fresh parsley

1. In a large stockpot or Dutch oven, heat the oil over medium heat. Add the onion, celery, and carrots and sauté for 4 to 5 minutes, until the onion becomes translucent. Add the garlic and sauté 1 minute more.

2. Add the broth to the pot, along with the chicken, ginger, turmeric, coriander, salt, and pepper. Bring to a boil, then reduce the heat to low and cover the pot. Simmer the soup for 15 minutes, or until the chicken is cooked through.

3. With tongs, remove the chicken to a cutting board and shred with two forks, then return to the pot. Stir in the spiralized zucchini and parsley and simmer for an additional minute. Divide among bowls and serve.

Serving size:
2 cups (440g)

Calories: 182
Fat: 7g
Saturated fat: 1g
Carbs: 10g
Fiber: 2g
Sugar: 5g
Protein: 20g
Cholesterol: 56mg
Sodium: 297mg

honey citrus chicken breasts

Chicken breasts make for a perfect weeknight meal—they're healthy, cook quickly, and are especially economical when purchased in family-size packs. But they can be bland and boring. This recipe changes that! Juicy chicken breasts are cooked to perfection, then drenched in a sweet, honey citrus glaze full of pungent garlic and shallot. Serve alongside my Roasted Green Beans Almondine (page 244) or on top of my Lemon Herb Rice (page 243) and you've got a deliciously filling and sensational weeknight chicken dinner. **serves 4**

storage

Store in an airtight container in the fridge for 4 to 5 days, or in the freezer for up to 3 months.

to reheat

Once thawed, reheat in a pan on the stove or in the microwave for 1 to 2 minutes, until warmed through.

get creative

I use navel oranges, but you could also use Cara Cara or blood oranges for a deeper orange or red color. If you prefer dark meat, boneless, skinless chicken thighs also work great in this recipe.

2 tablespoons olive oil

4 boneless, skinless chicken breasts (6 ounces/170g each), lightly pounded

1 teaspoon kosher salt

½ teaspoon freshly ground black pepper

3 tablespoons finely chopped shallot

2 garlic cloves, minced

1 tablespoon orange zest

⅓ cup fresh orange juice (from about 1 orange)

3 tablespoons fresh lemon juice (from about 1 lemon)

3 tablespoons honey

1 teaspoon arrowroot powder

2 teaspoons water

1 orange, peeled, sectioned, and diced

1. In a large skillet, heat the oil over medium heat. Season both sides of the chicken breasts with the salt and pepper. Place in the skillet and cook for 5 to 7 minutes on each side, until lightly golden and the chicken has reached an internal temperature of 160°F (71°C). Remove the chicken to a plate.

2. Place the shallot and garlic in the skillet and sauté for about 1 minute, until the shallot has softened. Stir in the orange zest, orange juice, lemon juice, and honey, simmering until it reduces slightly, about 2 minutes.

3. Meanwhile, in a small bowl, stir together the arrowroot powder and water to create a slurry. Pour the slurry into the pan and immediately whisk into the pan juices. Add the diced orange to the pan and stir with the sauce.

4. Make room in the pan by pushing the orange slices to the side and return the chicken to the pan. Turn the chicken to coat in the sauce and warm through, plate the chicken, and pour extra sauce on top.

Serving size:
1 chicken breast

Calories: 350

Fat: 11g

Saturated fat: 2g

Carbs: 22g

Fiber: 1g

Sugar: 19g

Protein: 39g

Cholesterol: 124mg

Sodium: 359mg

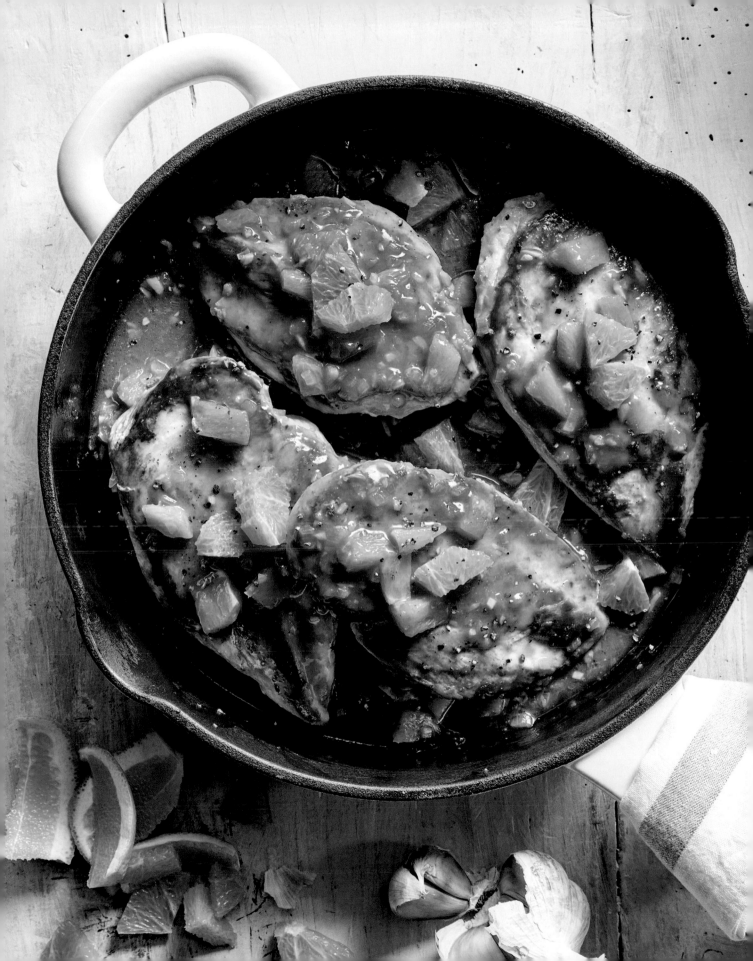

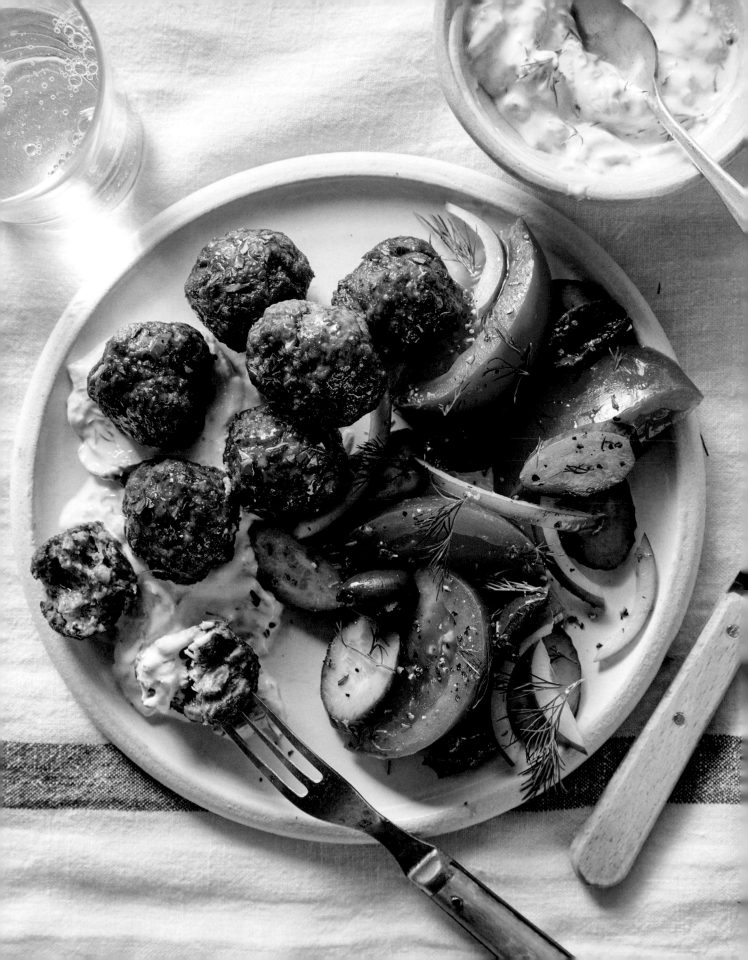

mediterranean lamb meatballs

Made with ground lamb, these meatballs are packed with a good amount of both fresh and dried Mediterranean herbs for the most mouthwatering flavor. Every time I make them, the aroma that wafts from my oven has me counting down the minutes until they're done. I'm such a lover of lamb (I guess it's in the Kiwi blood), but I doubt many will be able to resist popping these meatballs in their mouth. Serve them over a bed of mixed greens, with a side of Tzatziki (page 253), tomatoes, cucumber, olives, and bell pepper (or a variety of other vegetables). They're also great on top of my Garlicky Root Vegetable Mash (page 247). **makes 30 meatballs, to serve 6**

storage

Store in an airtight container in the fridge for 3 to 4 days, or in the freezer for up to 3 months.

storage

Store in an airtight container in the fridge for 3 to 4 days, or in the freezer for up to 3 months.

to reheat

If frozen, thaw in the fridge overnight. Place them in a single layer on a rimmed baking sheet in a 300°F (150°C) oven for 10 to 15 minutes, or microwave in 30-second increments, until warmed through.

dietary swaps

If you're not a fan of lamb, you can swap in ground pork or beef as well (or a use a mix of ground meats).

1½ pounds (680g) ground lamb

1 large egg

¼ cup (32g) finely chopped red onion

¼ cup (30g) almond flour

2 garlic cloves, minced

¼ cup (15g) finely chopped fresh parsley

2 tablespoons finely chopped fresh mint

2 teaspoons dried oregano

½ teaspoon ground cumin

2 teaspoons lemon zest

1 teaspoon kosher salt

½ teaspoon freshly ground black pepper

1. Preheat the oven to 400°F (200°C). Line a rimmed baking sheet with parchment paper.

2. In a medium bowl, combine the lamb, egg, onion, flour, garlic, parsley, mint, oregano, cumin, lemon zest, salt, and pepper. Using your hands, mix the ingredients together until well combined.

3. Measure out 1½ tablespoons (27g) of the mixture (or use a medium cookie scoop) and roll the mixture between your hands, forming about 30 meatballs. Place the meatballs on the prepared baking sheet and bake for 25 to 30 minutes, until browned on the outside and cooked through.

Serving size:
5 meatballs

Calories: 361
Fat: 26g
Saturated fat: 10g
Carbs: 3g
Fiber: 1g
Sugar: 1g
Protein: 28g
Cholesterol: 135mg
Sodium: 276mg

chicken breasts with tarragon cream sauce

Tarragon may be an underused herb, but the impact it has on chicken dishes is next level. In this astoundingly easy recipe, chicken breasts are seared until golden, then simmered in a creamy, garlicky tarragon-mustard sauce. It's an easy weeknight meal that comes together in less than 20 minutes, though it's reminiscent of a classic French restaurant dish (albeit healthier) that might have taken hours. I serve the chicken with rice to soak up all the sauce and steamed or roasted veggies, like Balsamic Roasted Mushrooms (page 235). **serves 4**

2 tablespoons extra-virgin olive oil

4 boneless, skinless chicken breasts (6 ounces/170g), lightly pounded

1 teaspoon kosher salt

½ teaspoon freshly ground black pepper

3 tablespoons finely diced shallot

4 garlic cloves, minced

¾ cup (180ml) low-sodium chicken broth

½ cup (114g) plain Greek yogurt (dairy or dairy-free)

1 tablespoon Dijon mustard

1 tablespoon roughly chopped fresh tarragon, plus more for garnish

Zest and juice of ½ lemon (about ½ tablespoon zest + 1½ tablespoons juice)

1 teaspoon arrowroot powder

2 teaspoons water

1. In a large skillet over medium heat, heat the oil. Season both sides of the chicken breasts with the salt and pepper, then place in the skillet. Cook for 5 to 7 minutes on each side, until lightly golden, and the chicken has reached an internal temperature of 160°F (71°C). Remove the chicken to a plate.

2. Reduce the heat to medium-low, add the shallot and garlic, and sauté for 1 minute. Add the broth and yogurt, then whisk to remove any clumps. Add the mustard, tarragon, and lemon zest and juice and stir until the sauce is smooth.

3. In a small bowl, stir together the arrowroot powder and water to create a slurry. Add it to the pan and immediately whisk together with the pan juices. Return the chicken back to the skillet and spoon some of the sauce on top, simmering until the chicken is warmed through. Garnish with more tarragon.

storage
Store in an airtight container in the fridge for 3 to 4 days. I don't recommend freezing, as cream-based sauces have a tendency to separate.

to reheat
Place in a small baking dish, cover with aluminum foil, and reheat in a 350°F (180°C) oven for 10 to 15 minutes. You can also reheat in the microwave for 1 to 2 minutes, until warmed through.

helpful tip
If you'd like a thicker sauce, add another teaspoon of arrowroot powder mixed with water. Just don't add too much or the sauce will become gloppy.

Serving size: 1 chicken breast with sauce

Calories: 310
Fat: 12g
Saturated fat: 2g
Carbs: 5g
Fiber: 1g
Sugar: 2g
Protein: 42g
Cholesterol: 127mg
Sodium: 420mg

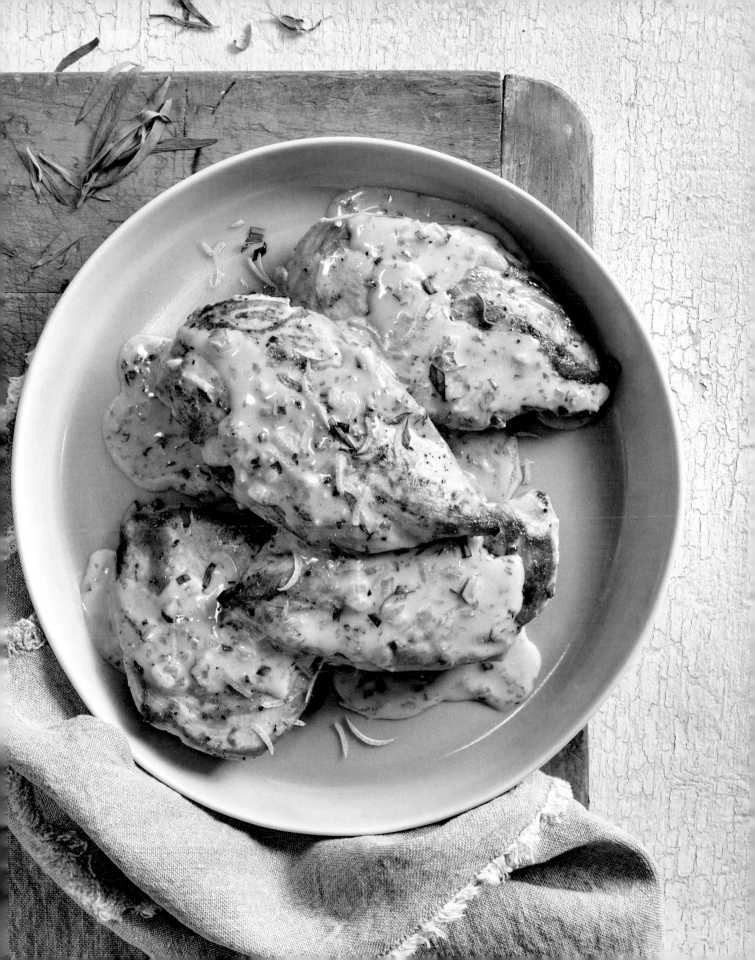

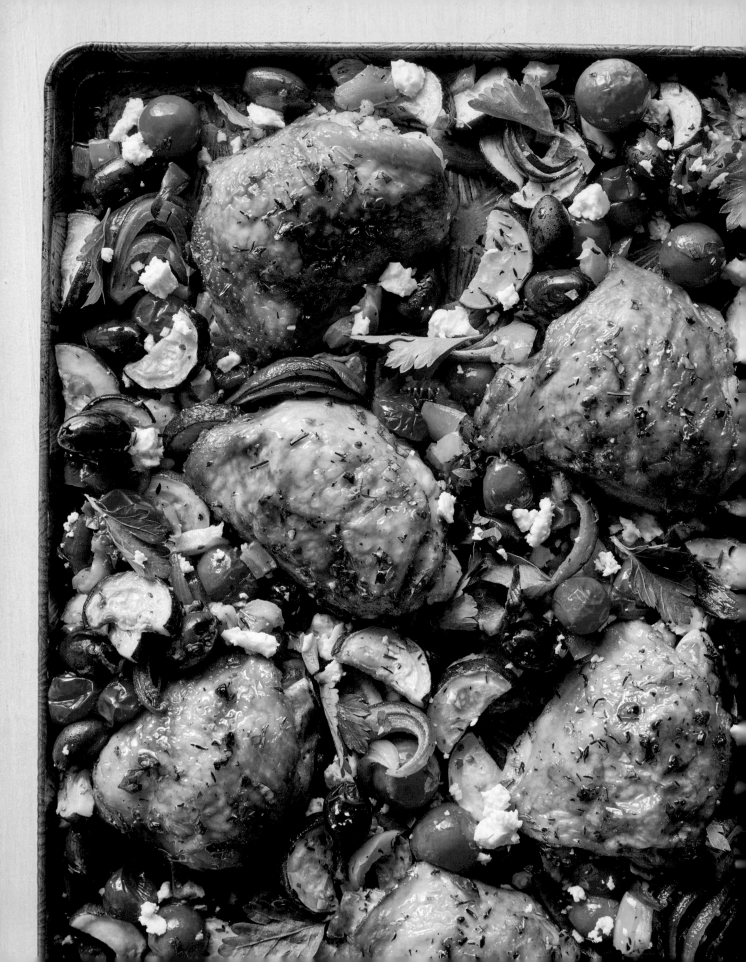

greek sheet pan chicken

This recipe has been a reader favorite on the website, and for good reason. It's the ultimate combination of vibrant summer vegetables paired with juicy, golden chicken thighs. But the best part is that everything is doused in Greek flavors—I'm talking oregano, thyme, garlic, zesty lemon, and, of course, pops of olives and feta cheese. **serves 6**

½ cup (120ml) extra-virgin olive oil

Juice of 1 lemon (about 3 tablespoons)

4 garlic cloves, minced

2 teaspoons dried oregano

1 teaspoon dried thyme

1 teaspoon Dijon mustard

1 teaspoon kosher salt

½ teaspoon freshly ground black pepper

6 bone-in chicken thighs (28.5 ounces/810g total)

1 medium zucchini, halved lengthwise and thickly sliced

1 yellow bell pepper, seeded and diced

½ large red onion, thinly sliced into wedges

2 cups (300g) cherry or grape tomatoes

½ cup (85g) kalamata olives, pitted

¼ cup (35g) feta cheese

2 tablespoons finely chopped fresh parsley, for garnish

1. Preheat the oven to 425°F (220°C).

2. In a small bowl, whisk together the oil, lemon juice, garlic, oregano, thyme, mustard, salt, and pepper.

3. In a large bowl, use your hands to thoroughly coat the chicken thighs with two-thirds of the marinade. Marinate the chicken for 10 to 15 minutes on the counter.

4. While the chicken is marinating, spread the zucchini, bell pepper, red onion, and cherry tomatoes in an even layer on a rimmed baking sheet. Drizzle the remaining marinade on top and toss together to coat the vegetables. Add the chicken thighs to the baking sheet, nestling them around the veggies, and bake for 30 minutes.

5. Remove the baking sheet from the oven and add the olives and feta. Return the baking sheet to the oven for another 10 to 15 minutes, or until the vegetables are softened and the chicken is cooked through. Sprinkle with chopped parsley before serving.

Serving size:
1 chicken thigh +
⅙ portion of veggies

Calories: 257
Fat: 17g
Saturated fat: 1g
Carbs: 9g
Fiber: 2g
Sugar: 4g
Protein: 20g
Cholesterol: 94mg
Sodium: 624g

slow-cooker maple mustard pulled pork

Something beautiful happens when you slather a pork shoulder with maple syrup, whole grain mustard, and a little seasoning—you end up with a tasty, giant mound of juicy, succulent shreds of meat that's a little bit sweet and a little bit tangy. Pop the pork shoulder in your slow cooker first thing in the morning for an almost effortless dinner that's perfect for the fall and winter months when you're curling up in front of a fireplace. **serves 12**

storage

Store in an airtight container in the fridge for 3 to 4 days, or in the freezer for up to 3 months.

to reheat

Thaw in the fridge overnight, then reheat in the oven at 250°F (120°C) in a covered pan for about 30 minutes, or in the microwave for 1 to 2 minutes, until warmed through.

FOR THE PORK SHOULDER

1 tablespoon dried oregano

1 tablespoon ground mustard

1 teaspoon kosher salt

½ teaspoon freshly ground black pepper

4½ pounds (2.25kg) pork shoulder or pork butt

1 medium yellow onion, finely diced

4 garlic cloves, minced

FOR THE SAUCE

½ cup (160ml) pure maple syrup

⅓ cup (80g) whole grain mustard

½ teaspoon dried oregano

¼ teaspoon kosher salt

Pinch of freshly ground black pepper

1. To make the pork shoulder: In a small bowl, stir together the oregano, ground mustard, salt, and pepper. Trim any excess fat from the pork shoulder (but remember that some fat is good), then rub the spice mixture generously over the entire pork. Place the pork in the slow cooker and add the onion and garlic around it.

2. To make the sauce: In a medium bowl, stir together the maple syrup, whole grain mustard, oregano, salt, and pepper. Pour half the sauce all over the pork. Use your hands to make sure the meat is coated on all sides except the bottom. Reserve the other half of the sauce. Secure the lid on the slow cooker and cook on the low setting for 8 to 10 hours, or on the high setting for 5 to 6 hours, until the meat is fall-apart tender.

3. Remove the pork from the slow cooker to a large cutting board and use two forks to shred the meat. Using a slotted spoon or small fine-mesh sieve, scoop up some of the onions from the slow cooker, letting the liquid drain, and add to the shredded meat. Pour the remaining sauce over the meat and stir it together.

Serving size:
1 cup (185g)

Calories: 300

Fat: 12g

Saturated fat: 4g

Carbs: 11g

Fiber: 0g

Sugar: 9g

Protein: 36g

Cholesterol: 113mg

Sodium: 349mg

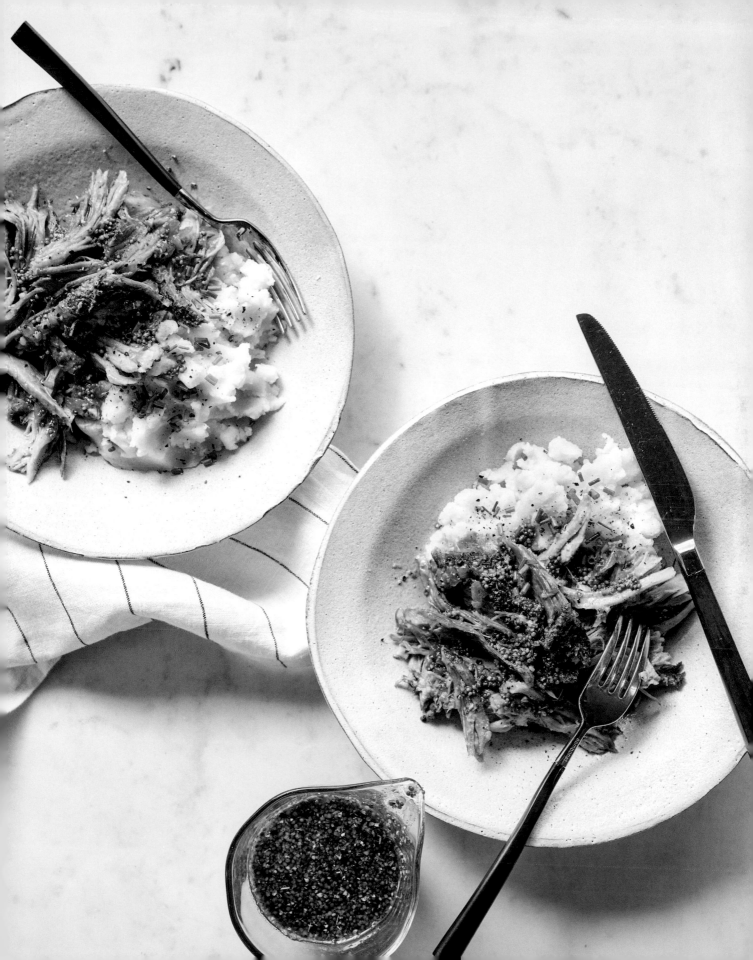

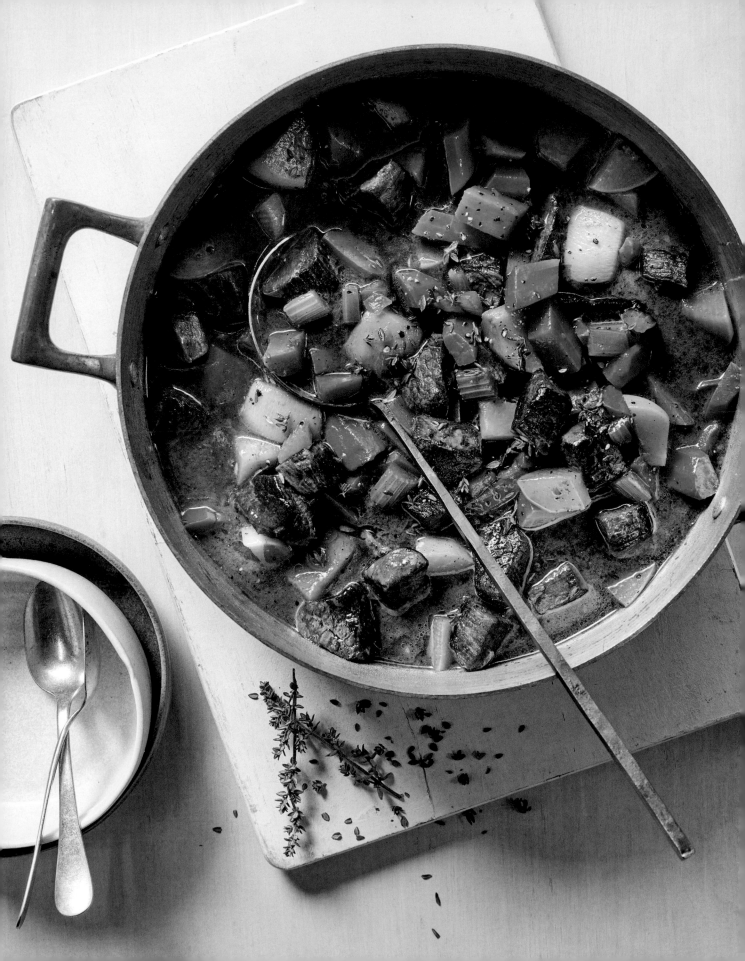

apple cider beef stew

storage

Store in an airtight container in the fridge for 3 to 4 days, or in the freezer for up to 3 months.

to reheat

If frozen, thaw in the fridge overnight, then microwave for 1 to 2 minutes or heat on the stove over medium heat, until hot.

It's hard to beat beef stew during the cold-weather months for a hearty and satisfying meal, and this version hits all the right seasonal notes. Tender beef and root vegetables simmer in aromatic apple cider for a subtle sweetness that'll make you think you're meandering apple orchards while scooping the stew into your mouth. The broth itself is lighter than the classic tomato-based version, and turnips rather than potatoes help create a stew that won't weigh you down—that is, you'll have room for seconds. **serves 4**

2 pounds (908g) beef stew meat, cut into 1-inch cubes

1½ teaspoons kosher salt

½ teaspoon freshly ground black pepper

2 tablespoons avocado oil or extra-virgin olive oil

1 large yellow onion, cut into chunks

1 tablespoon apple cider vinegar

2 tablespoons arrowroot powder

2 cups (480ml) apple cider juice

2 cups (480ml) low-sodium beef broth

½ teaspoon dried thyme

1 bay leaf

1 large or 2 small-to-medium turnips, chopped

4 medium carrots, sliced

3 celery ribs, chopped

Fresh thyme sprigs, for garnish (optional)

1. Pat the beef dry with paper towels. Season with salt and pepper.

2. In a large stockpot or Dutch oven, heat the oil over medium-high heat. Working in batches, place the beef in the pot and sear on all sides until golden, 2 to 3 minutes per side, then remove to a plate.

3. Place the onion in the pot and pour in the vinegar (which will help loosen the browned bits from the bottom of the pan) and cook for 3 to 4 minutes, until the onion is softened. Return the beef to the pot and stir in the arrowroot powder, coating the beef and vegetables, until fully dissolved.

4. Add the cider, broth, thyme, and bay leaf. Use a large spoon or spatula to stir everything together. Bring the broth to a boil, then reduce the heat to low and simmer partially covered for 1 hour.

5. Add the turnips, carrots, and celery. Cook for an additional 20 to 30 minutes, or until the vegetables are fork-tender. Remove the bay leaf and, if you'd like, garnish with fresh thyme.

Serving size:
2 cups (522g)

Calories: 765
Fat: 42g
Saturated fat: 14g
Carbs: 32g
Fiber: 4g
Sugar: 19g
Protein: 64g
Cholesterol: 179g
Sodium: 716g

garlic rosemary turkey breast

When you're craving turkey but don't want to roast an entire bird, this garlic rosemary turkey breast is the perfect alternative. It's the ideal size for family dinners, and I love to serve it up for informal dinner parties because most of the work is done before the guests arrive (which gives me ample time to chitchat). After a couple of hours in the oven, the skin is flawlessly crispy and the white meat is truly moist and tender. Just remove the meat from the bone and slice it up. No complicated carving required. **serves 6**

2 medium yellow onions, sliced into wedges

1 whole bone-in turkey breast (6½ pounds/3kg)

2 tablespoons extra-virgin olive oil

6 garlic cloves, minced

1½ tablespoons finely chopped fresh rosemary

2 tablespoons fresh lemon juice

2 teaspoons kosher salt

1 teaspoon freshly ground black pepper

1 cup (240ml) low-sodium turkey or chicken broth

1. Preheat the oven to 325°F (160°C). Arrange the onions in a roasting pan and place the turkey breast on top, skin side up.

2. In a small bowl, stir together the oil, garlic, rosemary, lemon juice, salt, and pepper.

3. With your fingers, gently loosen the skin from both halves of the turkey breast. Spread half of the garlic mixture under the skin, all over the turkey breast, then smooth the skin and spread the remaining mixture evenly on top of the skin. Pour the broth into the pan.

4. Roast the turkey uncovered for 1¾ to 2 hours, until the skin is golden brown and an instant-read thermometer reaches 160°F (71°C) when inserted into the thickest part of the breast. Remove the turkey from the oven and let it rest, covered with foil, for 15 minutes (the temperature will rise to 165°F/74°C). Slice the turkey away from the bone, then slice it crosswise on a cutting board.

storage

Store in an airtight container in the fridge for 3 to 4 days, or in the freezer for up to 3 months.

to reheat

If frozen, thaw in the fridge overnight. Then reheat in a 325°F (165°C) oven with a splash of broth in a pan covered with aluminum foil for 15 to 20 minutes. You can also reheat in the microwave for 1 to 2 minutes, until warmed through.

get creative

Once thawed, reheat the turkey for dicing and adding to garden salads, stuffing into sandwiches or wraps, tossing into casseroles, or subbing for chicken in a classic creamy chicken salad recipe.

helpful tip

If the skin is browning too quickly, you can cover it with aluminum foil in the oven. Alternatively, you can increase the oven temperature to 350°F (177°C) for the last 30 minutes to crisp up the skin even more.

Serving size: 6 ounces (170g) turkey meat

Calories: 298

Fat: 8g

Saturated fat: 2g

Carbs: 2g

Fiber: 0g

Sugar: 0g

Protein: 51g

Cholesterol: 136mg

Sodium: 542mg

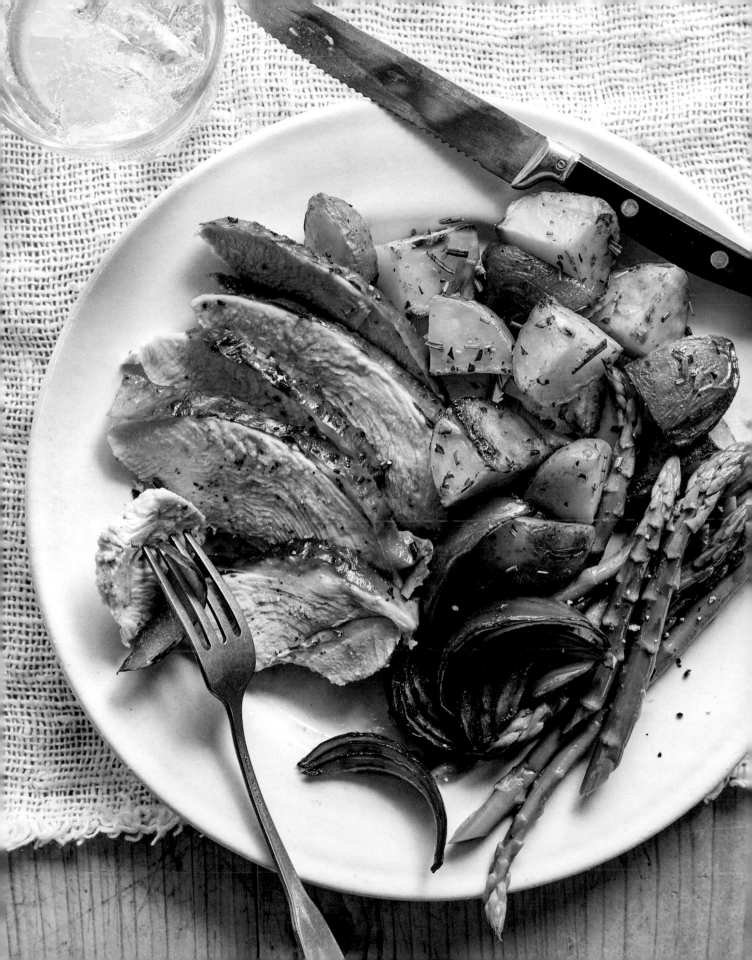

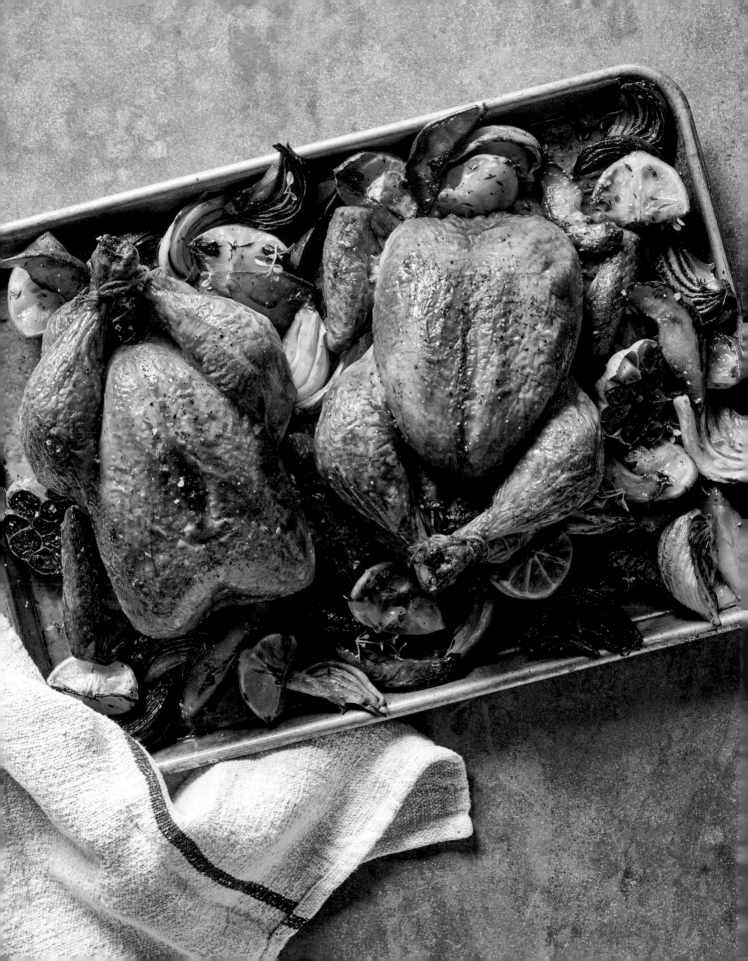

two whole roasted chickens with fennel, pear, and onion

If ever there was a recipe that screamed meal prep, it's this one. There's no additional work to roast two chickens instead of one, and the beauty of it is that you can eat one immediately and refrigerate (or freeze) the other for the future. The perfectly golden chicken is simply roasted with lemon, garlic, and thyme infusing the meat, while the veggies soak up all those same flavors, becoming incredibly tender and sweetly caramelized in the process. **serves 12**

2 Anjou or Bosc pears, cut into wedges and seeds removed

1 medium yellow onion, cut into wedges

1 large fennel bulb, leaves removed, cored, and cut into wedges

3 lemons, quartered

8 thyme sprigs

3 tablespoons extra-virgin olive oil

3½ teaspoons kosher salt

1¾ teaspoons freshly ground black pepper

2 whole chickens (5 pounds/ 2.3kg each), giblets removed

1 head garlic, cut in half crosswise

1. Preheat the oven to 425°F (220°C) and place a rack in the lower third of the oven.

2. Place the pears, onion, fennel, 8 of the lemon quarters, and 4 of the thyme sprigs in a large roasting pan. Drizzle with 1 tablespoon of the oil, season with ½ teaspoon of the salt and ¼ teaspoon of the pepper, then toss together.

3. Pat the chickens dry with paper towels. Rub 1 tablespoon oil each on the outside of the chickens. Season each chicken with 1 teaspoon of salt and ½ teaspoon of pepper, and the inside with ½ teaspoon of salt and ¼ teaspoon of pepper. Then stuff each chicken with 2 lemon quarters, the garlic, and 2 sprigs of thyme.

4. Place the chicken on top of the pears and vegetables, breast side up, and tuck the wings under. Tie the legs together with kitchen twine (you can also leave them untied if you wish).

5. Roast the chicken for 1¾ to 2 hours, or until an instant-read thermometer reads 160°F (71°C) at the thickest part of the breast (the juices should run clear when you cut between a leg and thigh). Let rest for 15 minutes, then slice and serve.

paprika rubbed pork tenderloin with shallot pan sauce

These juicy pork tenderloins are rubbed in a paprika spice blend that layers them in delicious flavor. Grab your favorite oven-safe skillet as you'll sear them on the stove first, then finish them in the oven. Once they're done, take advantage of the residual spices in the pan (and all those delicious browned bits), and whip up a quick and easy shallot pan sauce. There's a touch of sweetness in the pan sauce that perfectly balances the robust paprika flavor! **serves 6**

FOR THE TENDERLOIN

1 tablespoon sweet paprika

2 teaspoons smoked paprika

1 teaspoon garlic powder

1 teaspoon onion powder

1 teaspoon dried thyme

1 teaspoon kosher salt

½ teaspoon freshly ground black pepper

2 tablespoons avocado oil or extra-virgin olive oil

2 pork tenderloins (1 pound/454g each)

FOR THE SAUCE

1 small shallot, finely diced

½ cup (120ml) low-sodium chicken broth

2 teaspoons honey

1 tablespoon butter (optional)

1 teaspoon roughly chopped fresh thyme

Pinch of kosher salt and freshly ground black pepper

1. Preheat the oven to 375°F (190°C).

2. To make the tenderloin: In a small bowl, stir together the sweet paprika, smoked paprika, garlic powder, onion powder, dried thyme, salt, and pepper. Sprinkle the spice blend all over the tenderloins, then use your hands to rub it in.

3. In a large oven-safe skillet, heat the oil over medium-high heat. Add the pork and cook, turning occasionally, until seared and browned on all sides, about 4 minutes total. Transfer the pan to the oven and roast the pork tenderloin for 15 to 20 minutes, or until an instant-read thermometer reaches 140°F (60°C). Place the skillet back on the stove and remove the pork to a plate, cover with foil, and let rest for 10 minutes.

4. To make the sauce: Add the shallot to the skillet and stir for a minute over medium heat until softened. Pour the broth into

storage

Store in an airtight container in the fridge for 3 to 4 days, or in the freezer for up to 3 months.

to reheat

Add the slices to a skillet on medium heat, cover the skillet, and flip after a minute or so. You can also reheat in the microwave for 1 to 2 minutes, until warmed through.

helpful tips

Remember that pork is a lean cut of meat, and when it's overcooked it becomes dry, which isn't very tasty. It's always best to double-check the doneness with an instant-read thermometer rather than eyeball it. Slightly pink in the middle is okay, and don't forget there's carry-over cooking while it rests.

Serving size: 4 slices

Calories: 224

Fat: 8g

Saturated fat: 2g

Carbs: 5g

Fiber: 1g

Sugar: 3g

Protein: 32g

Cholesterol: 98mg

Sodium: 281mg

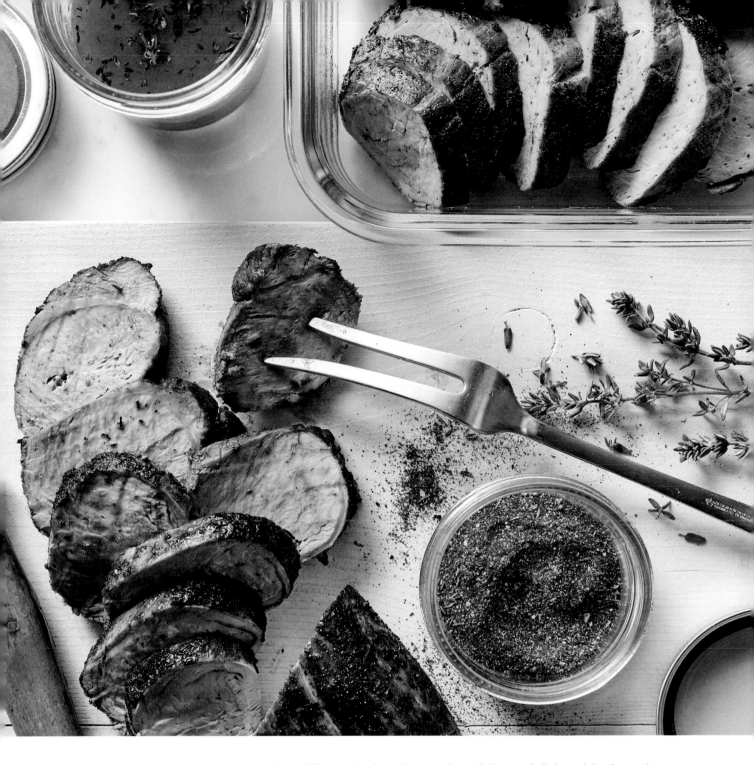

the skillet to deglaze it, scraping all those delicious bits from the bottom, and simmer for 2 minutes, until slightly reduced. Add the honey and, if desired, the butter (for a richer sauce) and stir together. Remove from the heat and stir in the thyme. Taste and season with salt and pepper.

5. Cut the pork tenderloin across into ½-inch (1.3cm) slices and arrange on a platter. Spoon the shallot sauce over the pork.

seafood mains

Living in coastal Southern California I realize that I'm spoiled with many things, including beautiful sunny weather, access to year-round farmers' markets, and some of the best seafood anywhere. Every week I hit up my local fishmonger for fresh catches (yes, just off the shores of Newport Beach) of tuna, halibut, and sea bass. And then I'll peruse the fish market for a global supply of Alaskan salmon, shrimp from the Gulf of Mexico, North American trout, and Pacific cod, among other seafood delights.

But I'll let you in on a little secret—even if you're in a land-locked seafood desert, you can still benefit from the health-boosting nutrients and omega-3s of the following pescatarian recipes—just buy frozen fish! (In case you missed it, I mention how to buy the best seafood on page 62.)

When it comes to meal prep, most people bypass seafood, thinking that it can only be eaten the day it's cooked, but that's simply not true. Fish and other seafood may be a bit more delicate than, say, chicken or beef, so you don't want to store it for 5 days in the fridge. But you can most definitely enjoy it for a couple of days, and in certain cases it freezes well! The most important thing is to be gentle when reheating. If you follow that basic rule, seafood delights like Cilantro Lime Shrimp (page 187) and Pan-Seared Cod in Romesco Sauce (page 195) can be enjoyed again and again!

spicy shrimp and parsnip noodles

Spiralized parsnip noodles make a great substitute for spaghetti noodles. If you lightly sauté them, they become crisp-tender, almost the same texture as pasta, *and* with an uncanny resemblance due to parsnip's bright white color. They also make a great substitute for rice noodles, which means they work beautifully in this grain-free, pad Thai–inspired recipe. The parsnip noodles soak up the spicy, umami-rich sauce, and when they're tossed with aromatics like garlic, ginger, and green onion, plus crisp mung bean sprouts and perfectly pink shrimp, you'll honestly feel like you're eating pad Thai. Just make sure you have everything prepped in small bowls before you get started, as this recipe moves fast. **serves 4**

FOR THE SPICY SAUCE

3 tablespoons coconut sugar

3 tablespoons fish sauce

2 tablespoons water

2 tablespoons tamarind paste or fresh lime juice

1 tablespoon low-sodium tamari soy sauce

½ teaspoon cayenne pepper

FOR THE SHRIMP AND NOODLE STIR-FRY

2 tablespoons avocado oil or extra-virgin olive oil

8 ounces (226g) extra-large shrimp, peeled and deveined

2 teaspoons finely grated peeled fresh ginger

3 garlic cloves, minced

3 green onions, thinly sliced and separated into white and green parts

2 medium parsnips, peeled and spiralized

2 large eggs, lightly beaten

2 cups (208g) mung bean sprouts

⅓ cup (47g) raw cashews, roughly chopped, for garnish

2 tablespoons roughly chopped fresh cilantro, for garnish

1. To make the sauce: In a medium bowl, stir together the coconut sugar, fish sauce, water, tamarind paste, tamari, and cayenne pepper. Set aside.

2. To make the stir-fry: In a large skillet or wok, heat 1 tablespoon of the oil on medium-high heat and swirl the pan to coat the bottom. Arrange the shrimp in a single flat layer. Cook the shrimp for 1 minute, then flip and cook another 30 seconds, until lightly pink but not quite cooked all the way through. Use tongs to remove the shrimp to a plate.

Serving size:
1½ cups (215g)

Calories: 310

Fat: 15g

Saturated fat: 3g

Carbs: 28g

Fiber: 4g

Sugar: 14g

Protein: 19g

Cholesterol: 165mg

Sodium: 1,675mg

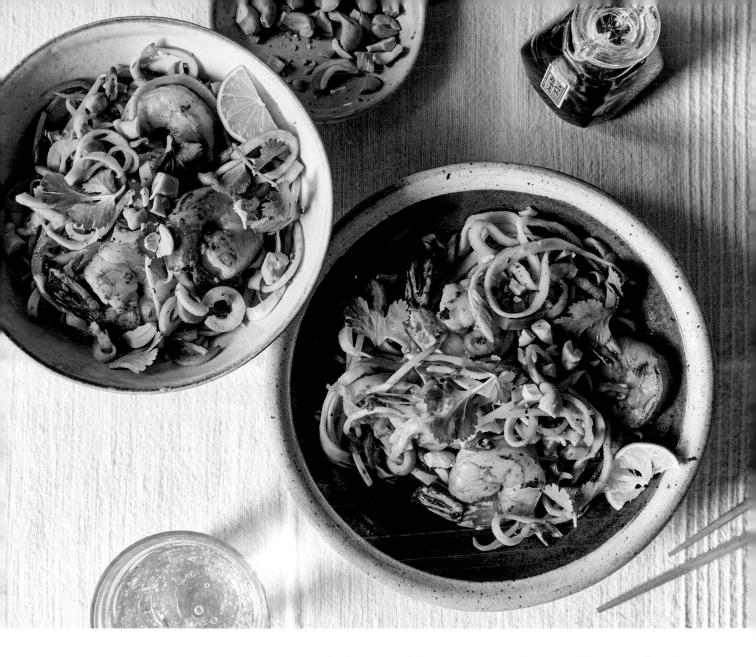

3. In the same skillet, add the remaining 1 tablespoon oil and sauté the ginger, garlic, and white parts of the green onion for 30 seconds. Add the parsnip noodles and use tongs to stir the noodles with the aromatics. Pour the sauce on top of the noodles and stir-fry for another 2 to 3 minutes, until the sauce has reduced and the noodles have softened.

4. Push the noodles to the side of the skillet, pour in the beaten eggs, and push them around until soft curds form, then incorporate the eggs with the noodles.

5. Return the shrimp to the skillet, add the bean sprouts, and stir-fry for 30 seconds until warmed through. Turn off the heat, stir in the green parts of the green onions, and garnish with the cashews and cilantro before serving.

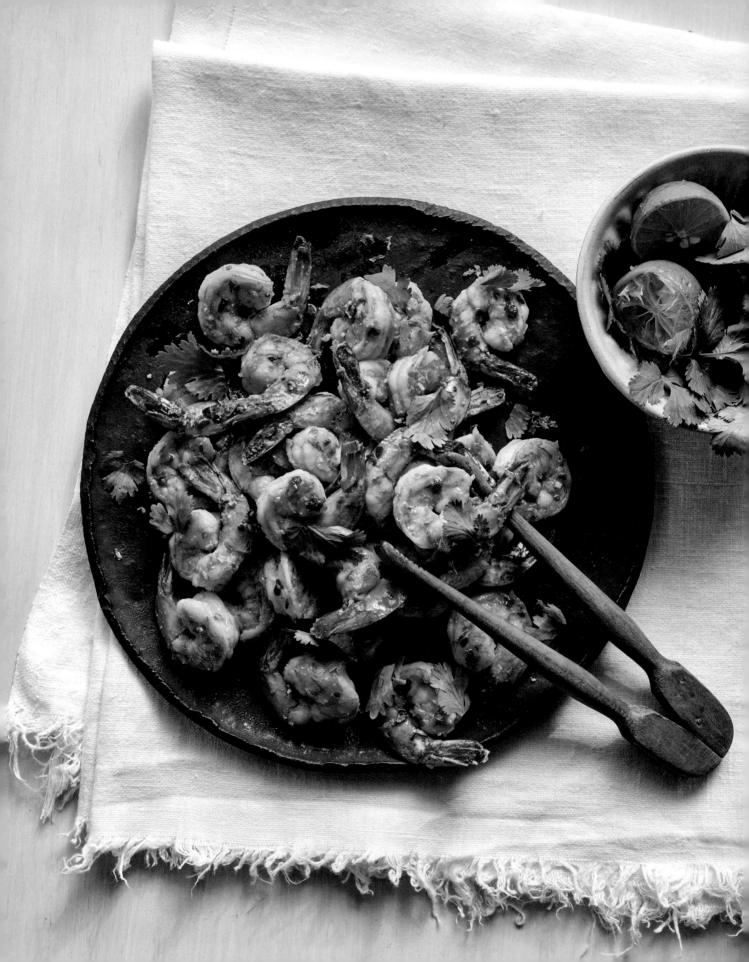

cilantro lime shrimp

When it comes to incredibly easy weeknight dinners, it's hard to beat shrimp. In about 10 minutes you can sauté shrimp with garlicky, zesty cilantro and lime—add a pinch of red pepper flakes for a kick of heat. I frequently use cilantro and lime together because the combination is light, bright, and fresh. Serve the shrimp over zucchini noodles or rice, with extra liquid from the pan drizzled on top. You could also top them on tortillas with avocado slices for tasty shrimp fajitas or assemble a quick Mexican-inspired salad. **serves 4**

storage

Store in an airtight container in the fridge for 3 to 4 days.

to reheat

Heat in a sauté pan on the stove or in the microwave in 30-second increments, until just warmed through. You can also enjoy them cold topped on a salad—no reheating necessary.

helpful tip

While you may be tempted to marinate the shrimp for a couple of hours, avoid doing so as the lime juice can start to denature and "cook" the shrimp (similar to ceviche), making the shrimp a bit rubbery after it's cooked.

1 pound (454g) extra-large shrimp, peeled and deveined

½ teaspoon ground cumin

¼ teaspoon kosher salt

2 tablespoons extra-virgin olive oil

4 cloves garlic, minced

1 teaspoon lime zest

¼ cup (60ml) fresh lime juice (from about 2 limes)

Pinch of crushed red pepper flakes (optional)

2 tablespoons roughly chopped fresh cilantro

1. In a large bowl, toss together the shrimp, cumin, and salt until well coated.

2. In a large skillet, heat the oil over medium heat. Add the garlic and stir for 30 seconds.

3. Add the shrimp to the pan and arrange in a single flat layer. Cook the shrimp for 1 to 2 minutes undisturbed. Flip the shrimp, cook for 1 minute more, then add the lime zest, lime juice, red pepper flakes (if using), and cilantro. Stir for another minute, or until the shrimp is cooked through.

Serving size:
About 8 shrimp (95g)

Calories: 150
Fat: 8g
Saturated fat: 1g
Carbs: 3g
Fiber: 0g
Sugar: 0g
Protein: 16g
Cholesterol: 143mg
Sodium: 713mg

grilled halibut skewers with orange chimichurri

When I was a kid, I visited relatives in Alaska for a couple of weeks of endless fishing adventures. It was a phenomenal trip, set among the most majestic scenery possible, and I proudly caught a ten-pound halibut just off the coast of Ketchikan. Admittedly, I never liked fish much prior to that trip, but catching my own dinner in Alaska was life-changing. Halibut has since had a special place in my heart, and the thick, meaty, mild-flavored white fish pairs beautifully with light and fresh flavors, like this orange chimichurri. A very quick sear on the grill is all you need! **serves 4**

½ cup (30g) finely chopped fresh parsley

1 garlic clove, minced

¼ cup (60ml) extra-virgin olive oil

½ teaspoon orange zest

¼ cup (60ml) fresh orange juice (from about 1 orange)

2 tablespoons fresh lemon juice

¼ teaspoon kosher salt

¼ teaspoon freshly ground black pepper

1½ pounds (680g) halibut, cut into small cubes

2 medium zucchini, thinly sliced lengthwise with a mandoline

Avocado oil or other high-heat cooking oil, for greasing

1. In a medium bowl, whisk together the parsley, garlic, olive oil, orange zest, orange juice, lemon juice, salt, and pepper.

2. In a separate medium bowl, gently toss the cubed halibut and two-thirds of the orange chimichurri (reserve the rest to drizzle at the end) until fully coated. Marinate for 30 minutes in the fridge.

3. Preheat a grill or stovetop grill pan to medium-high heat.

4. Thread pieces of halibut and zucchini on skewers, alternating a piece of halibut with a slice of zucchini that's folded back on itself like a ribbon, until you have about 4 pieces of halibut on each skewer.

5. Moisten a paper towel with a little avocado oil and pinch it between tongs, then carefully but quickly wipe the grates of the grill until coated and glossy, to prevent sticking.

storage

Store in an airtight container in the fridge for 2 to 3 days.

to reheat

Place on a rimmed baking sheet and cover with aluminum foil (to prevent drying out), then reheat in a 275°F (140°C) oven for 10 to 15 minutes. Or microwave in 30-second increments, until warmed through. You can also enjoy the halibut cold, flaked into a salad.

helpful tip

Since fish is more likely to stick to grills than chicken or beef, it's important to ensure your grill is clean, well-oiled, and hot. If you notice the halibut sticking, gently slide a spatula underneath to loosen it, rather than by pulling up on the skewers. I recommend using flat metal skewers or double skewers, which prevent the fish from rotating around the skewer as you flip.

Serving size: 2 skewers

Calories: 350

Fat: 17g

Saturated fat: 3g

Carbs: 8g

Fiber: 2g

Sugar: 6g

Protein: 41g

Cholesterol: 102mg

Sodium: 175mg

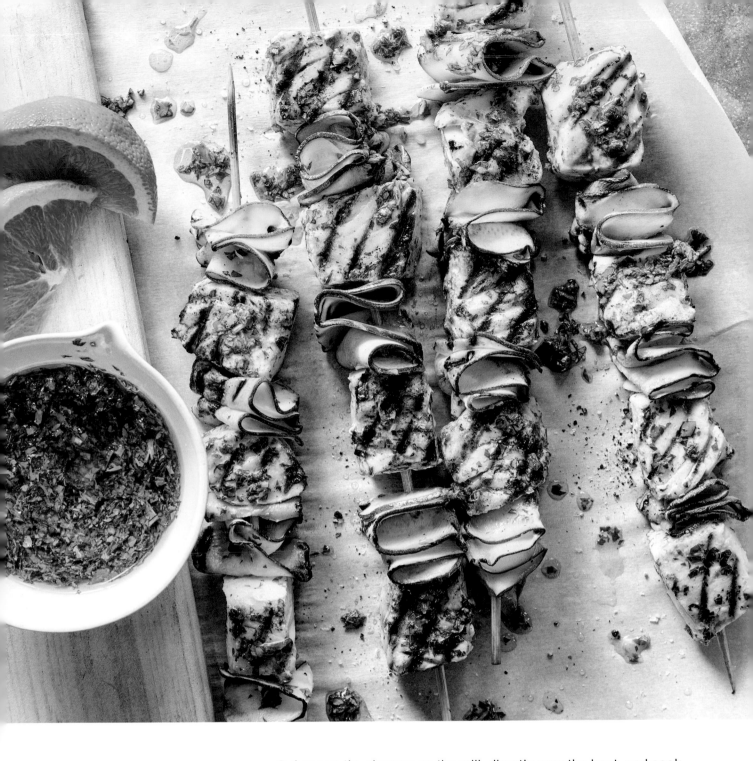

6. Arrange the skewers on the grill, directly over the heat, and cook for 2 to 2½ minutes, then turn just once, and cook another 2 to 2½ minutes, until no longer translucent. Halibut cooks quickly, so do keep an eye on it, as you don't want it to overcook. Transfer the skewers to a plate and accompany with the remaining orange chimichurri.

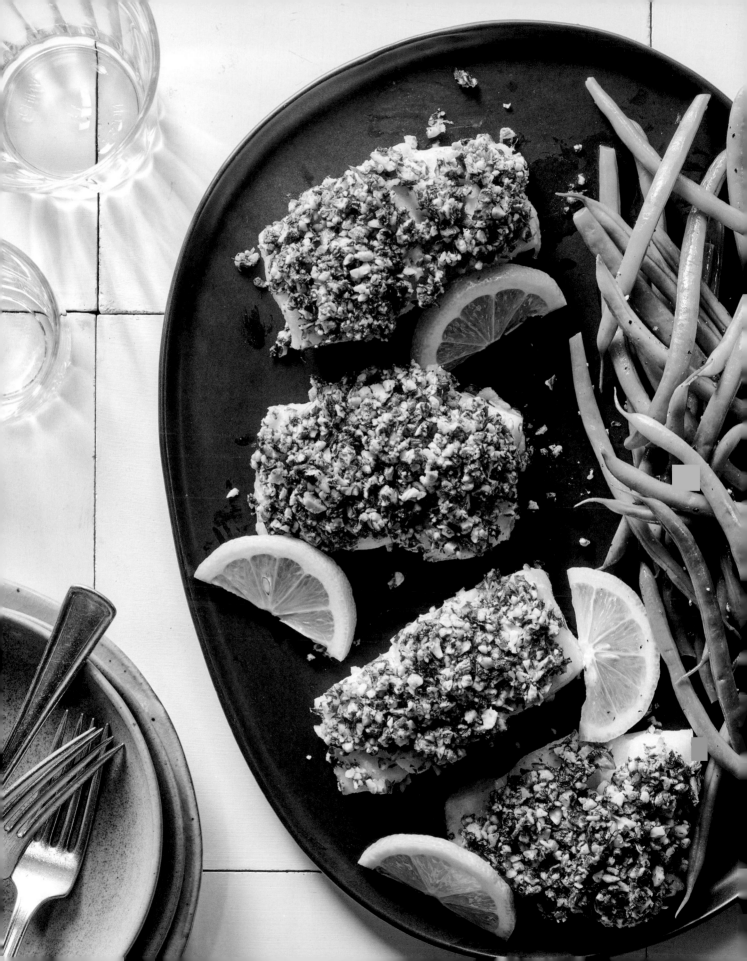

almond-herb crusted cod

Crusted seafood often contains bread crumbs, but this simple mix of roughly chopped almonds, garlic, lemon zest, and fresh herbs is just as satisfying, if not more so. I often think of cod as a great "gateway" fish—it's mild in flavor, with a light, flaky texture most people love, even seafood newbies. This recipe is a stand-out weeknight meal that's sort of fancy-ish with very little effort. I often serve it with steamed vegetables or sautéed greens, like my Garlic Sautéed Beet Greens (page 262). **serves 4**

½ cup raw almonds (70g), roughly chopped

1 tablespoon melted butter or extra-virgin olive oil

2 garlic cloves, minced

1 tablespoon lemon zest

3 tablespoons finely chopped fresh parsley

2 tablespoons finely chopped fresh chives

¼ teaspoon kosher salt

Pinch of freshly ground black pepper

4 cod fillets (6 ounces/170g each)

Lemon quarters, for serving

1. Preheat the oven to 400°F (200°C).

2. In a small bowl, stir together the almonds, butter, garlic, lemon zest, parsley, chives, salt, and pepper. Place the cod on a rimmed baking sheet and evenly spread the mixture on top of the cod, pressing down a little with your fingers to lightly compact it. Bake for 13 to 15 minutes, or until the fish is opaque and flakes easily with a fork and the top is lightly golden. Before serving, squeeze fresh lemon juice on top.

Serving size: 1 fillet

Calories: 261
Fat: 13g
Saturated fat: 3g
Carbs: 5g
Fiber: 3g
Sugar: 1g
Protein: 34g
Cholesterol: 96mg
Sodium: 227mg

blackened cajun trout

Years ago, back when I was in the corporate world, I'd meet up at my local Houston's Restaurant with a friend for a catch-up drink and dinner after work. They had a grilled Cajun trout on the menu that I'd invariably order (after perusing the menu for the umpteenth time, thinking I'd try something different). It was cooked simply, but with an abundance of bold flavor, and was served up with a side of steamed broccoli and creamy mashed potatoes. This trout replicates that satisfying flavor, though I broil it rather than bake it, and go a bit heavier on the blackened Cajun seasoning. It's perfect for those who love powerful, spicy flavors! **serves 4**

1 teaspoon sweet paprika

½ teaspoon kosher salt

½ teaspoon garlic powder

¼ teaspoon onion powder

¼ teaspoon dried oregano

¼ teaspoon dried thyme

¼ teaspoon cayenne pepper

¼ teaspoon freshly ground black pepper

1½ pounds (681g) steelhead trout

1 tablespoon olive oil

1. Preheat the oven broiler to high and set an oven rack 6 to 8 inches (20 to 25cm) below the top heating element.

2. In a small bowl, stir together the paprika, salt, garlic powder, onion powder, oregano, thyme, cayenne pepper, and black pepper.

3. Rub both sides of the trout with oil and place on a rimmed baking sheet (don't add parchment paper as it will burn when broiled). Sprinkle the seasoning evenly over the trout, rubbing it in with your fingers to make sure the trout is evenly coated.

4. Broil the trout for 5 to 8 minutes (depending on the thickness of your trout), or until it flakes easily with a fork.

storage

Store in an airtight container in the fridge for 3 to 4 days, or in the freezer for up to 3 months.

to reheat

If frozen, thaw in the fridge overnight. Place on a rimmed baking sheet and cover with aluminum foil (to prevent drying out), then reheat in a 275°F (140°C) oven for 10 to 15 minutes. Or microwave in 30-second increments, until warmed through. You can also turn leftover flaked trout into spicy fish cakes!

helpful tip

If you're worried about the level of spice, you can reduce the cayenne pepper to ⅛ teaspoon. Or you can just use less of the spice mix and save any leftovers in a small container for sprinkling on chicken, salmon, or other protein in the future.

Serving size:
6 ounces (170g)

Calories: 471

Fat: 38g

Saturated fat: 9g

Carbs: 1g

Fiber: 0g

Sugar: 0g

Protein: 30g

Cholesterol: 38mg

Sodium: 194mg

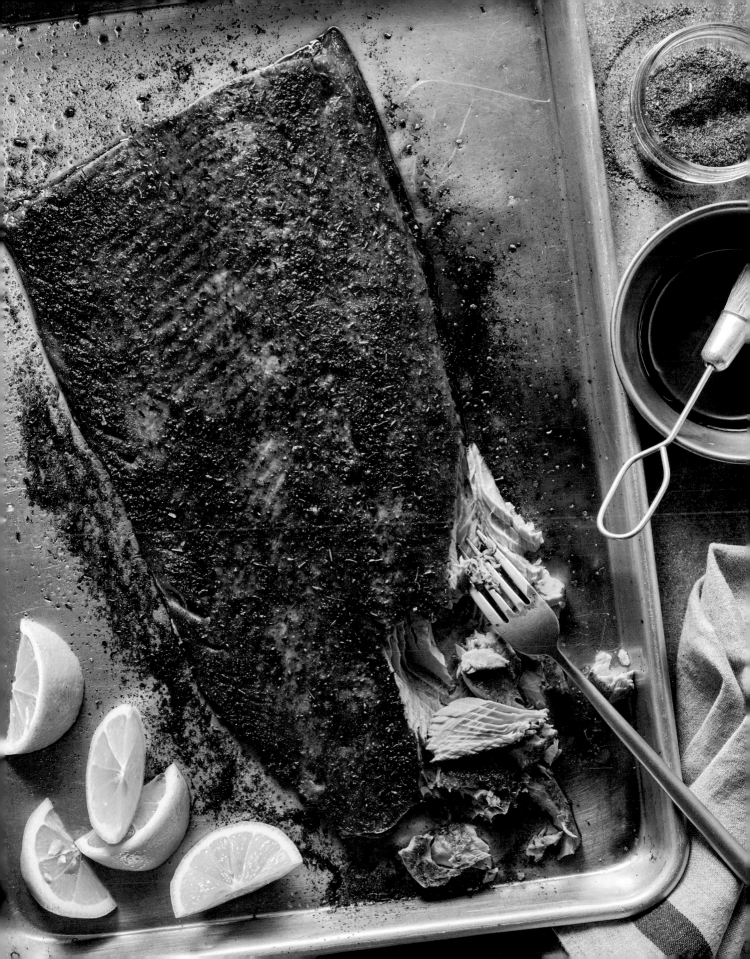

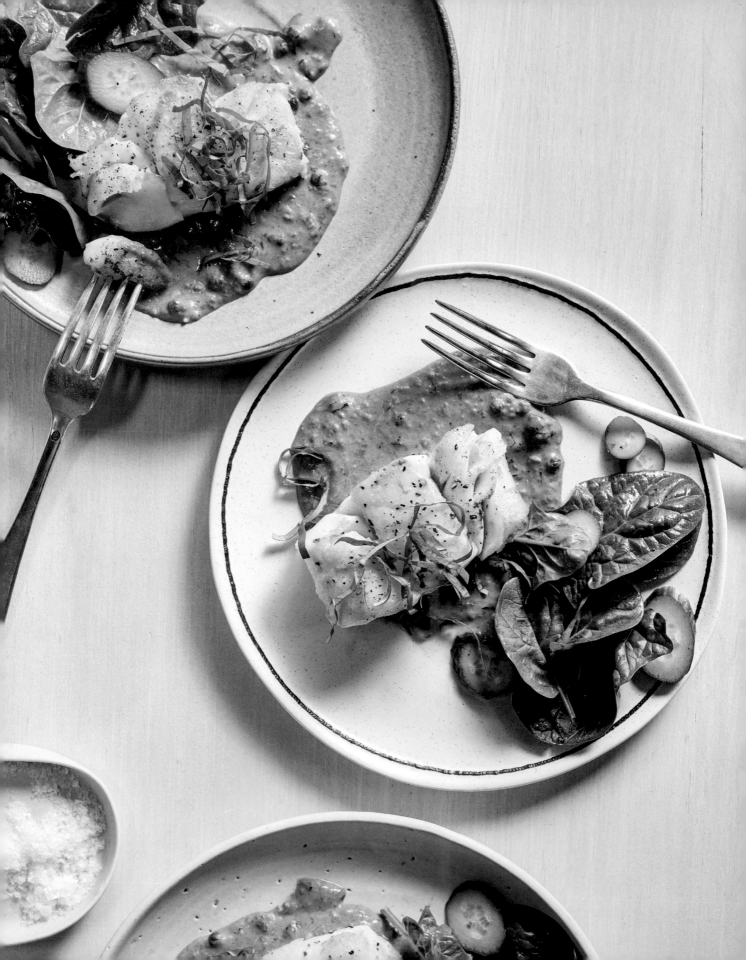

pan-seared cod in romesco sauce

storage

Store in an airtight container in the fridge for 2 to 3 days, or in the freezer for 3 months.

to reheat

If frozen, thaw in the fridge overnight, then place a piece of fish and some of the sauce in a pan on the stove over medium heat, or microwave in 30-second increments, until warmed through.

Smoky romesco sauce pairs beautifully with flaky cod. Here I add coconut cream to a classic romesco sauce for a luxuriously smooth texture, then simmer the fish in the sauce after quickly searing it. The capers add a salty, briny bite, and fresh herbs enhance the summertime tomato and roasted red pepper flavor. This recipe is utterly delicious served over Lemon Herb Rice (page 243), which soaks up all the creamy, smoky sauce! **serves 4**

2 tablespoons extra-virgin olive oil or an equal mix of butter and oil

4 cod fillets (6 ounces/170g each)

½ teaspoon kosher salt

¼ teaspoon freshly ground black pepper

1 cup (240g) Romesco Sauce (page 253)

1 cup (240g) coconut cream

3 tablespoons drained capers

2 tablespoons roughly chopped fresh parsley, plus more for garnish

2 tablespoons roughly chopped fresh basil, plus more for garnish

1. In a large pan, heat the oil over medium heat. Pat the cod dry with paper towels and season both sides with salt and pepper. Place the cod in the pan and cook 3 to 4 minutes, until lightly golden, then flip and cook an additional 3 minutes, until cooked through. Remove the fish to a plate.

2. Stir together the romesco sauce and coconut cream in the pan and bring to a simmer. Stir in the capers, parsley, and basil. Return the cod to the pan and continue simmering until heated through. Garnish with extra herbs.

Serving size:
1 fillet + sauce

Calories: 409
Fat: 29g
Saturated fat: 12g
Carbs: 5g
Fiber: 2g
Sugar: 3g
Protein: 28g
Cholesterol: 80mg
Sodium: 1,080mg

spicy shrimp with tomatoes and feta

This is my take on a traditional Greek shrimp saganaki, which is tender shrimp nestled in a spicy tomato sauce and topped with feta and parsley. In Greece, it's served as an appetizer, or meze, with crusty bread, and it often has ouzo or white wine in it. I've swapped the alcohol for tomato sauce, which makes it extra saucy and perfect for topping on rice, cauliflower rice, mashed potatoes, or my Garlicky Root Vegetable Mash (page 247). **serves 4**

3 tablespoons extra-virgin olive oil

½ medium yellow onion, finely diced

2 cups (285g) grape or cherry tomatoes

6 garlic cloves, roughly chopped

1 teaspoon dried oregano

½ teaspoon crushed red pepper flakes

¼ teaspoon sweet or smoked paprika

1 (8-ounce/227g) can tomato sauce

1 teaspoon kosher salt

¼ teaspoon freshly ground black pepper

1½ pounds (681g) extra-large shrimp, peeled and deveined

¼ cup (28g) crumbled feta cheese

2 tablespoons roughly chopped fresh parsley, for garnish

1. In a large pan, heat the oil over medium heat. Add the onion and grape tomatoes and sauté for 4 to 5 minutes, until the onions start to soften and the tomatoes start to blister.

2. Add the garlic, oregano, red pepper flakes, and paprika and sauté for an additional 1 to 2 minutes, stirring frequently.

3. Add the tomato sauce, salt, and pepper, stir everything together, then add the shrimp, and stir again, making sure the shrimp are coated in the sauce and evenly distributed throughout the pan. Cover the pan, reduce the temperature to medium-low, and cook the shrimp for 5 minutes.

4. Remove the lid, sprinkle the feta on top, and simmer for an additional 2 to 3 minutes uncovered, to warm the feta and thicken the sauce.

5. Remove the pan from the heat and sprinkle with chopped parsley.

storage
Store in an airtight container in the fridge for 3 to 4 days, or in the freezer for up to 3 months.

to reheat
If frozen, thaw in the fridge overnight, then place the shrimp and sauce in a pan on the stove over medium heat. You can also microwave in 30-second increments, until warmed through.

helpful tips
Double-check the ingredients on your tomato sauce to make sure there's no added sugar, corn syrup, or other sweeteners. Also, heads-up that this is a moderately spicy dish; if you'd like it less spicy, reduce the amount of red pepper flakes.

get creative
This recipe also works well with cod or halibut. Just cut the fish into smaller portions and nestle it into the sauce. The fish may break up a bit when stirring, but that's okay; it'll still be delicious!

Serving size: 1¼ cups (290g)

Calories: 276
Fat: 14g
Saturated fat: 3g
Carbs: 11g
Fiber: 2g
Sugar: 5g
Protein: 26g
Cholesterol: 223mg
Sodium: 1,624mg

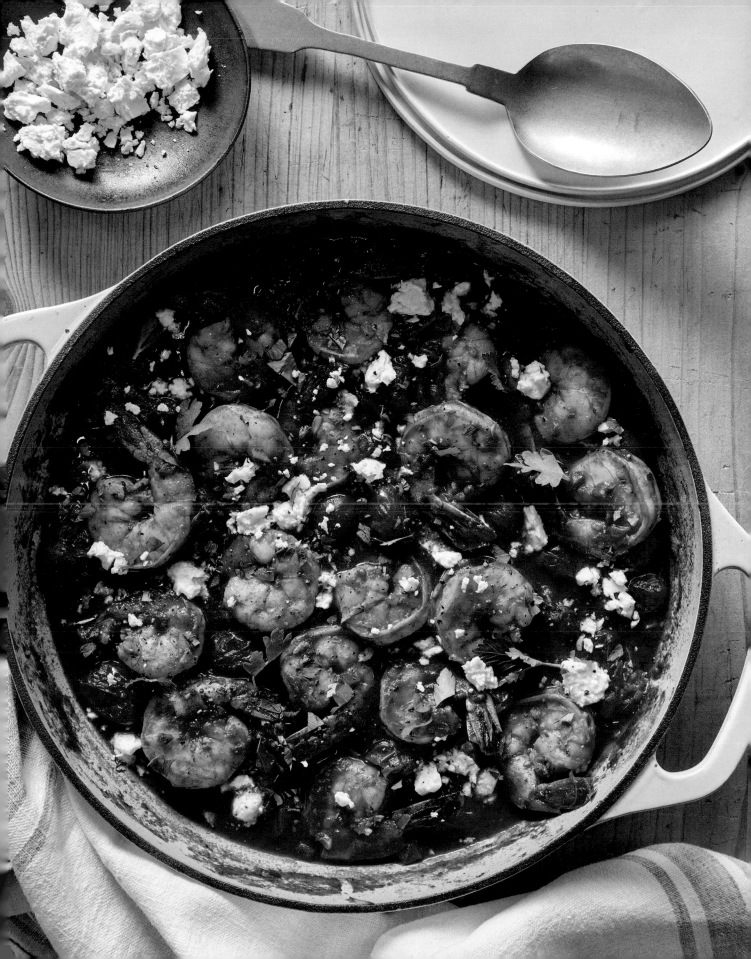

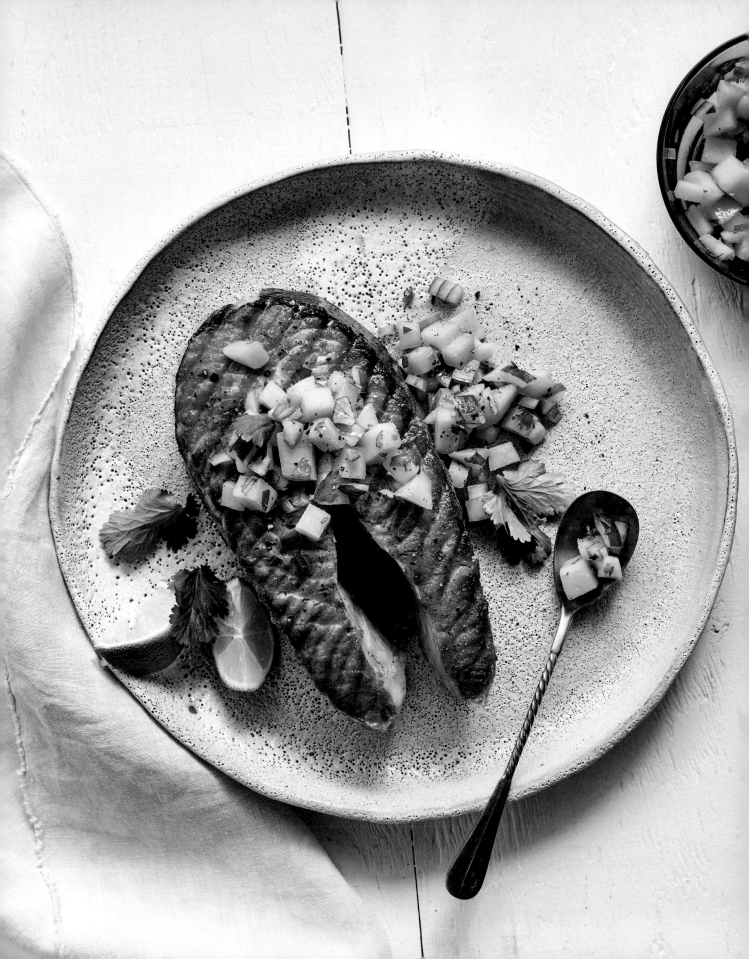

grilled salmon steaks with fruit salsa

Serving size: 1 salmon steak + fruit salsa

Calories: 374
Fat: 18g
Saturated fat: 3g
Carbs: 4g
Fiber: 1g
Sugar: 3g
Protein: 50g
Cholesterol: 115mg
Sodium: 428mg

Salmon steaks really are perfect for the grill because they're cut perpendicular to the spine, and the bone structure, thickness, and skin all help hold the salmon together as it cooks. This recipe is a summertime favorite of mine that looks fancy (very SoCal wouldn't you say?), but it's incredibly easy to make. The salmon just needs a quick flip on a hot grill to get that deliciously smoky char, and then it's topped with your favorite fruit salsa. If you're making this for an outdoor party, make a few different fruit salsa flavors and let people choose!

serves 4

4 salmon steaks (10 ounces/ 284g each), pin bones removed

2 tablespoons avocado oil or extra-virgin olive oil

1 teaspoon kosher salt

½ teaspoon freshly ground black pepper

1 cup (240g) Fruit Salsa (page 232)

1. Preheat a grill or stovetop grill pan to medium-high heat. Brush both sides of the salmon steaks with oil, then season with the salt and pepper. Moisten a paper towel with a little avocado oil and pinch it between tongs, then carefully but quickly wipe the grates of the grill until coated and glossy, to prevent sticking.

2. Grill the salmon for 5 to 7 minutes each side, depending on thickness. To flip, use a spatula underneath the fish rather than grabbing from the side with tongs (which may cause the salmon to fall apart).

3. Top each salmon steak with a portion of fruit salsa before serving.

tuna zoodle casserole with lemon cashew alfredo

The classic tuna noodle casserole is completely revamped and flipped upside down in this light and fresh veggie-forward, gluten-free, *and* dairy-free version. Pasta noodles are replaced with zucchini "noodles," and the traditional cheesy sauce is replaced with a lemony, cashew-based alfredo. The extra boost of lemon pairs beautifully with the zucchini and tuna, and the cashew alfredo helps keep you full in this lighter, healthier take on the classic one-dish meal.

serves 6

FOR THE LEMON CASHEW ALFREDO

1 cup (140g) raw cashews, soaked overnight, drained, and rinsed

½ small yellow onion, finely diced

2 garlic cloves

½ cup (120ml) fresh lemon juice (from about 4 lemons)

½ cup (120ml) low-sodium vegetable broth, chicken broth, or water

2 tablespoons nutritional yeast

¼ teaspoon dried thyme

1 teaspoon kosher salt

¼ teaspoon freshly ground black pepper

FOR THE CASSEROLE

2 large zucchini

1 tablespoon extra-virgin olive oil

½ small yellow onion, finely diced

2 celery ribs, diced

1 cup (130g) frozen peas

2 (5-ounce/142g) cans tuna, drained

2 tablespoons finely chopped fresh parsley, plus more for garnish

2 tablespoons finely chopped fresh dill, plus more for garnish

Lemon slices, for serving

storage

Store in an airtight container in the fridge for 4 to 5 days.

to reheat

Reheat in a 325°F (160°C) oven for about 8 to 10 minutes, or in the microwave for 1 to 2 minutes, until warmed through. I don't recommend freezing the casserole, as the zucchini will become thin and watery when thawed.

helpful tip

You can use tuna in oil or water (I prefer water). I also recommend Wild Planet or Safe Catch brands because the meat is more chunky and flaky rather than mushy.

1. Preheat the oven to 350°F (177°C).

2. To make the alfredo sauce: In a high-powered blender on high speed, blend the cashews, onion, garlic, lemon juice, broth, nutritional yeast, thyme, salt, and pepper for 30 seconds, or until smooth and creamy.

3. To make the casserole: Spiralize the zucchini into ribbons or noodles and place them in a large mixing bowl.

Serving size:
1½ cups (216g)

Calories: 264

Fat: 14g

Saturated fat: 3g

Carbs: 18g

Fiber: 4g

Sugar: 6g

Protein: 19g

Cholesterol: 19mg

Sodium: 258mg

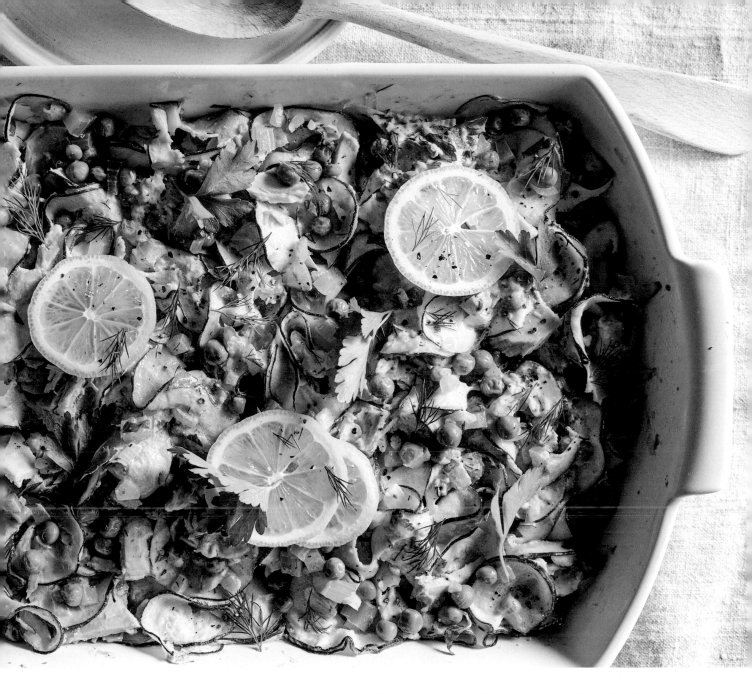

4. In a medium pan over medium heat, heat the oil and sauté the onion and celery for 4 to 5 minutes, until softened and translucent. Add the frozen peas and stir for another minute, until thawed. Transfer the veggies to the bowl with the zucchini.

5. Flake the tuna into the bowl and add the parsley, dill, and alfredo sauce. Stir together until well combined and creamy, then scrape the mixture into a 13 × 9-inch (23 × 33cm) casserole dish and bake for 15 to 20 minutes, until warmed through and the top starts to turn lightly golden. Garnish with parsley and dill and serve with lemon slices.

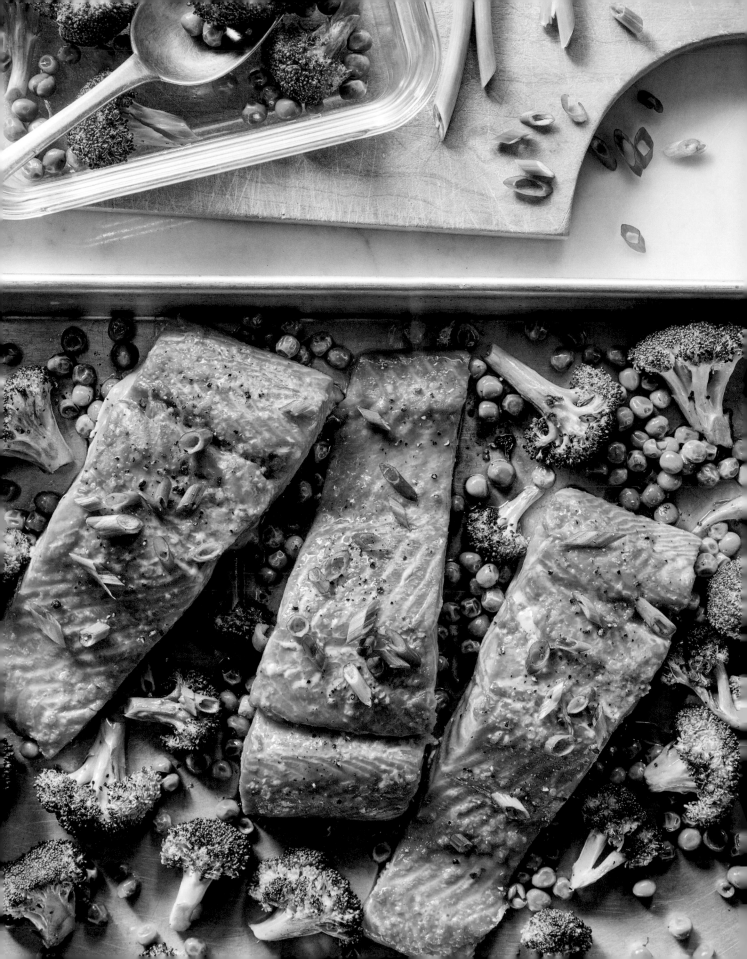

honey-ginger sheet pan salmon

storage

Store in an airtight container in the fridge for 3 to 4 days, or in the freezer for up to 3 months.

to reheat

If frozen, thaw in the fridge overnight. Place on a rimmed baking sheet and cover with aluminum foil (to prevent drying out), then reheat in a 275°F (140°C) oven for 10 to 15 minutes. Or microwave in 30-second increments, until warmed through.

get creative

To switch up leftovers, I'll often eat this dish on subsequent nights as part of a macro bowl by flaking the cold salmon on top of some rice with the roasted broccoli and peas. To that I'll add grated carrots, diced cucumber, red onion, avocado slices, and a sprinkle of finely chopped fresh cilantro.

Serving size: 1 salmon fillet + ¼ portion of veggies

Calories: 377
Fat: 12g
Saturated fat: 3g
Carbs: 22g
Fiber: 4g
Sugar: 12g
Protein: 45g
Cholesterol: 94mg
Sodium: 654mg

For all my sheet pan recipe lovers, I'm serving up a new quick-and-easy favorite with this Asian-inspired honey-ginger salmon. After a quick toss with olive oil, salt, and pepper, the broccoli roasts on its own for a bit, giving you time to stir together the sweet and gingery marinade. Then all you've got to do is place the salmon on the sheet pan, add some frozen peas, drizzle with the marinade, and cook another few minutes. Healthy weeknight dinner—done! **serves 4**

1 head of broccoli, florets removed

1 tablespoon extra-virgin olive oil

1 teaspoon kosher salt

½ teaspoon freshly ground black pepper

2 garlic cloves, minced

1 tablespoon minced peeled fresh ginger

2 tablespoons honey

1 tablespoon low-sodium tamari soy sauce or coconut aminos

1 teaspoon sesame oil

4 salmon fillets (6 ounces/170g each)

1 cup (170g) frozen peas

2 green onions (white and green parts), thinly sliced, for garnish

1. Preheat the oven to 375°F (190°C).

2. On a rimmed baking sheet, drizzle the broccoli florets with the olive oil and sprinkle with ½ teaspoon of the salt and ¼ teaspoon of the pepper. Toss together, then roast for 10 minutes.

3. In a small bowl, stir together the garlic, ginger, honey, tamari, sesame oil, and the remaining ½ teaspoon salt and ¼ teaspoon pepper.

4. Pat the salmon dry with a paper towel. Remove the baking sheet from the oven, push the broccoli and cauliflower to the outer edges, add the peas, and place the salmon on the sheet pan. Drizzle the marinade evenly on top of the salmon, then place the sheet pan back in the oven for another 12 to 15 minutes, until the salmon flakes easily. Remove from the oven, then sprinkle the green onions on top before serving.

veggie mains

Gone are the days when vegetables were relegated to "supporting character" roles. Today's vegetarian and vegan mains 100 percent hold their own as satisfying fill-you-up main dishes worthy of center stage. And the beauty is that you don't have to consider yourself vegetarian or vegan to enjoy them—they're just all-around delicious no matter your dietary preference. So, omnivores, dig in!

When it comes to meal prepping vegetarian dishes, the added bonus is that they tend to keep longer than animal-based mains. And reheating is a breeze, without the concern of accidentally turning your leftovers into something rubbery or dry. Simple plant-based proteins such as lentils, chickpeas, nuts, beans, and chia seeds were quite frankly made for meal prep!

In this chapter, you'll find an assortment of naturally gluten-free, veggie-forward meals, like my Lemony Lentil and Chickpea Soup (page 213), Zucchini Rollatini with Spinach Cashew Ricotta (page 218), and White Gazpacho (page 217). And while there may be sprinkles of cheese here and there, as with the Spiralized Sweet Potato "Burrito" Bake (page 214), dairy is not a requirement on any of these dishes, so feel free to leave it off!

falafel

I've had my fair share of falafel on travels through Egypt, Israel, and Jordan. I've had them in restaurants and on street corners (about as authentic as they come). I've had them stuffed in gluten-free pita and on salads. After eating so many, I've realized that what makes the best falafel is tons of herbs (double the typical amount) and a small amount of green chile pepper. This makes for an addictive flavor that's "a little something extra" but not spicy. Just insanely delicious, especially when paired with my Tahini Sauce (page 250). In this recipe, don't use canned chickpeas, because the falafels will turn out far too soft. Dried and soaked chickpeas are the way to go. **makes 18 falafel balls, to serve 6**

1 cup (200g) dried chickpeas, soaked overnight

½ cup (95g) medium yellow onion, roughly chopped

1 large bunch of fresh parsley, roughly chopped

1 large bunch of fresh cilantro, roughly chopped

1 small green chile pepper, such as serrano or jalapeño

3 garlic cloves

1 teaspoon ground cumin

½ teaspoon ground cardamom

1 teaspoon kosher salt

¼ teaspoon freshly ground black pepper

2 tablespoons chickpea flour, plus more as needed

½ teaspoon baking soda

1 or 2 teaspoons water or lemon juice, as needed

Avocado oil or another high-heat oil, for frying or baking

1. Drain and rinse the chickpeas, then place them in a food processor. Add the onion, parsley, cilantro, chile pepper, garlic, cumin, cardamom, salt, and pepper. Pulse several times until the mixture resembles the texture of coarse sand.

2. Transfer the falafel mixture to a large bowl. Stir in the flour and baking soda. Cover and refrigerate the mixture for 30 to 60 minutes.

3. Use your hands or an ice cream or falafel scoop to form the falafel into balls or patties. If you find the dough is too wet, you can add another tablespoon of flour. If it's too dry and crumbly, add the water a little at a time.

storage
Store in an airtight container in the fridge for 3 to 4 days.

to reheat
Reheat in a 350°F (180°C) oven for 5 to 10 minutes, or in a skillet until warmed through, to retain the crispy outside texture.

helpful tip
The beauty of this recipe is that you can make the falafel dough ahead of time and freeze it for up to 3 months. When you're ready, thaw the dough in the fridge overnight, give it a stir, then form into balls or patties and cook.

Serving size:
3 falafel balls

Calories: 143
Fat: 2g
Saturated fat: 0g
Carbs: 26g
Fiber: 7g
Sugar: 2g
Protein: 8g
Cholesterol: 0g
Sodium: 303g

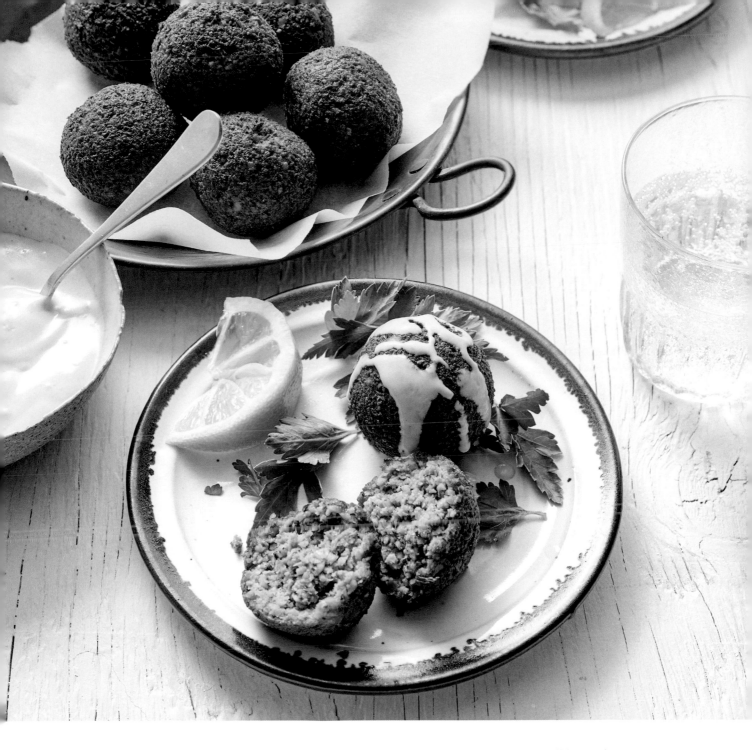

4. To deep-fry the falafel: Pour about 3 inches oil into a large pot over medium heat. Heat the oil to 350°F (180°C). Cook the falafel in batches (about 6 to 8 at a time) for 1 to 2 minutes, until golden. Then use a skimmer to remove them to a paper towel–lined plate.

5. To bake the falafel: Preheat the oven to 425°F (220°C). Lightly spray or brush a rimmed baking sheet with oil. Arrange the falafel on the baking sheet and lightly spray or brush the top side with oil. Bake for 25 to 30 minutes, flipping halfway through.

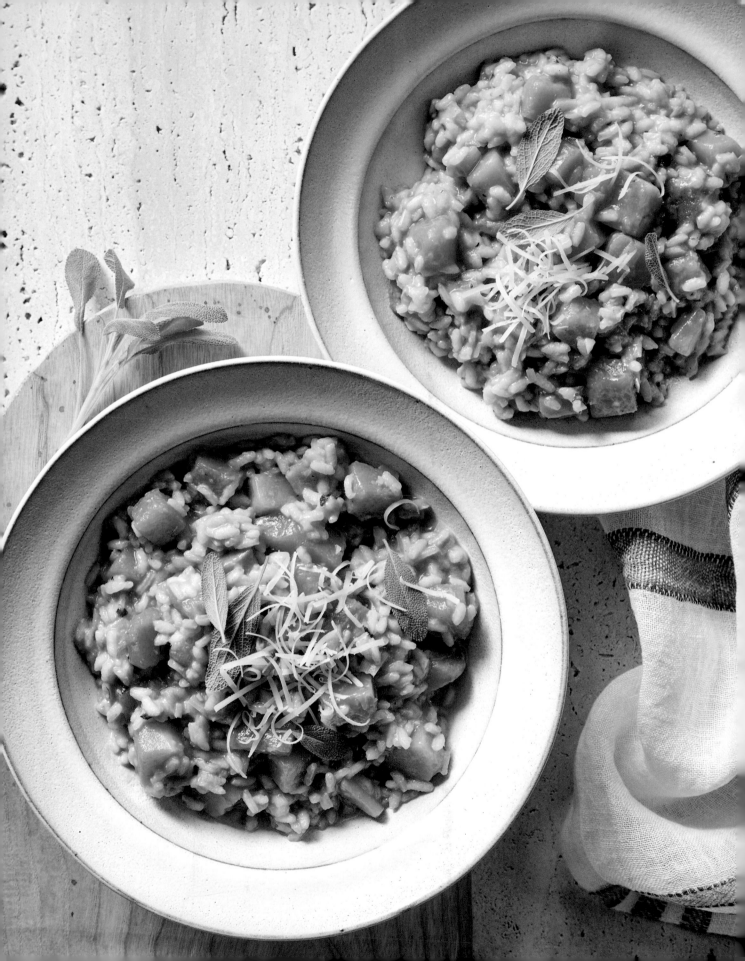

leek, sage, and butternut squash risotto

In the fall and winter when it's cold and drizzly outside, there's nothing better than a warm, comforting bowl of creamy risotto. The butternut squash gets slightly caramelized on the stove, imparting a subtle sweetness, and little flecks of sage infuse earthy, savory goodness. I add just a bit of cheese, but in all honesty, you could leave it off if you're dairy-free. It will still be ultra-creamy thanks to the higher starch content of the arborio rice. **serves 6**

Serving size:
1½ cups (320g)

Calories: 383
Fat: 10g
Saturated fat: 2g
Carbs: 67g
Fiber: 6g
Sugar: 4g
Protein: 9g
Cholesterol: 7g
Sodium: 502g

7 cups (1.7L) low-sodium vegetable broth

3 tablespoons extra-virgin olive oil

4 cups (540g) cubed butternut squash (from 2¼ pounds/1kg squash)

1 teaspoon kosher salt

½ teaspoon freshly ground black pepper

1 leek (white and light green parts only), roughly chopped

4 garlic cloves, minced

2 tablespoons finely chopped fresh sage

2 cups (380g) arborio rice

½ cup (50g) freshly grated Parmesan

1. In a medium saucepan over low heat, bring the broth to a simmer.

2. Heat 2 tablespoons of the oil in a large, high-sided pan or Dutch oven over medium heat. Add the squash, ½ teaspoon of the salt, and ¼ teaspoon of the pepper and sauté for 8 to 10 minutes, until the squash begins to soften and caramelize around the edges. Transfer the squash to a large bowl.

3. Pour the remaining 1 tablespoon oil in the pan, add the leeks, and sauté for 5 minutes, until softened. Stir in the garlic and sage, then the rice, and stir another minute.

4. Add 1 cup (240ml) of the heated broth and simmer until it's absorbed, stirring constantly for 3 to 4 minutes. Continue adding the broth, a cup at a time, simmering until fully absorbed before adding more. Stir constantly throughout this process, about 15 minutes.

5. Return the squash to the pot and stir in the remaining ½ teaspoon salt and ¼ teaspoon pepper. Continue cooking until the rice is creamy and has the consistency of thick porridge, about 5 minutes longer. Remove from the heat, stir in the cheese, and serve.

coconut chickpea curry

This one-pan coconut chickpea curry is a healthy, budget-friendly meal with bold Indian-inspired flavor. A simple blend of warming spices—garlic, ginger, curry powder, garam masala, and cumin—meld together with creamy coconut milk, chickpeas, cilantro, and lime juice. It's a quick-cooking dish full of hearty, plant-based protein, perfect for meatless Monday (or any day of the week), and it's just begging to be served over rice. If you want, you can also stir in a handful or two of roughly chopped spinach, kale, or chard in the last few minutes of cooking. **serves 4**

1 tablespoon coconut oil

1 large medium yellow onion, diced

4 garlic cloves, minced

1 tablespoon grated peeled fresh ginger

2 (15.5-ounce/439g) cans chickpeas, drained and rinsed

1 (13.5-ounce/398ml) can full-fat coconut milk

1 cup (240ml) low-sodium vegetable broth

2 tablespoons curry powder, or more to taste

1½ teaspoons garam masala

1 teaspoon ground cumin

1 teaspoon kosher salt

1 bunch of cilantro, roughly chopped, plus more for garnish

Juice of 1 lime (about 2 tablespoons)

Cooked rice, for serving

Lime slices, for serving

1. In a large skillet, heat the oil over medium-high heat. Add the onion and sauté for 4 to 5 minutes, until softened. Add the garlic and ginger and stir together for another minute, until fragrant.

2. Add the chickpeas, coconut milk, broth, curry powder, garam masala, cumin, and salt. Stir everything together, bring to a boil, then reduce the heat to medium-low and simmer for 10 minutes, so that the flavors can meld.

3. Remove from the heat and stir in the cilantro and lime juice. Serve the curry over plain rice, Coconut Rice (page 240), or cauliflower rice. Garnish with more cilantro and lime slices.

storage

Store in an airtight container in the fridge for 4 to 5 days, or in the freezer for 3 months. You can store the curry by itself or with leftover rice.

to reheat

If frozen, thaw in the fridge overnight. Microwave the curry for 1 to 2 minutes, or cook on the stove, until warmed through.

helpful tip

Remember that curry powder, which contains turmeric, may stain plastic or silicone storage containers. To avoid this, use glass storage containers.

Serving size:
1 cup (220g)

Calories: 303

Fat: 15g

Saturated fat: 10g

Carbs: 35g

Fiber: 10g

Sugar: 2g

Protein: 14g

Cholesterol: 0mg

Sodium: 374mg

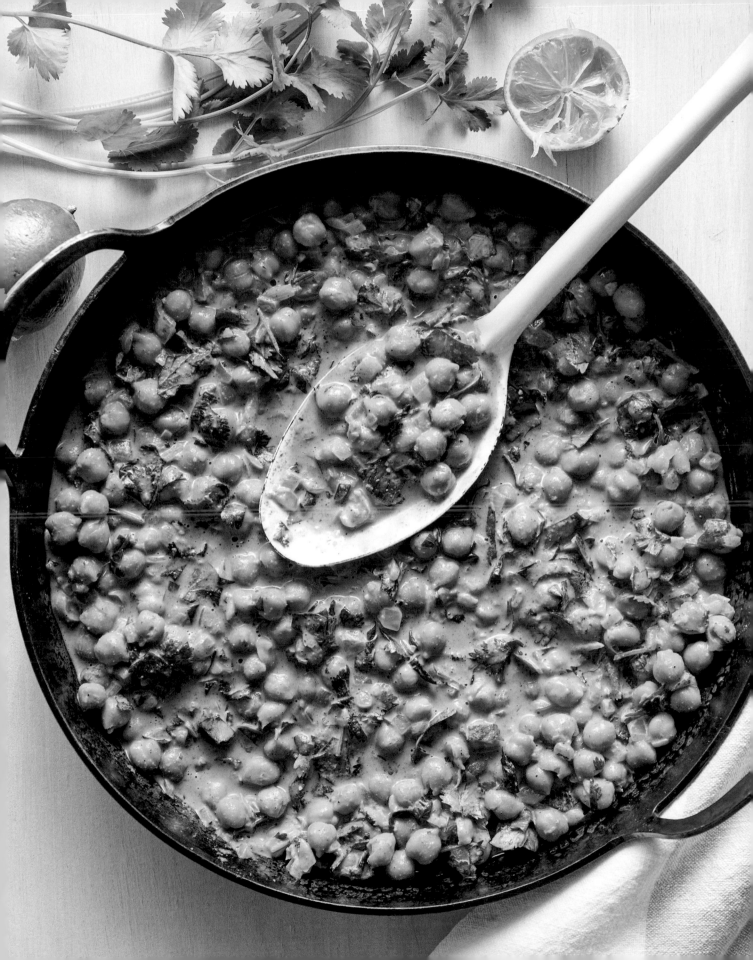

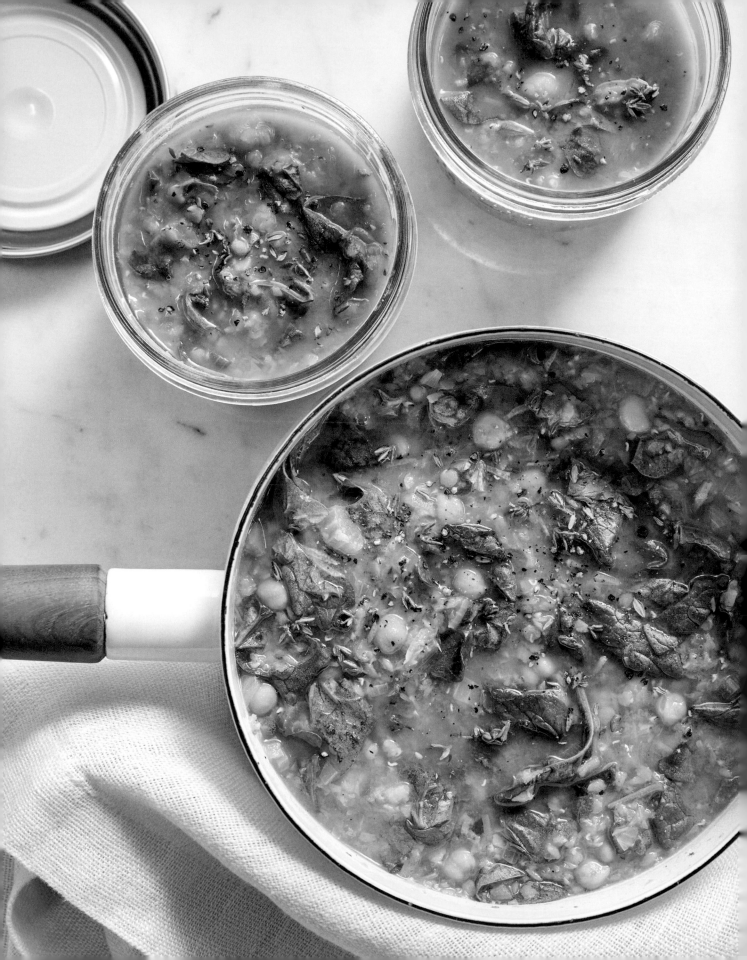

lemony lentil and chickpea soup

Lentil soups are my favorite—they're hearty, nourishing, and a full-meal kind of soup rather than a starter soup. This bright, lemony version begins with sautéed onion, celery, and garlic, which are then simmered with lentils and chickpeas, thyme, and oregano. The red lentils naturally break down into a soft texture that renders blending unnecessary (always a bonus). And a good amount of fresh lemon juice and zest is stirred in at the end along with chopped spinach. It's an uplifting, happy-inducing soup that's sure to become a family favorite—I promise! **serves 4**

2 tablespoons olive oil

1 medium yellow onion, diced

2 celery ribs, diced

3 garlic cloves, minced

6 cups (1.4L) low-sodium vegetable broth

1½ cups (300g) red lentils, rinsed and picked over

1 (15.5-ounce/439g) can chickpeas, drained and rinsed

1 teaspoon dried oregano

2 tablespoons roughly chopped fresh thyme, plus more for garnish

1 teaspoon kosher salt

½ teaspoon freshly ground black pepper, plus more for garnish

2 cups (90g) packed spinach or kale, roughly chopped

Zest and juice of 1 lemon (about 1 tablespoon zest + 3 tablespoons juice)

1. In a large stockpot or Dutch oven, heat the oil over medium heat. Add the onion and celery and sauté for 4 to 5 minutes, until the onion becomes translucent. Add the garlic and sauté 1 minute more.

2. Add the broth, lentils, chickpeas, oregano, thyme, salt, and pepper and bring to a simmer. Cover the pot and cook for 15 minutes, stirring occasionally. Stir in the spinach and cook for 5 to 8 minutes more, until the lentils are softened and starting to break apart.

3. Remove the soup from the heat and stir in the lemon juice and zest. Garnish with more thyme and pepper before serving.

Serving size: 2 cups (505g)

Calories: 465
Fat: 10g
Saturated fat: 2g
Carbs: 72g
Fiber: 15g
Sugar: 3g
Protein: 25g
Cholesterol: 0mg
Sodium: 595mg

spiralized sweet potato "burrito" bake

Burrito flavors in non-burrito form. Spiralized sweet potato provides a wholesome base for this one-dish meal. Just layer everything on top, including the rice, black beans, corn, bell pepper, and onion, plus the spicy tomato-based broth. After a pop in the oven, the rice soaks up the liquid and the veggies become saucy, tender, and packed with Mexican-inspired flavor—a guaranteed meal-prep favorite! **serves 6**

1 small sweet potato (about 12 ounces/340g), peeled, spiralized, and snipped into smaller pieces with kitchen shears

1 cup (185g) white rice, rinsed and drained

3 cups (720ml) low-sodium vegetable broth

1 (15-ounce/425g) can crushed tomatoes

3 teaspoons chili powder

2 teaspoons ground cumin

1 teaspoon dried oregano

1 teaspoon garlic powder

1 teaspoon kosher salt

½ teaspoon freshly ground black pepper

1 (15-ounce/425g) can black beans, drained and rinsed

1 (15-ounce/425g) can corn, drained and rinsed

1 green bell pepper, seeded and diced

½ medium yellow onion, diced

½ cup (50g) grated mozzarella cheese

1 medium avocado, pitted, peeled, and sliced, for garnish

Roughly chopped fresh cilantro, for garnish

storage

Store in an airtight container for 4 to 5 days in the fridge, or up to 3 months in the freezer.

to reheat

If frozen, thaw in the fridge overnight, then reheat in a 325°F (160°C) oven for 5 to 10 minutes, or in the microwave for 1 to 2 minutes.

1. Preheat the oven to 400°F (200°C).

2. Place the sweet potato and rice in a 13 × 9-inch (33 × 23cm) casserole dish and toss to combine.

3. In a large bowl, whisk together the broth, tomatoes, chili powder, cumin, oregano, garlic powder, salt, and pepper. Stir in the black beans, corn, bell pepper, and onion to combine, then pour on top of the sweet potato and rice.

4. Cover the casserole dish tightly with a lid or aluminum foil and bake for 40 to 45 minutes, until the sweet potato is tender and the rice is cooked through. Remove the lid, sprinkle the cheese on top, and bake uncovered another 5 minutes, until the cheese melts. Top with avocado slices and cilantro and serve.

Serving size:
1½ cups (240g)

Calories: 423

Fat: 8g

Saturated fat: 2g

Carbs: 77g

Fiber: 16g

Sugar: 11g

Protein: 16g

Cholesterol: 6g

Sodium: 945g

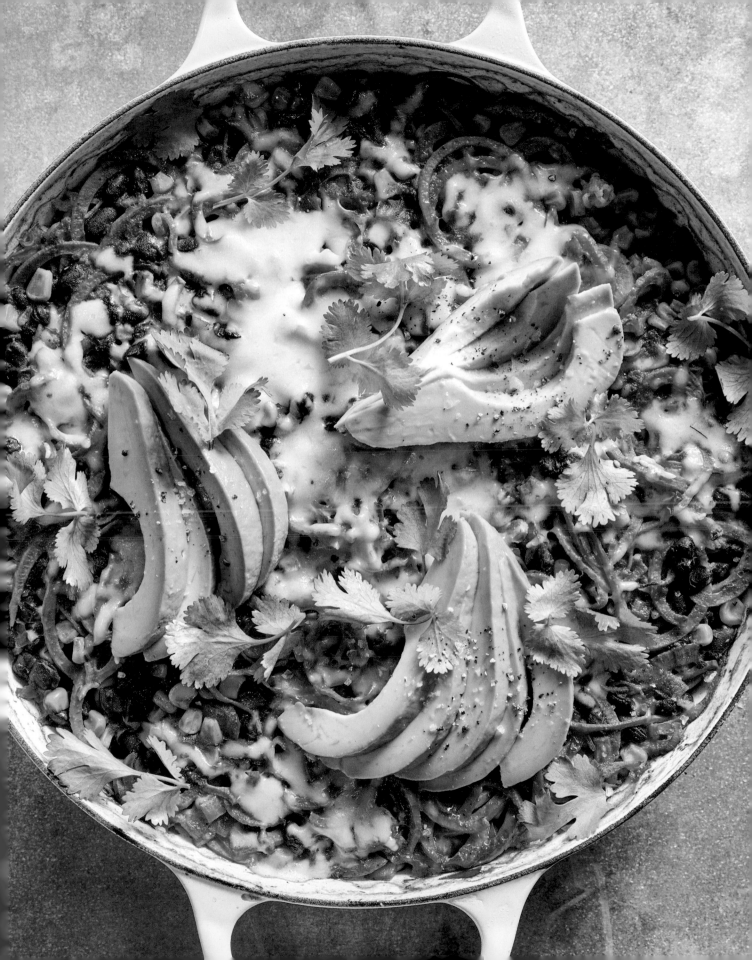

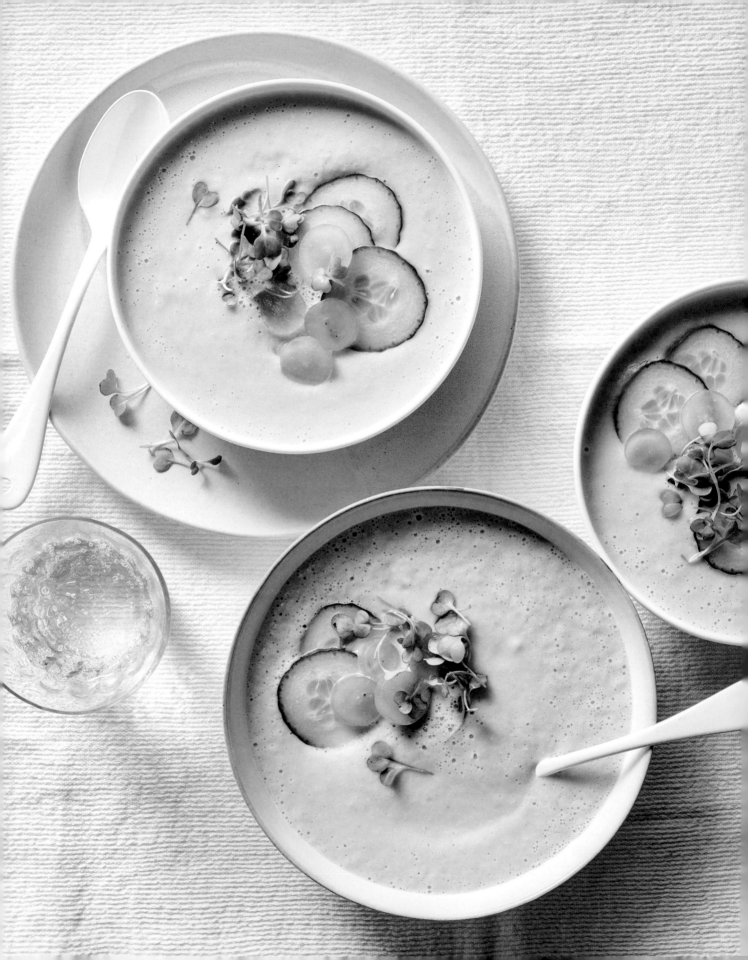

white gazpacho

Let's talk about recipes that stealthily contain gluten—I'm looking at you, gazpacho. Yes, it's the traditional Spanish way to put crusty day-old bread in this summertime vegetable soup and blend it up, but trust me, with a little recipe creativity you can render the gluten completely superfluous. This ajo blanco (white gazpacho) is filled with cooling cucumber, sweet grapes, and almonds for a little heft. Now *this* is how you cool down on hot summer days. To thicken it up, a little avocado does the trick! Anyone missing the bread now? Didn't think so. **serves 4**

2 English cucumbers, peeled, and diced, plus more for garnish

2 cups (200g) green grapes, plus more for garnish

½ cup (42g) slivered almonds

2 garlic cloves

¼ medium avocado, pitted and peeled

3 tablespoons olive oil

2 tablespoons white balsamic or sherry vinegar

1 teaspoon kosher salt

1½ cups (360ml) cold water

Microgreens, for garnish

1. In a high-powered blender on high speed, blend the cucumbers, grapes, almonds, garlic, avocado, oil, vinegar, salt, and water for 1 minute, or until creamy. Transfer the gazpacho to an airtight container and refrigerate for 3 to 4 hours.

2. To serve, divide the gazpacho among four bowls and garnish with diced cucumber, grapes, and microgreens.

Serving size:
2 cups (480ml)

Calories: 251
Fat: 20g
Saturated fat: 3g
Carbs: 18g
Fiber: 4g
Sugar: 13g
Protein: 5g
Cholesterol: 0mg
Sodium: 285mg

zucchini rollatini
with spinach cashew ricotta

These rollatini highlight the best of summertime zucchini in a light and fresh way. A spin on the classic Italian involtini de zucchini, they're filled with a vegan cashew ricotta rather than dairy ricotta and a bit of chopped spinach for good measure. The thin slices of zucchini are then rolled up and baked in a garlic basil marinara sauce for a surprisingly filling dish.

makes about 28, to serve 4

FOR THE RICOTTA

1½ cups (210g) raw cashews, soaked overnight and drained

½ cup (120ml) water

2 tablespoons fresh lemon juice

2 tablespoons nutritional yeast

1 small garlic clove

½ teaspoon kosher salt

Pinch of freshly ground black pepper

1 cup (35g) loosely packed baby spinach, roughly chopped

FOR THE ROLLATINI

1½ cups (375g) Marinara Sauce (page 252)

2 large zucchini

Kosher salt and freshly ground black pepper to taste

Fresh basil, for garnish

1. To make the ricotta: In a food processor, blend the cashews, water, lemon juice, nutritional yeast, garlic, salt, and pepper for about 1 minute, scraping down the sides as needed, until you've got an almost smooth, ricotta-like texture. Add the spinach and pulse again a few times to incorporate.

2. To make the rollatini: Preheat the oven to 400°F (200°C). Spread 1 cup (250g) of the marinara sauce onto the bottom of a 9-inch (23cm) square or round baking dish and set aside.

3. Trim the ends off the zucchini and thinly slice lengthwise, using a sharp knife or mandoline (if using a mandoline, set to the thinnest or second-thinnest setting). Season both sides of the zucchini strips with salt and pepper.

4. In a dry grill pan, grill the zucchini slices on medium-high heat just until softened with visible grill marks, 1 to 2 minutes each side. Remove the zucchini to a plate.

storage

Store in an airtight container in the fridge for up to 5 days, or in the freezer for up to 3 months. Just be aware that the zucchini will be more watery once it's thawed after frozen.

to reheat

Warm leftovers quickly in the microwave for 20 to 30 seconds or reheat in an oven-safe dish in a 350°F (180°C) oven for 5 to 10 minutes.

dietary swaps

If you're not vegan, you can swap the cashew ricotta with 2 cups (496g) regular or part-skim ricotta and sprinkle a little shredded Parmesan or mozzarella on top before baking.

Serving size:
About 7 zucchini rollatini with sauce

Calories: 395

Fat: 26g

Saturated fat: 5g

Carbs: 34g

Fiber: 6g

Sugar: 15g

Protein: 15g

Cholesterol: 0g

Sodium: 504g

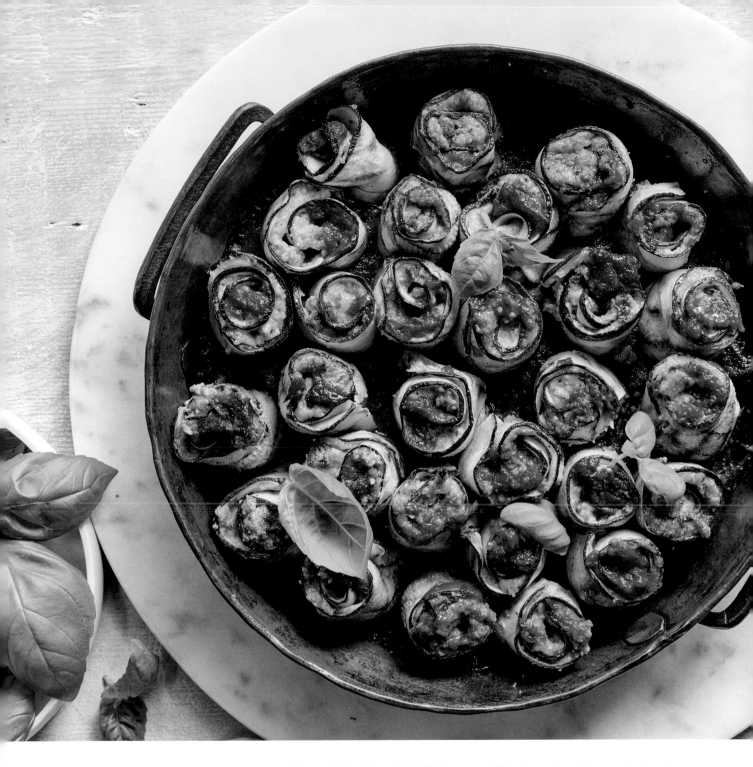

5. Lay a strip of zucchini flat on a cutting board and spread about 1 tablespoon of the cashew ricotta mixture evenly over it. Roll it up and place in the prepared baking dish. Continue with the remaining zucchini.

6. Top the zucchini with the remaining ½ cup (125g) marinara sauce and bake for 25 to 30 minutes, or until the rolls are heated through and lightly golden on top. Garnish with fresh basil, then serve.

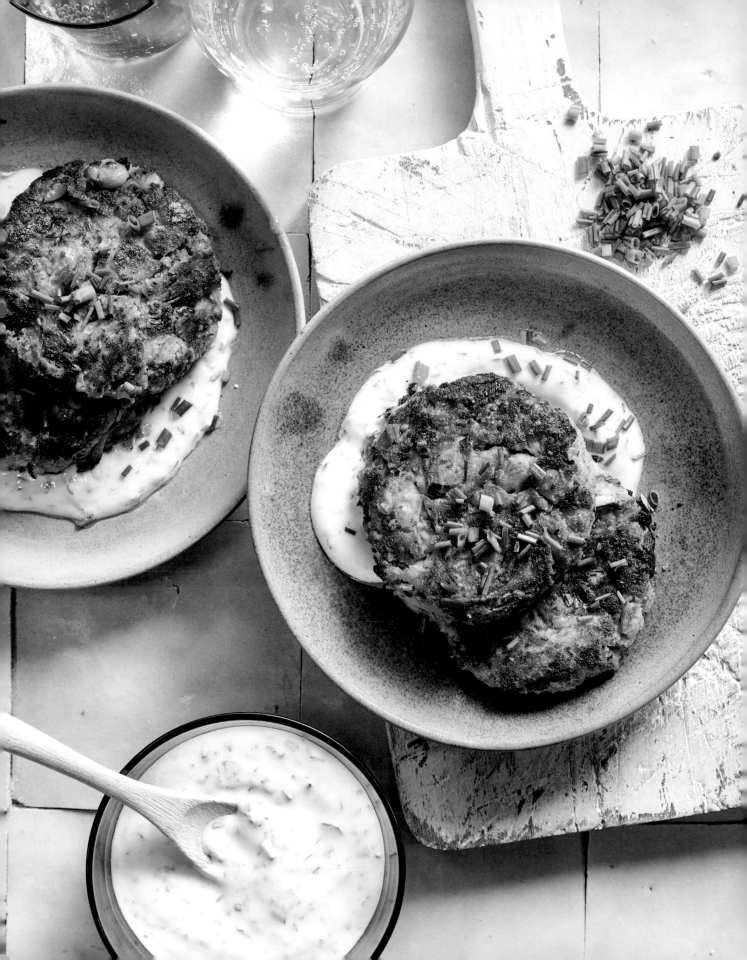

carrot and cannellini bean fritters with herb yogurt sauce

These golden crispy bean-based fritters use chia seeds as a binder and make for the perfect vegetarian meal. A dollop of the yogurt sauce adds that creamy herbaceous pop. Like most fritters, they're perfect for meal prep, so feel free to make a double batch! **serves 3**

storage

Let the fritters cool, then store in an airtight container in the fridge for 4 to 5 days, or in the freezer (with parchment paper in between) for up to 3 months.

to reheat

Place a thawed fritter in the microwave for 20 to 30 seconds, heat in a pan on the stove with a little bit of oil, or place in a 350°F (180°C) oven, until warmed through.

dietary swap

If you eat eggs you can swap the gelled chia seeds with 1 large egg.

FOR THE SAUCE

¾ cup (170g) plain Greek yogurt (dairy or dairy-free)

1 garlic clove, minced

1 tablespoon finely chopped fresh parsley

1 tablespoon finely chopped fresh chives

Juice of ½ lemon (about 1½ tablespoons)

Pinch of kosher salt

FOR THE FRITTERS

1 tablespoon chia seeds

3 tablespoons water

1 (15.5-ounce/439g) can cannellini beans, drained and rinsed

1½ cups (135g) grated carrot (about 2 medium carrots)

3 green onions (white and green parts), thinly sliced

¼ cup (30g) almond flour

2 tablespoons roughly chopped fresh parsley

1 garlic clove, minced

1 teaspoon kosher salt

½ teaspoon freshly ground black pepper

2 tablespoons extra-virgin olive oil

1. To make the sauce: In a small bowl, stir together the yogurt, garlic, parsley, chives, lemon juice, and salt. Cover and refrigerate until ready to use.

2. To make the fritters: In a small bowl, stir together chia seeds and water and set aside for 15 minutes to let the chia seeds gel up.

3. Meanwhile, place the cannellini beans in a medium bowl and roughly mash them with the back of a fork. Add the carrots, green onions, flour, parsley, garlic, gelled chia seeds, salt, and pepper and stir together until well combined.

4. In a large pan, heat the oil over medium heat. Scoop out 3 tablespoons of mixture and form into a fritter. Fry for 2 to 3 minutes each side, until golden brown, then remove to a paper towel–lined plate to absorb any excess oil. Serve with the herb yogurt sauce.

Serving size: 2 fritters + 3 tablespoons sauce

Calories: 447
Fat: 18g
Saturated fat: 3g
Carbs: 51g
Fiber: 5g
Sugar: 8g
Protein: 23g
Cholesterol: 5mg
Sodium: 565mg

creamy white bean, artichoke, and kale soup

While I consider this soup creamy, you can actually make it as brothy or creamy as you'd like. A simple mirepoix base is layered with garlic, dried herbs, and a touch of crushed red pepper flakes. After the beans have simmered, take a few ladles out and blend them up, for a naturally creamy base. Blend up a bit more for a creamier base. **serves 5**

2 tablespoons extra-virgin olive oil

1 medium yellow onion, diced

2 celery ribs, diced

2 medium carrots, diced

4 cloves garlic, minced

½ teaspoon dried thyme

½ teaspoon dried oregano

¼ teaspoon crushed red pepper flakes, or more to taste

5 cups (1.2L) low-sodium vegetable broth

2 (15.5-ounce/439g) cans white beans, such as cannellini, great northern, or navy, drained and rinsed

1 teaspoon kosher salt

½ teaspoon freshly ground black pepper

1 (14-ounce/400g) can artichoke hearts, drained and roughly chopped

3 cups (95g) packed roughly chopped kale leaves (from about 1 bunch)

3 tablespoons lemon juice (from about 1 lemon)

2 tablespoons roughly chopped fresh parsley

Grated Parmesan, for garnish (optional)

1. In a large pot, heat the oil over medium heat. Add the onion, celery, and carrots and stir for 4 to 5 minutes, until softened. Add the garlic, thyme, oregano, and red pepper flakes and stir for an additional 30 seconds.

2. Pour in the broth and add the white beans, salt, and pepper. Bring the soup to a boil. Add a few ladles of the soup to a blender or food processor and, using caution, blend until creamy, then pour it back into the pot. You can also use an immersion blender to puree some of the soup until creamy.

3. Add the artichoke hearts and kale. Stir together for a couple of minutes, until the kale is slightly wilted. Stir in the lemon juice and parsley. Taste for seasoning and add any additional salt and pepper. If you'd like, garnish with fresh Parmesan before serving.

storage

Store in an airtight container in the fridge for 4 to 5 days, or in the freezer for up to 3 months.

to reheat

Reheat from thawed or frozen. Add a portion to a pot on the stove or heat in the microwave for a few minutes, until warmed through.

helpful tip

As this soup sits in the fridge, it will thicken up a bit from all the starch in the white beans. You can always add a splash of water or broth to thin it before reheating.

Serving size:
2 cups (450g)

Calories: 268

Fat: 7g

Saturated fat: 1g

Carbs: 42g

Fiber: 13g

Sugar: 7g

Protein: 12g

Cholesterol: 0mg

Sodium: 666mg

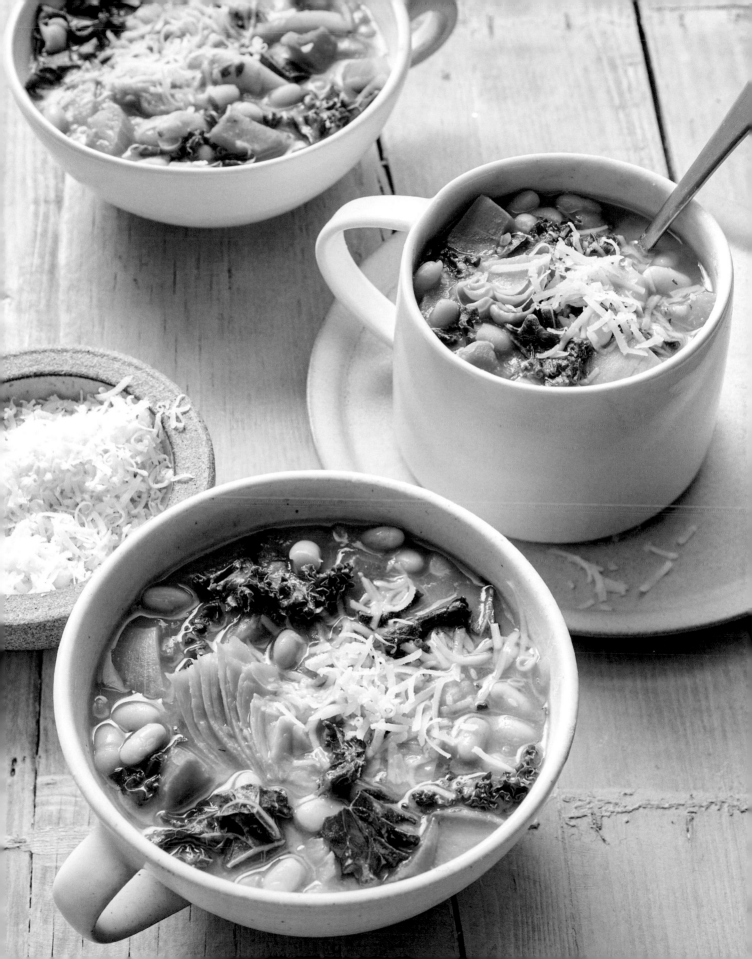

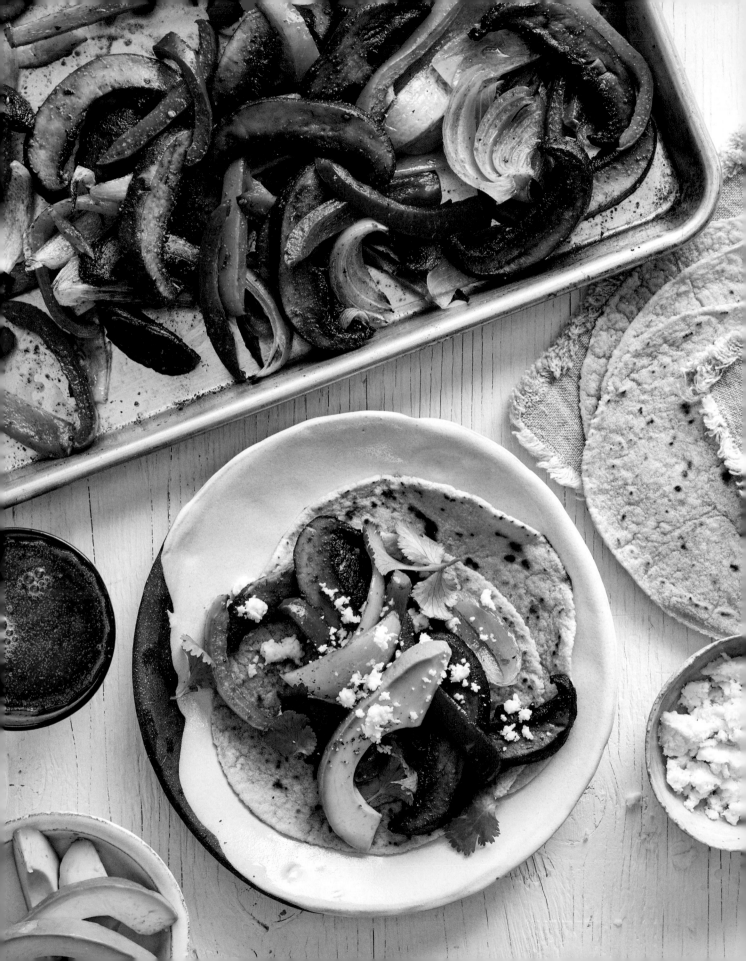

portobello mushroom sheet pan fajitas

storage

Store the mushroom, onions, and bell peppers in an airtight container in the fridge for 4 to 5 days. Store the tortillas and other ingredients in separate airtight containers in the fridge.

to reheat

Warm the mushroom, onions, and bell peppers in a pan on the stove, or in a 350°F (180°C) oven for 5 to 10 minutes, until warmed through.

These vegetarian sheet pan fajitas are outright delicious and seriously foolproof! Portobello mushrooms provide the "meaty" filling and are roasted alongside thinly sliced onion and bell peppers that have been tossed with those classic fajita spices. Warm the tortillas in a skillet (or with tongs over a gas stove burner) while the filling gets nicely charred in the oven. **serves 6**

FOR THE SEASONING

½ tablespoon chili powder

½ tablespoon ground cumin

1 teaspoon garlic powder

½ teaspoon sweet paprika

½ teaspoon oregano

½ teaspoon kosher salt

¼ teaspoon freshly ground black pepper

FOR THE FILLING

4 portobello mushroom caps, sliced about ½ inch (1.3cm) thick

1 medium yellow onion, halved and thinly sliced

2 medium bell peppers (any color), seeded and thinly sliced

2 tablespoons avocado oil or extra-virgin olive oil

6 Cassava Flour Tortillas (page 265) or gluten-free store-bought, warmed

1 medium avocado, peeled, pitted, and thinly sliced, for garnish

2 limes, cut into wedges, for squeezing

Roughly chopped cilantro, for garnish

½ cup (56g) crumbled queso fresco, for garnish

1. Preheat the oven to 450°F (230°C).

2. To make the seasoning: In a small bowl, stir together the chili powder, cumin, garlic powder, paprika, oregano, salt, and pepper.

3. To make the filling: On one rimmed baking sheet, place the sliced mushrooms. On a second rimmed baking sheet, place the sliced onion and bell peppers. Drizzle the oil over both baking sheets, then sprinkle the seasoning on top. Toss the vegetables with the oil and spices and bake for 20 to 25 minutes, until the vegetables are softened and nicely roasted.

4. Assemble the fajitas by placing a portion of the mushrooms, onions, and bell peppers on a warmed tortilla. Garnish with avocado, a squeeze of lime juice, cilantro, and queso fresco.

Serving size: 2 fajitas

Calories: 544

Fat: 30g

Saturated fat: 6g

Carbs: 65g

Fiber: 12g

Sugar: 5g

Protein: 12g

Cholesterol: 13mg

Sodium: 595mg

cauliflower and chickpea stuffed eggplant with turmeric tahini

I'm a big fan of stuffing wholesome veggies with *even more* wholesome ingredients. It just creates layer upon layer of appetizing flavor and texture. For this recipe, you'll simply score the eggplant (no need to scoop it out ahead of time, it gets perfectly soft and scoopable after roasting), then top with a warming spiced chickpea filling. Before serving, a drizzle of turmeric tahini gives the stuffed eggplant a pop of golden color and that unmistakable earthy-bitter-peppery taste for yet one more layer of flavor. **serves 4**

storage

Store in an airtight container in the fridge for 4 to 5 days, or up to 3 months in the freezer.

to reheat

If frozen, thaw in the fridge overnight. Place the stuffed eggplant on a rimmed baking sheet in a 350°F (180°C) oven for 5 to 10 minutes or reheat in the microwave for 1 to 2 minutes, until warmed through.

FOR THE STUFFED EGGPLANTS

2 medium eggplants

2 tablespoons extra-virgin olive oil

1 teaspoon kosher salt

½ teaspoon freshly ground black pepper

1 (15.5-ounce/439g) can chickpeas, drained and rinsed

1 cup (100g) cauliflower rice

¼ cup (35g) pine nuts

¼ cup (25g) grated Parmesan cheese

Juice of ½ lemon (about 1½ tablespoons)

1 garlic clove, minced

1 teaspoon ground cumin

1 teaspoon ground coriander

½ teaspoon smoked paprika

½ teaspoon dried thyme

Fresh thyme, for garnish

FOR THE TURMERIC TAHINI

⅓ cup (80g) Tahini Sauce (page 250)

½ teaspoon ground turmeric

Pinch of cayenne pepper

1. Preheat the oven to 400°F (200°C).

2. To prepare the eggplant: Cut the eggplants in half lengthwise and then score the flesh in a crosshatch pattern, slicing deeply. Be careful not to cut through the skin. Place it cut side up on a rimmed baking sheet, drizzle with oil, and season with ½ teaspoon of the salt and ¼ teaspoon of the black pepper. Roast 20 minutes to soften the eggplant.

3. Meanwhile, in a medium bowl, stir together the chickpeas, cauliflower, pine nuts, Parmesan cheese, lemon juice, garlic, cumin, coriander, paprika, thyme, and the remaining ½ teaspoon salt and ¼ teaspoon black pepper.

Serving size: 1 stuffed eggplant half

Calories: 400

Fat: 23g

Saturated fat: 3g

Carbs: 41g

Fiber: 16g

Sugar: 12g

Protein: 15g

Cholesterol: 5g

Sodium: 467g

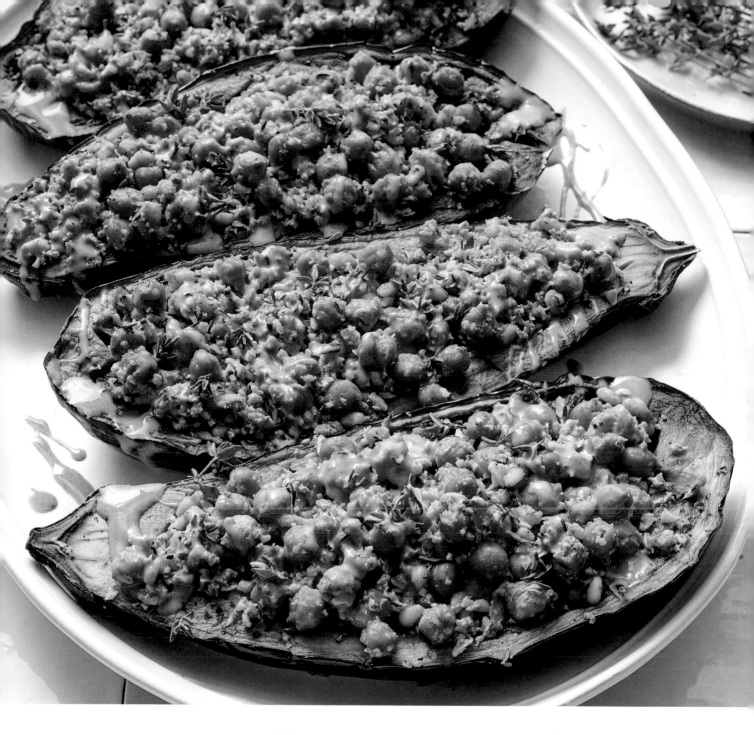

4. Remove the eggplants from the oven, spoon the chickpea mixture over the eggplants, then place them back in the oven and cook for another 10 to 15 minutes, until the eggplant is tender and the filling is lightly golden.

5. To make the turmeric tahini: In a small bowl, stir together the tahini sauce, turmeric, and cayenne pepper until smooth.

6. Drizzle each stuffed eggplant with turmeric tahini and garnish with fresh thyme before serving.

side dishes and building blocks

You've probably gathered by now that side dishes, sauces, and other "components," which I like to call building blocks, are anything *but* afterthoughts in my mind. Nope! They're critical pieces that equip you with the most robust arsenal of nourishing, feel-good ingredients in your fridge. That's why they often show up in my quick-assembly meals.

The reality is that I often think of the pieces before I think of the whole. What am I craving for the base of a protein or grain bowl—maybe Lemon Herb Rice (page 243)? What dressings will complement the veggies I want to eat this week—maybe a Balsamic Vinaigrette (page 260)? What in-season produce can I meal prep that will help to round out the "buffet bar" in my fridge—maybe Fruit Salsa (page 232)? What can I drizzle or dollop for a flavor boost or added texture—maybe Green Tahini Sauce (see page 236)? Those are the questions that constantly go through my mind. Because at the end of the day, sides, small dishes, and sauces are quick and easy recipes to layer and assemble with *other* recipes in the book to create complete meals that taste pretty darn fantastic.

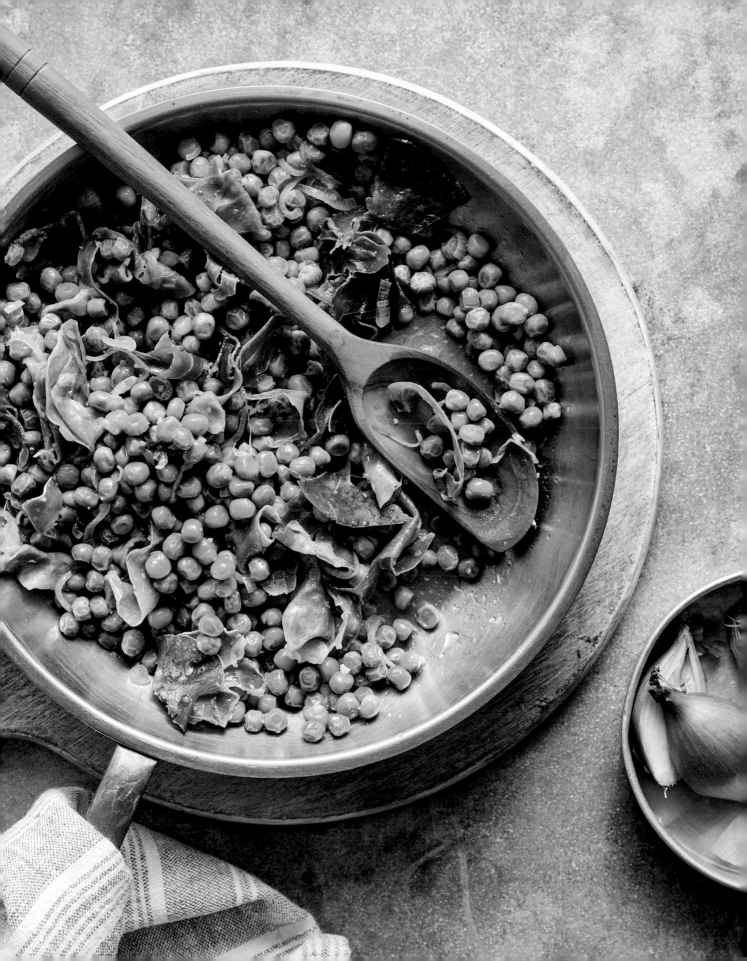

peas and prosciutto

storage

Store in an airtight container in the fridge for 4 to 5 days.

to reheat

Sauté in a pan for 2 to 3 minutes, or heat in the microwave for 1 minute, until warmed through.

Sautéed shallots and garlic along with diced prosciutto instantly elevates your supermarket bag of frozen peas to a restaurant-quality side dish. Pair this with grilled or roasted meat, use it as a base for a breakfast salad with a soft-boiled egg, or make a double batch and serve it up as a holiday side (it's always a favorite). **serves 6**

2 tablespoons olive oil

2 shallots, halved lengthwise and thinly sliced

2 garlic cloves, minced

1 (16-ounce/454g) bag frozen peas

¼ teaspoon kosher salt, plus more to taste

¼ teaspoon freshly ground black pepper, plus more to taste

4 ounces (113g) prosciutto, diced or torn into small pieces

1. In a large pan, heat the oil over medium heat. Add the shallots and garlic and sauté for 1 minute, until softened.

2. Add the peas, salt, and pepper and sauté for 5 minutes, until the peas are warmed through.

3. Add the prosciutto and sauté for another 1 to 2 minutes. Season to taste with additional salt and pepper before serving.

Serving size:
⅔ cup (109g)

Calories: 144
Fat: 6g
Saturated fat: 1g
Carbs: 13g
Fiber: 4g
Sugar: 4g
Protein: 9g
Cholesterol: 11mg
Sodium: 386mg

fruit salsa—any which way

I was going to give you a few recipes for fruit salsa but then decided it's probably smarter if I just give you this foolproof base recipe for salsa *any which way*. Once you've got the ratios down, you can combine various in-season fruits and different types of onions—white onions, yellow onions, red onions, shallots, and green onions all work—into tasty combinations (see Best Fruits to Use and Fruits to Avoid). Three fruit salsa combinations that are perennial winners are cantaloupe and cucumber with red onion, strawberries with white onion, and nectarines with green onion. **makes about 2½ cups (560g)**

2 cups (320g) finely diced fruit

½ cup (96g) finely chopped onion

1 jalapeño, seeded and finely diced

¼ cup (12g) finely chopped fresh cilantro

2 tablespoons fresh lime juice (from 1 to 2 limes)

¼ teaspoon kosher salt

In a medium bowl, stir together the fruit, onion, jalapeño, cilantro, lime juice, and salt.

storage
Store in an airtight container in the fridge for 3 to 4 days.

best fruits to use
You can use a wide variety, including mango, pineapple, strawberries, peaches, nectarines, plums, oranges, tangerines, cantaloupe, honeydew melon, kiwi fruit, cucumber, cherries, and watermelon.

fruits to avoid
Apples and pears are too firm and will discolor, and bananas, raspberries, and other very soft fruits have a tendency to go mushy.

Serving size: ¼ cup (30g) (nutrition info for cantaloupe salsa)

Calories: 16
Fat: 0g
Saturated fat: 0g
Carbs: 4g
Fiber: 1g
Sugar: 3g
Protein: 0g
Cholesterol: 0mg
Sodium: 34mg

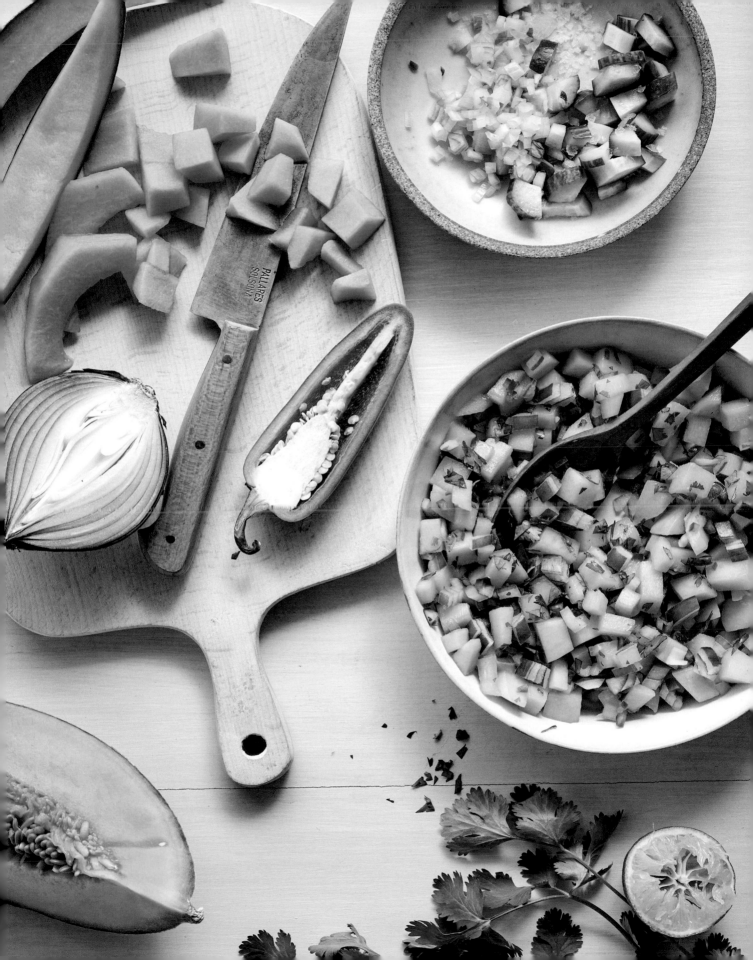

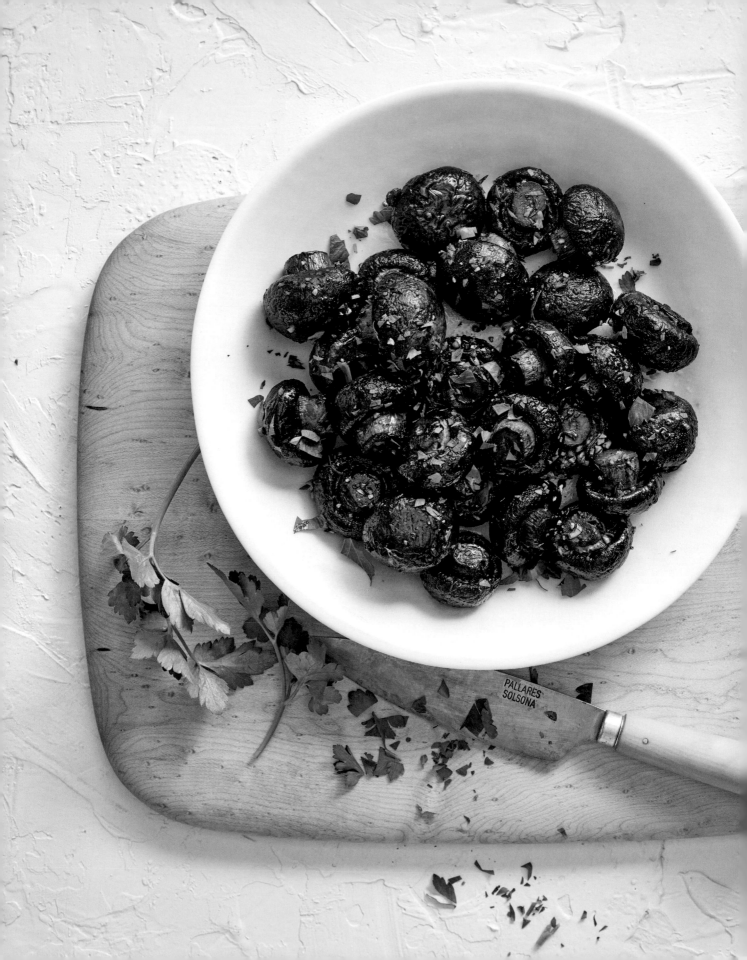

balsamic roasted mushrooms

Truth: Up until fairly recently, I was never a fan of mushrooms. Probably something to do with my older brother always calling them "fungus" as kids, but this recipe is what converted me into a steadfast mushroom lover. These are garlicky with a pop of fresh herbs, and both the balsamic vinegar and maple syrup add a touch of sweetness. They're fab served up alongside the Paprika Rubbed Pork Tenderloin with Shallot Pan Sauce (page 180). **serves 4**

(page 180)

storage

Store in an airtight container in the fridge for 4 to 5 days, or in the freezer for up to 3 months.

to reheat

If frozen, thaw in the fridge overnight. Reheat the mushrooms in the microwave for 1 to 2 minutes or gently toss them in a skillet, until warmed through.

helpful tip

Leftovers can be added to veggie noodle dishes, casseroles, soups, and stews. You can also chop them up and add them to a breakfast scramble, omelet, or egg muffin for a punch of savory flavor!

1 pound (454g) cremini or baby bell mushrooms, stems lightly trimmed

1 tablespoon extra-virgin olive oil

3 tablespoons balsamic vinegar

2 teaspoons pure maple syrup

3 garlic cloves, minced

1 teaspoon roughly chopped fresh thyme

1 teaspoon roughly chopped fresh parsley, plus more for garnish

¼ teaspoon kosher salt

Freshly ground black pepper to taste

1. Preheat the oven to 425°F (220°C).

2. In a large bowl, gently toss together the mushrooms, oil, vinegar, maple syrup, garlic, thyme, parsley, salt, and pepper to evenly coat the mushrooms.

3. Arrange the mushrooms in a single layer on a rimmed baking sheet or in a casserole dish, pouring any liquid on top.

4. Roast the mushrooms for 20 to 25 minutes, stirring two or three times, until tender. Garnish with extra parsley before serving.

Serving size:
¾ cup (107g)

Calories: 78

Fat: 4g

Saturated fat: 1g

Carbs: 9g

Fiber: 1g

Sugar: 6g

Protein: 4g

Cholesterol: 0mg

Sodium: 156mg

spicy roasted cauliflower steaks with green tahini

Embrace cauliflower for the mighty vegetable that it is! Cauliflower steaks, with their beautifully thick tree-like slices, can be served up as a spicy side dish or turned into a stand-alone vegetarian meal with a few toppings (see how I transformed them in Meal Prep Ideas #4, page 86). All they need is a simple dusting of garlic, paprika, and cayenne pepper and a quick roast until the cauliflower steak's edges are crisp and the core is tender. Drizzle with some herby green tahini and slice into them just as you would a steak. **serves 4**

storage

Store in an airtight container in the fridge for 3 to 4 days, or in the freezer for up to 3 months.

to reheat

Reheat in a 400°F (200°C) oven for 5 to 10 minutes, or in the microwave for 1 to 2 minutes, until warmed through.

helpful tip

You really only get two clean, whole slices from one cauliflower head because the edges tend to fall apart. So grab 2 heads for 4 even slices. And dice up all those leftover cauliflower bits and pieces and save them for breakfast hashes or power bowls.

FOR THE CAULIFLOWER STEAKS

2 large heads of cauliflower

1 teaspoon kosher salt

1 teaspoon garlic powder

1 teaspoon sweet paprika

½ teaspoon freshly ground black pepper

Pinch of cayenne pepper

2 tablespoons extra-virgin olive oil

FOR THE GREEN TAHINI SAUCE

½ cup (116g) Tahini Sauce (page 250)

½ cup roughly chopped tender herbs, such as parsley, cilantro, dill, basil, mint, or a combination, plus more for garnish

1 to 2 tablespoons water, as needed

1. Preheat the oven to 450°F (230°C). Remove the outer leaves from the cauliflower head. Cut the cauliflower in half through the stem and slice 1-inch (2.5cm) pieces from each half. Then place the cauliflower steaks on a rimmed baking sheet.

2. In a small bowl, stir together the salt, garlic powder, paprika, black pepper, and cayenne pepper. Brush the oil on each side of the cauliflower steaks and evenly sprinkle the seasoning mixture on top.

3. Roast the cauliflower steaks in the oven for 15 minutes, then use a spatula to carefully flip them over. Roast another 10 to 15 minutes, until golden and the stems are tender.

4. While the steaks are roasting, in a food processor blend the tahini sauce with the chopped herbs. If you'd like a thinner sauce, add the water a little at a time until you've reached the desired consistency.

5. Remove the cauliflower steaks from the oven. Drizzle the green tahini sauce over them and garnish with a sprinkle of herbs.

Serving size: 1 slice + 2 tablespoons sauce

Calories: 348
Fat: 26g
Saturated fat: 4g
Carbs: 26g
Fiber: 10g
Sugar: 7g
Protein: 12g
Cholesterol: 0mg
Sodium: 725mg

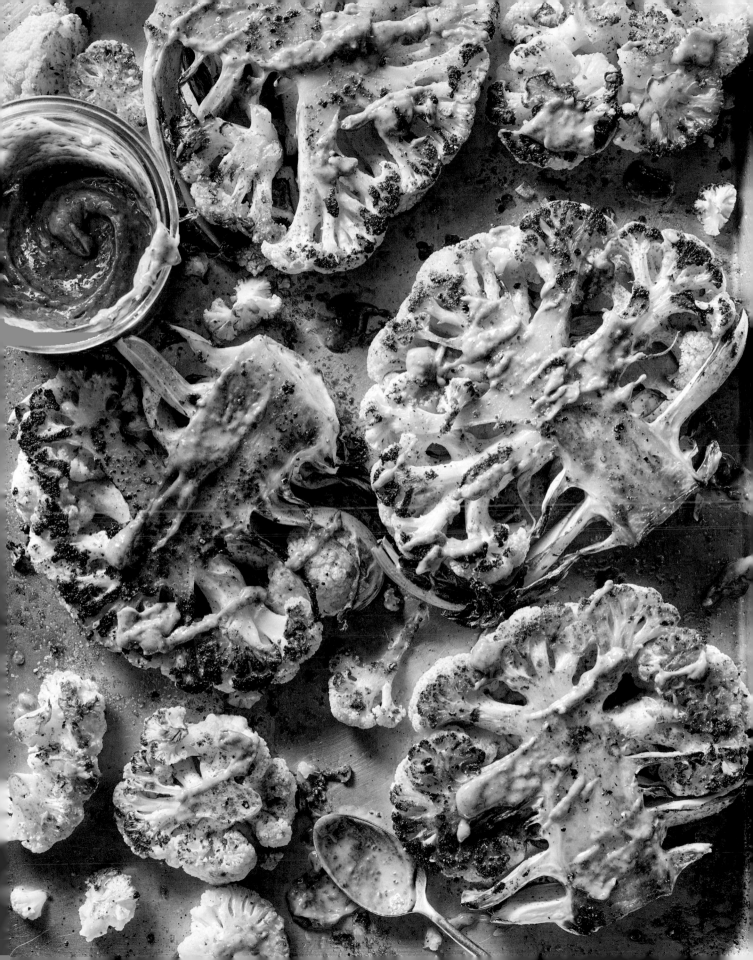

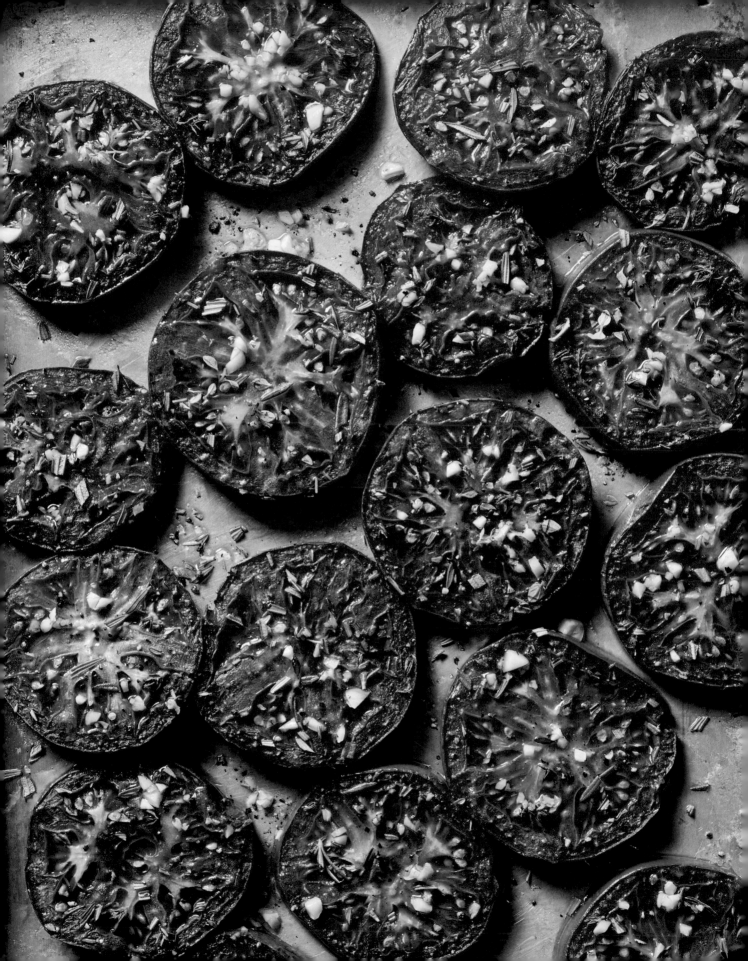

garlic herb roasted tomatoes

storage

Store in an airtight container in the fridge for 4 to 5 days.

helpful tip

While any tomatoes will work in this recipe, including Roma or even cherry tomatoes, I prefer large vine-ripened tomatoes, as they're naturally sweeter.

In-season ripe tomatoes don't need a lot of adornment. A couple of finely chopped garlic cloves and fresh herbs do the trick. The beauty of this recipe really lies in its simplicity, where roasting intensifies the tomato flavor and turns it into a succulent and juicy side dish. **serves 6**

2 tablespoons extra-virgin olive oil

4 large tomatoes

2 garlic cloves, finely chopped

½ teaspoon finely chopped fresh thyme

½ teaspoon finely chopped fresh rosemary

½ teaspoon kosher salt

¼ teaspoon freshly ground black pepper

1. Preheat the oven to 400°F (200°C).

2. Lightly coat a rimmed baking sheet with 1 tablespoon of the oil.

3. Cut the tomatoes into ½-inch (1.3cm) slices (I usually get 4 or 5 slices per tomato) and arrange them in a single layer on the prepared baking sheet. Sprinkle the garlic, thyme, rosemary, salt, and pepper on top. Drizzle the remaining 1 tablespoon oil on top of the tomatoes. Roast for 15 to 20 minutes, or until the tomatoes have softened.

Serving size:
About 3 slices (105g)

Calories: 64
Fat: 5g
Saturated fat: 1g
Carbs: 5g
Fiber: 2g
Sugar: 3g
Protein: 1g
Cholesterol: 0mg
Sodium: 99mg

coconut rice

When you're whipping up bold-flavored Thai- or Asian-inspired recipes, it only makes sense to have a batch of coconut rice on hand. It's richer and creamier than plain rice with that subtle tropical flavor (thanks to coconut milk), and it has just a hint of sweetness. It perfectly balances the spiciness in stir-fries and curries, but you can't go wrong serving it up as a simple, yet exciting side dish to baked fish or chicken either. **serves 8**

1 (13.5-ounce/398ml) can full-fat coconut milk

1¼ cups (300ml) water

1 tablespoon honey

2 cups (360g) long-grain white rice, rinsed and drained

½ teaspoon kosher salt

1. In a medium pot over high heat, stir together the coconut milk, water, honey, rice, and salt. Bring it to a boil, then reduce the heat to low, add a lid, and simmer for 12 to 15 minutes, until the liquid is absorbed and the rice is tender. If bubbles start to come out of the pot, adjust the lid so that steam can escape.

2. Remove the rice from the heat and let it rest covered for a couple of minutes. Fluff with a fork before serving.

storage

Store in an airtight container in the fridge for 4 to 5 days, or in the freezer for up to 3 months. Make sure to read the tips in the Individual Meal Prep Ingredients chapter on safely storing rice after cooking (see page 60).

to reheat

If frozen, thaw in the fridge overnight. Rice has a tendency to dry out, so sprinkle a tablespoon or two of water on it before reheating. Reheat thawed rice in a covered pot on the stove, or in the microwave for 1 minute, or until warmed through.

helpful tip

I use regular full-fat coconut milk for a creamier texture, but you could use light coconut milk as well.

Serving size:
1 cup (152g)

Calories: 252

Fat: 8g

Saturated fat: 7g

Carbs: 40g

Fiber: 1g

Sugar: 4g

Protein: 4g

Cholesterol: 0mg

Sodium: 89mg

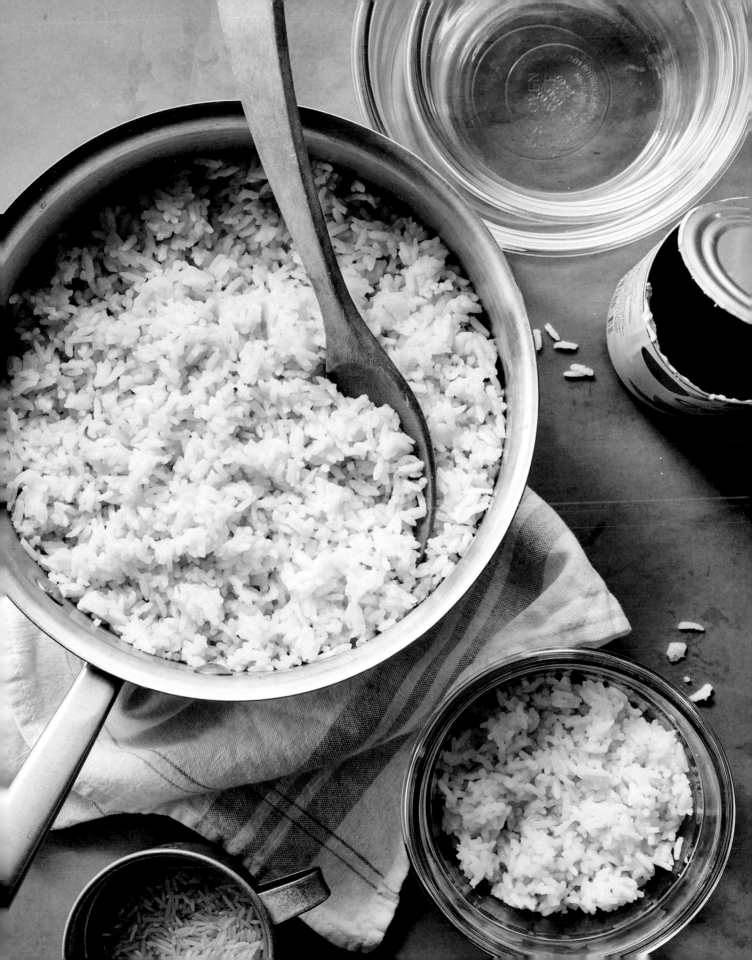

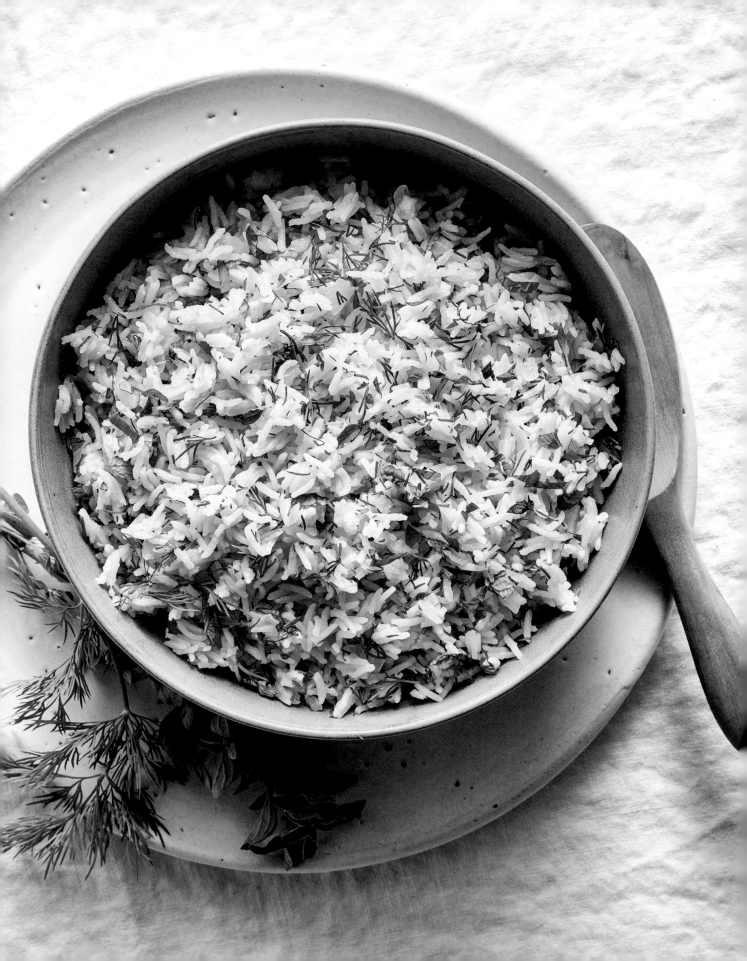

lemon herb rice

This Greek-inspired rice shines bright with fresh, zingy flavor thanks to a zested and juiced lemon (zest + juice = more lemony flavor) plus a good handful of tender herbs. This is one of those recipes where you can just walk into your herb garden, pick a few herbs, and chop them together into this dish. I use basmati rice for this recipe because it stays light and fluffy and won't clump. Serve it with grilled chicken or fish, sautéed shrimp, or really any recipe you'd like to impart a fresh Mediterranean flair. **serves 6**

2 tablespoons extra-virgin olive oil

½ medium yellow onion, diced

2 garlic cloves, minced

Zest of 1 lemon (about 1 tablespoon)

1½ cups (270g) basmati rice, well rinsed and drained

2½ cups (620ml) low-sodium chicken broth

Juice of 1 lemon (about 3 tablespoons)

½ teaspoon kosher salt

¼ cup (15g) finely chopped fresh herbs, such as any 2- or 3-herb combination of parsley, cilantro, dill, mint, tarragon, basil, thyme, and oregano

1. In a large pan on medium heat, heat the oil and sauté the onion for 3 to 4 minutes, until softened and translucent. Add the garlic, lemon zest, and rice and sauté another minute.

2. Add the broth, lemon juice, and salt. Bring to a boil, then reduce the heat to low, cover with a lid, and cook for 12 to 15 minutes, until the liquid is absorbed and the rice is tender. If bubbles start to come out of the pot, adjust the lid so that steam can escape.

3. Remove the rice from the heat and let it rest covered another 4 to 5 minutes. Stir in the fresh herbs and serve.

storage

Store in an airtight container in the fridge for 4 to 5 days, or in the freezer for up to 3 months. Make sure to read the tips in the Individual Meal Prep Ingredients chapter on safely storing rice after cooking (see page 60).

to reheat

If frozen, thaw in the fridge overnight. Rice has a tendency to dry out, so sprinkle a tablespoon or two of water on it before reheating. Reheat in a covered pot on the stove or in the microwave for 1 minute, or until warmed through.

helpful tip

I use parsley and dill in this recipe, but you could use a single herb or combine two or three of your favorite herbs. Other combinations that work great are tarragon-thyme, cilantro-mint, parsley-oregano-basil, and parsley-mint-dill.

Serving size:
1 cup (163g)

Calories: 207
Fat: 5g
Saturated fat: 1g
Carbs: 38g
Fiber: 1g
Sugar: 1g
Protein: 5g
Cholesterol: 1mg
Sodium: 143mg

roasted green beans almondine

Have you ever tried roasting your green beans? It's one of the easiest ways to prepare green beans, and like most roasted vegetables, the flavor gains depth and intensity. Fresh, snappy green beans (make sure to grab haricots verts) turn slightly blistered, perfectly tender, and almost fancy when topped with crunchy, toasted almonds and a good amount of roasted garlic. This simple side dish looks decidedly elegant, which makes it perfect for the holidays or a dinner party. Yet it's simple enough to enjoy in your weekly dinner rotation.

serves 4

1 pound (454g) French haricots verts, trimmed

4 garlic cloves, minced

⅓ cup (28g) sliced almonds

2 tablespoons olive oil

½ teaspoon kosher salt

¼ teaspoon freshly ground black pepper

1. Preheat the oven to 425°F (220°C). In a medium bowl, toss the green beans with the garlic, sliced almonds, oil, salt, and pepper.

2. Spread the green beans out onto a rimmed baking sheet and bake for 15 to 18 minutes, stirring once, until the beans are softened and slightly blistered.

storage

Store in an airtight container in the fridge for 4 to 5 days, or in the freezer for up to 3 months.

to reheat

If frozen, thaw in the fridge overnight. Quickly sauté in a pan over medium-high heat or reheat in the microwave for 30 to 45 seconds, until warmed through.

helpful tip

Haricots verts are French green beans. They're slightly longer, skinnier, and more tender than regular green beans. You might find them loose or pretrimmed at the market in packaged bags. If not pretrimmed, make sure to trim the ends.

Serving size: 1 cup (96g)

Calories: 158
Fat: 12g
Saturated fat: 1g
Carbs: 11g
Fiber: 5g
Sugar: 4g
Protein: 5g
Cholesterol: 0g
Sodium: 148g

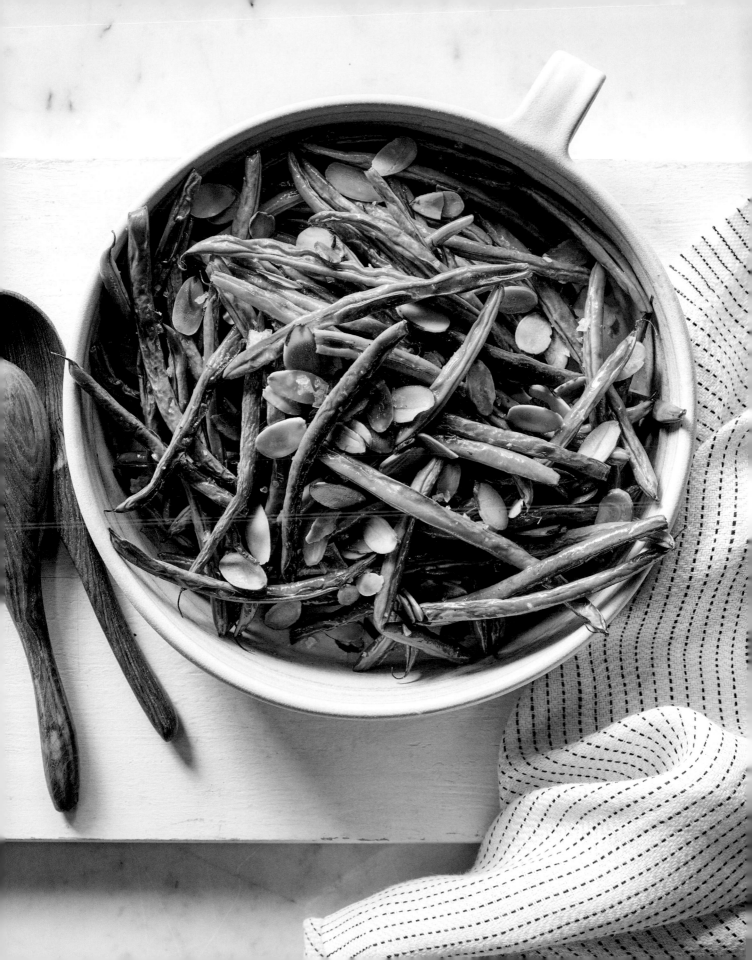

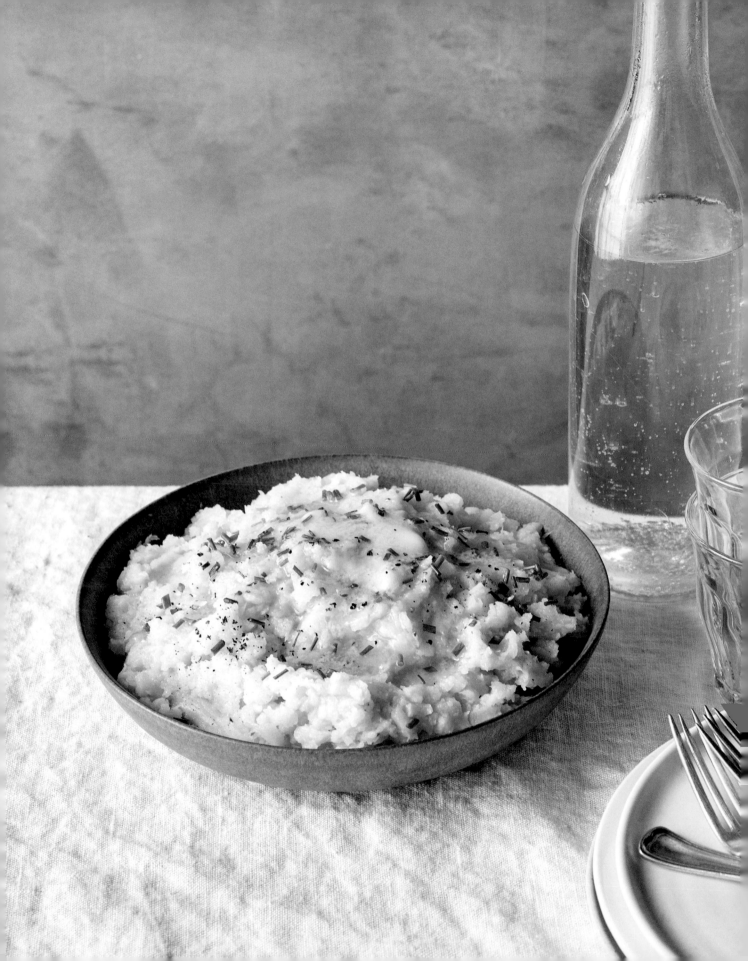

garlicky root vegetable mash

Switch up your mashed potatoes with these garlicky and creamy mashed root vegetables. This simple blend of parsnips, turnip, and celeriac (celery root) is naturally lower in carbs than mashed potatoes, plus a serious amount of garlic and chives turns it into one tasty side dish. Funky-shaped root vegetables are often underappreciated in the market, so it's time to give them a little love! serves 8

2 large parsnips, peeled and cut into chunks

1 large turnip, peeled and cut into chunks

1 medium celeriac, peeled and cut into chunks

1 tablespoon extra-virgin olive oil

6 garlic cloves, minced

3 tablespoons unsalted butter, plus a few pats to finish

1 teaspoon kosher salt

¼ teaspoon freshly ground black pepper

2 tablespoons finely chopped chives, plus more for garnish

1. Bring a large pot of water to a boil. Add the root vegetables and cook for 15 minutes, or until tender when pierced with a fork. Drain the root vegetables in a colander.

2. In the same large pot used for the vegetables, heat the oil over medium heat, then add the garlic, stirring for 1 minute.

3. Remove the pot from the heat and place the butter in it. Return the root vegetables to the pot and mash with a potato masher. Stir in the salt, pepper, and chives. Add a few pats of butter to the top, garnish with chives, and serve.

storage

Store in an airtight container in the fridge for 4 to 5 days, or in the freezer for up to 3 months.

to reheat

If frozen, thaw in the fridge overnight. Reheat in a covered baking dish in a 350°F (180°C) oven for 20 to 30 minutes, on the stove until warmed through, or in the microwave for 1 to 2 minutes.

helpful tips

If you can't find a certain root vegetable, feel free to swap in any other light-colored root vegetable. Rutabaga, white sweet potato, jicama, and yuca work as well!

Serving size:
¾ cup (167g)

Calories: 109
Fat: 6g
Saturated fat: 3g
Carbs: 13g
Fiber: 3g
Sugar: 3g
Protein: 1g
Cholesterol: 11mg
Sodium: 199mg

sautéed red cabbage

This antioxidant-rich, colorful side dish is the perfect accompaniment to roast chicken, pork, duck, or just about anything, really. It's tender and sweet yet has a punch of tartness from the apple cider vinegar. I love to use my mandoline to slice up the onion and cabbage quickly! This is a great freezer-friendly recipe so make a big batch, then freeze in individual portions for the future. **serves 8**

2 tablespoons extra-virgin olive oil, or a blend of butter and oil

1 small yellow onion, halved and thinly sliced

2 garlic cloves, minced

½ medium red cabbage, halved, cored, and thinly sliced

3 tablespoons apple cider vinegar

2 tablespoons honey

½ teaspoon kosher salt

¼ teaspoon freshly ground black pepper

1. In a large pan or Dutch oven, heat the oil over medium-high heat. Sauté the onion for 1 to 2 minutes, or until just starting to soften. Add the minced garlic and stir for another minute.

2. Add the cabbage and let it wilt for 4 to 5 minutes, using tongs to turn it in the pan. Add the vinegar, honey, salt, and pepper, and continue sautéing for 8 to 10 minutes, stirring occasionally, until the cabbage becomes soft and caramelized.

storage

Store in an airtight container in the fridge for 4 to 5 days, or in the freezer for up to 3 months.

to reheat

Thaw frozen cabbage in the fridge overnight and reheat in a skillet or in the microwave for 1 to 2 minutes, until warmed through.

ways to serve

Sautéed cabbage can be added to virtually anything! Add it chilled to salads or use it as a simple side dish. It's also great in casseroles, stir-fries, soups, veggie bowls, and wraps.

Serving size:
½ cup (75g)

Calories: 68

Fat: 4g

Saturated fat: 1g

Carbs: 9g

Fiber: 1g

Sugar: 7g

Protein: 1g

Cholesterol: 0g

Sodium: 85g

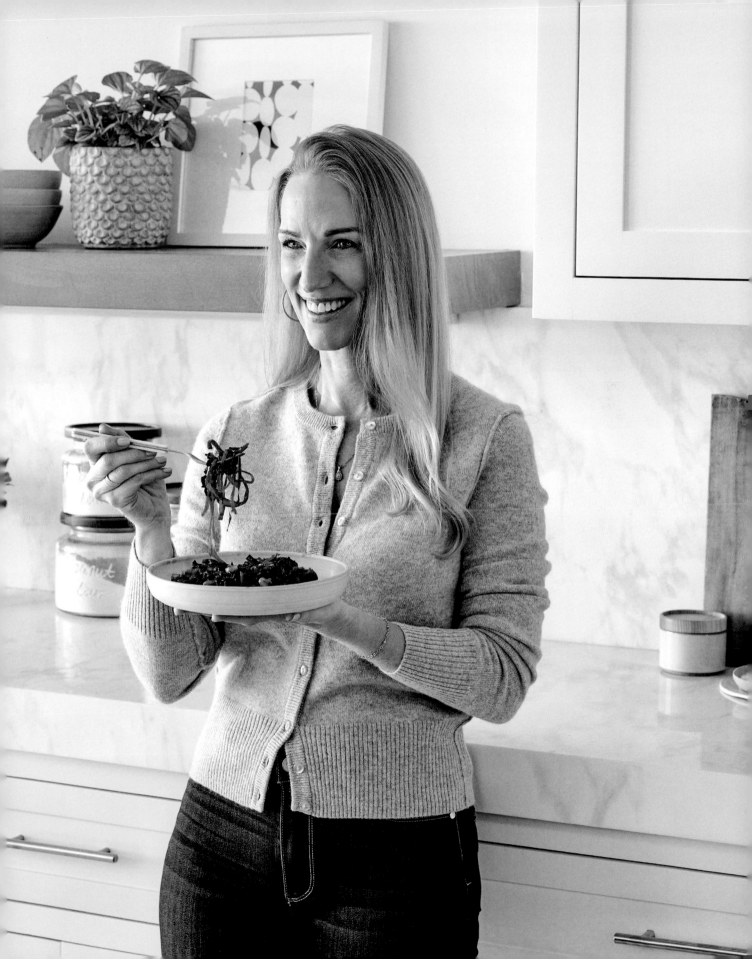

simple sauces

There's really no comparison between homemade and store-bought sauces—homemade *always* tastes a million times better! Make a big batch of your favorite sauce and freeze in smaller portions. For the perfect single serving, I love to freeze these sauces in ice cube trays. All these sauces will last for 4 to 5 days in the fridge, or up to 3 months in the freezer.

tahini sauce

makes 1 cup (240g)

½ cup (120g) tahini

¼ cup (60ml) water, or more for a thinner consistency

¼ cup (60ml) fresh lemon juice (from about 2 lemons)

2 garlic cloves, minced

½ teaspoon kosher salt

¼ teaspoon ground cumin

In a medium bowl, whisk together the tahini, water, lemon juice, garlic, salt, and cumin. It may look a bit separated at first but keep whisking until it's creamy. Alternatively, blend all the ingredients in a food processor. For a thinner consistency, add a little more water.

Serving size:
2 tablespoons

Calories: 92
Fat: 8g
Saturated fat: 1g
Carbs: 4g
Fiber: 1g
Sugar: 1g
Protein: 3g
Cholesterol: 0g
Sodium: 157g

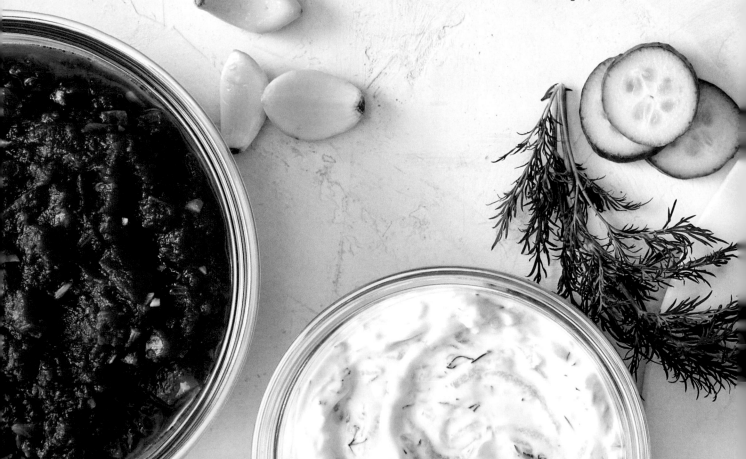

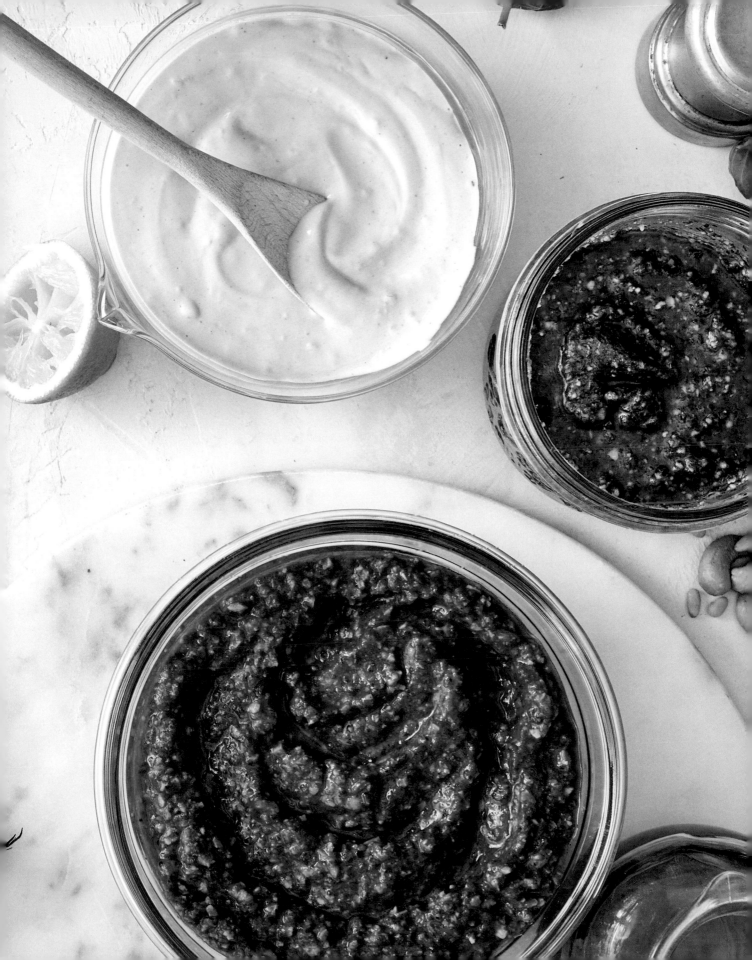

basil pesto

makes 1¼ cups (300g)

¼ cup (35g) raw pine nuts

¼ cup (35g) raw cashews

⅔ cup (150g) extra-virgin olive oil, or more as needed

2 teaspoons fresh lemon juice

2 cups (90g) packed fresh basil

3 garlic cloves

½ teaspoon kosher salt

Freshly ground black pepper to taste

¼ cup (25g) freshly grated Parmesan cheese

1. In a medium skillet, toast the pine nuts and cashews on medium-low heat for 5 minutes, tossing gently until lightly golden. Transfer them to a food processor.

2. Add the oil, lemon juice, basil, garlic, salt, pepper, and Parmesan to the food processor and pulse until the pesto is smooth. Add more oil as needed for a thinner texture.

marinara sauce

makes 4 cups (896g)

1 tablespoon extra-virgin olive oil

1 small yellow onion, finely diced

4 garlic cloves, minced

1 (28-ounce/793g) can crushed tomatoes

½ teaspoon kosher salt

1 tablespoon roughly chopped fresh thyme

1 tablespoon roughly chopped fresh basil

1. In a medium pot, heat the oil over medium-high heat. Add the onion and sauté for 3 to 4 minutes, until softened and translucent. Add the garlic and sauté for 30 seconds more.

2. Add the crushed tomatoes, salt, and thyme. Once the tomatoes have started to boil, reduce the heat to a simmer. Simmer for 20 to 25 minutes, or until the sauce has slightly thickened.

3. Remove the sauce from the heat and stir in the basil.

Serving size:
¼ cup (60g)

Calories: 367
Fat: 38g
Saturated fat: 6g
Carbs: 5g
Fiber: 1g
Sugar: 1g
Protein: 4g
Cholesterol: 4mg
Sodium: 204mg

Serving size:
½ cup (125g)

Calories: 53
Fat: 2g
Saturated fat: 0g
Carbs: 9g
Fiber: 2g
Sugar: 5g
Protein: 2g
Cholesterol: 0g
Sodium: 255g

tzatziki

makes 2 cups (448g)

1 medium cucumber, peeled and grated

1½ cups (342g) plain Greek yogurt

2 tablespoons finely chopped fresh dill

2 garlic cloves, minced

2 tablespoons extra-virgin olive oil

1 tablespoon fresh lemon juice

½ teaspoon kosher salt

1. Place the grated cucumber in a fine-mesh sieve over a bowl and press down on it to drain. Alternatively, place the cucumber in a nut milk bag or cheesecloth and gently squeeze all the moisture out. Transfer to a medium bowl.

2. Add yogurt, dill, garlic, oil, lemon juice, and salt to the bowl and stir until creamy.

Serving size:
¼ cup (56g)

Calories: 70
Fat: 4g
Saturated fat: 1g
Carbs: 3g
Fiber: 0g
Sugar: 2g
Protein: 5g
Cholesterol: 4g
Sodium: 87g

romesco sauce

makes 3¼ cups (785g)

½ cup (62g) raw hazelnuts

½ cup (42g) slivered almonds

1 (14.5-ounce/411g) can diced fire-roasted tomatoes, drained

1 (11.5-ounce/325g) jar roasted red peppers, drained (about 5 peppers)

3 garlic cloves, peeled

2 tablespoons red wine vinegar or sherry vinegar

1 teaspoon smoked paprika

1 teaspoon kosher salt

¼ cup (60ml) extra-virgin olive oil, or more for a thinner texture

1. In a small pan over medium heat, toast the hazelnuts for 5 to 8 minutes, stirring occasionally. Transfer them to a plate to cool.

2. In the same small pan, toast the almonds for 3 to 4 minutes, stirring occasionally, until lightly golden and fragrant. Place in a high-powered blender or food processor.

3. Once the hazelnuts are cool to the touch, rub them together with your hands or a kitchen towel to remove their skins. Add them to the almonds in the blender along with the tomatoes, red peppers, garlic, vinegar, paprika, salt, and oil. Blend on high speed for 1 minute, or until smooth.

Serving size:
¼ cup (56g)

Calories: 104
Fat: 9g
Saturated fat: 1g
Carbs: 4g
Fiber: 2g
Sugar: 3g
Protein: 2g
Cholesterol: 0mg
Sodium: 240mg

hummus

No doubt about it, I have a hummus obsession. Once I figured out how incredibly easy it was to make hummus in my Vitamix blender (literally just a couple of minutes), I started whipping up *all* the flavors. Similar to sauces, you can store hummus in the fridge for 4 to 5 days, or freeze it for up to 3 months, then thaw on demand—now how wonderful is that?

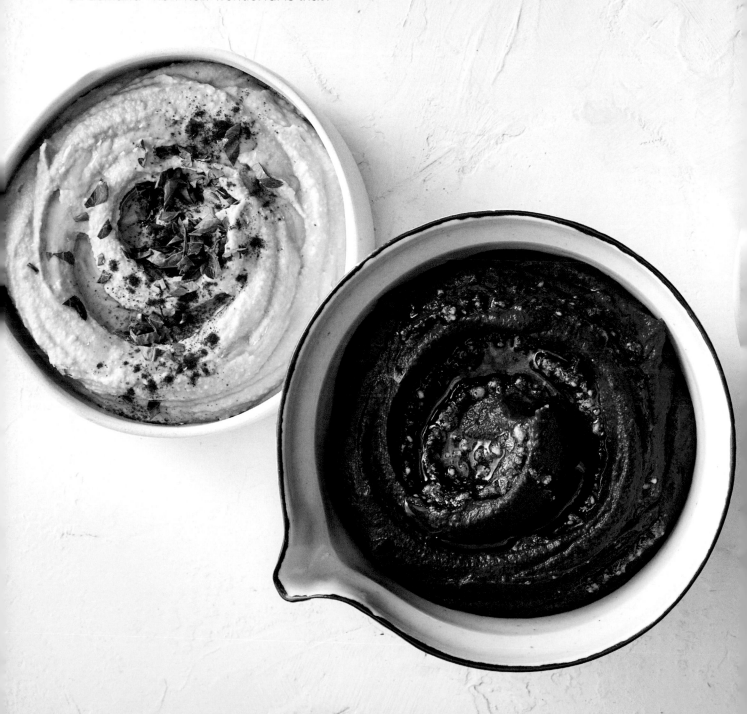

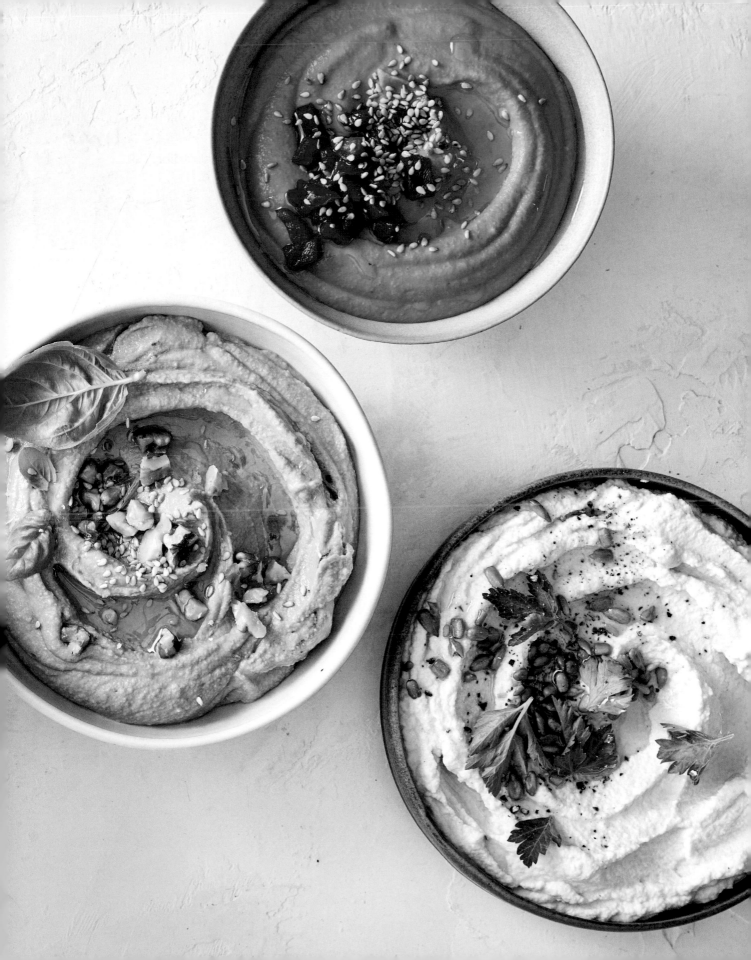

classic hummus

makes about 4 cups (896g)

2 (15.5-ounce/439g) cans chickpeas, drained with all liquid reserved

½ cup (120g) tahini

¼ cup (60ml) extra-virgin olive oil, plus more for drizzling

¼ cup (60ml) fresh lemon juice (from about 2 lemons)

2 garlic cloves

1 teaspoon ground cumin

½ teaspoon kosher salt

Sweet paprika, for garnish

Roughly chopped fresh parsley, for garnish

1. Place the chickpeas, ⅓ cup (75ml) of the reserved chickpea liquid, the tahini, oil, lemon juice, garlic, cumin, and salt in a high-powered blender. Remove the lid cap and insert the tamper. Blend on high speed for 30 seconds (or longer for a creamier texture). Use the tamper to push the hummus into the blades. Add more chickpea liquid, if desired, for a softer hummus.

2. Remove to a serving bowl. Drizzle with oil and garnish with a sprinkle of paprika and some parsley.

Serving size:
¼ cup (56g)

Calories: 128
Fat: 8g
Saturated fat: 1g
Carbs: 11g
Fiber: 3g
Sugar: 0g
Protein: 3g
Cholesterol: 0mg
Sodium: 82mg

roasted red pepper hummus

makes about 4 cups (896g)

2 (15.5-ounce/439 g) cans chickpeas, drained with all liquid reserved

1 (8-ounce/227g) jar of roasted red peppers, drained (about 3 peppers)

½ cup (120g) tahini

¼ cup (60ml) extra-virgin olive oil, plus more for drizzling

¼ cup (60ml) fresh lemon juice (from about 2 lemons)

1 garlic clove

1 teaspoon ground cumin

½ teaspoon kosher salt

Diced roasted red pepper, for garnish

Sesame seeds, for garnish

1. Place the chickpeas, ¼ cup (60ml) of the reserved chickpea liquid, the roasted peppers, tahini, oil, lemon juice, garlic, cumin, and salt in a high-powered blender. Remove the lid cap and insert the tamper. Blend on high for 30 seconds (or longer for a creamier texture). Use the tamper to push the hummus into the blades. Add more chickpea liquid, if desired, for a softer hummus.

2. Remove to a serving bowl. Drizzle with oil and garnish with diced roasted pepper and a sprinkle of sesame seeds.

Serving size:
¼ cup (56g)

Calories: 131
Fat: 8g
Saturated fat: 1g
Carbs: 11g
Fiber: 4g
Sugar: 1g
Protein: 4g
Cholesterol: 0mg
Sodium: 157mg

green goddess hummus

makes about 4 cups (896g)

2 (15.5-ounce/439g) cans chickpeas, drained with all liquid reserved

½ cup (120g) tahini

¼ cup (60ml) extra-virgin olive oil, plus more for drizzling

¼ cup (60ml) fresh lemon juice (from about 2 lemons)

1 cup (35g) loosely packed baby spinach

½ cup (30g) roughly chopped parsley

1 green onion (white and green parts), roughly chopped

1 garlic clove

1 teaspoon ground cumin

½ teaspoon kosher salt

Roughly chopped walnuts, for garnish

Sesame seeds, for garnish

1. Place the chickpeas, ⅓ cup (75ml) of the reserved chickpea liquid, the tahini, oil, lemon juice, spinach, parsley, green onion, garlic, cumin, and salt in a high-powered blender. Remove the lid cap and insert the tamper. Blend on high speed for 30 seconds (or longer for a creamier texture). Use the tamper to push the hummus into the blades. Add more chickpea liquid, if desired, for a softer hummus.

2. Remove to a serving bowl. Drizzle with oil and garnish with chopped walnuts, sesame seeds, and some herbs.

Serving size:
¼ cup (56g)

Calories: 130
Fat: 8g
Saturated fat: 1g
Carbs: 11g
Fiber: 4g
Sugar: 0g
Protein: 5g
Cholesterol: 0mg
Sodium: 85mg

roasted beet hummus

makes about 4 cups (896g)

2 medium beets, ends trimmed

¼ cup (60ml) + 1 teaspoon extra-virgin olive oil, plus more for drizzling

2 (15.5-ounce/439g) cans chickpeas, drained with all liquid reserved

½ cup (120g) tahini

¼ cup (60ml) fresh lemon juice (from about 2 lemons)

1 garlic clove

1 teaspoon ground cumin

½ teaspoon kosher salt

Basil Pesto (page 252), for garnish

Roughly chopped fresh parsley, for garnish

1. Preheat the oven to 400°F (200°C).

2. Lightly coat the beets with 1 teaspoon of the oil, place in a covered Dutch oven or other baking dish, and roast in the oven for 50 to 60 minutes. Remove the beets from the oven and let cool for 5 minutes.

3. Place the chickpeas, ⅓ cup (80ml) of the reserved chickpea liquid, the tahini, the remaining ¼ cup oil, lemon juice, garlic, cumin, salt, and beets in a high-powered blender. Remove the lid cap and insert the tamper. Blender on high speed for 30 seconds (or longer for a creamier texture). Use the tamper to push the hummus into the blades. Add more chickpea liquid, if desired, for a softer hummus.

4. Remove to a serving bowl. Drizzle with oil and garnish with a little pesto and some parsley.

Serving size:
¼ cup (56g)

Calories: 135

Fat: 9g

Saturated fat: 1g

Carbs: 12g

Fiber: 4g

Sugar: 1g

Protein: 5g

Cholesterol: 0mg

Sodium: 93mg

cauliflower hummus

makes about 3 cups (672g)

1 large head of cauliflower

3 tablespoons extra-virgin olive oil, plus more for drizzling

¼ cup (60g) tahini

3 tablespoons fresh lemon juice (from about 1 lemon)

2 tablespoons water, or more for desired consistency

1 garlic clove

¼ teaspoon ground cumin

Pinch of ground coriander

¼ teaspoon kosher salt

Sunflower seeds, for garnish

Roughly chopped fresh parsley, for garnish

Freshly ground black pepper, for garnish

1. Preheat the oven to 400°F (200°C).

2. Remove the florets from the head of cauliflower and place on a rimmed baking sheet. Drizzle with 1 tablespoon of the oil and toss to combine. Roast for 20 minutes.

3. Place the cauliflower, the remaining 2 tablespoons oil, the tahini, lemon juice, water, garlic, cumin, coriander, and salt in a high-powered blender. Remove the lid cap and insert the tamper. Blend on high speed for 30 seconds (or longer for a creamier texture). Use the tamper to push the hummus into the blades. Add more water, if desired, for a softer hummus.

4. Remove to a serving bowl. Drizzle with oil and garnish with a sprinkle of sunflower seeds, some parsley, and a few grinds of pepper.

Serving size:
¼ cup (56g)

Calories: 79
Fat: 6g
Saturated fat: 1g
Carbs: 5g
Fiber: 2g
Sugar: 1g
Protein: 2g
Cholesterol: 0g
Sodium: 74g

vinaigrettes

Truth be told, 99 percent of the time I just drizzle extra-virgin olive oil and balsamic vinegar onto my salads and macro bowls, but if I've got company visiting or want to feel a little fancy, I'll whip up one of these three staple vinaigrettes: balsamic, lemon, and apple cider. They're bright, zingy, and will last for about a week in the fridge. Just give them a quick shake if they separate.

balsamic vinaigrette
makes about ½ cup (130ml)

¼ cup (60ml) extra-virgin olive oil

¼ cup (60ml) balsamic vinegar

1 tablespoon honey

2 teaspoons Dijon mustard

¼ teaspoon kosher salt

1 garlic clove, minced

Pinch of freshly ground black pepper

In a small bowl, whisk together the oil, vinegar, honey, mustard, salt, garlic, and pepper.

lemon vinaigrette
makes about ⅔ cup (148ml)

⅓ cup (75ml) extra-virgin olive oil

¼ cup (60ml) fresh lemon juice (from about 2 lemons)

1 teaspoon Dijon mustard

½ teaspoon honey

1 garlic clove, minced

¼ teaspoon kosher salt

Pinch of freshly ground black pepper

In a small bowl, whisk together the oil, lemon juice, mustard, honey, garlic, salt, and pepper.

Balsamic Vinaigrette
Serving size:
2 tablespoons

Calories: 166
Fat: 11g
Saturated fat: 2g
Carbs: 7g
Fiber: 0g
Sugar: 7g
Protein: 0g
Cholesterol: 0g
Sodium: 134g

Lemon Vinaigrette
Serving size:
2 tablespoons

Calories: 184
Fat: 19g
Saturated fat: 3g
Carbs: 5g
Fiber: 1g
Sugar: 2g
Protein: 1g
Cholesterol: 0g
Sodium: 101g

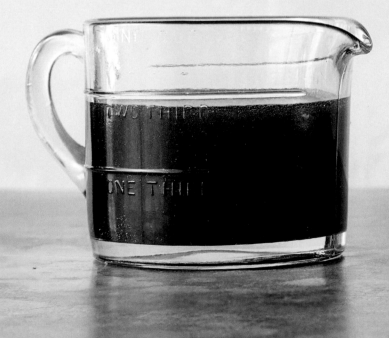

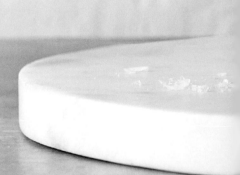

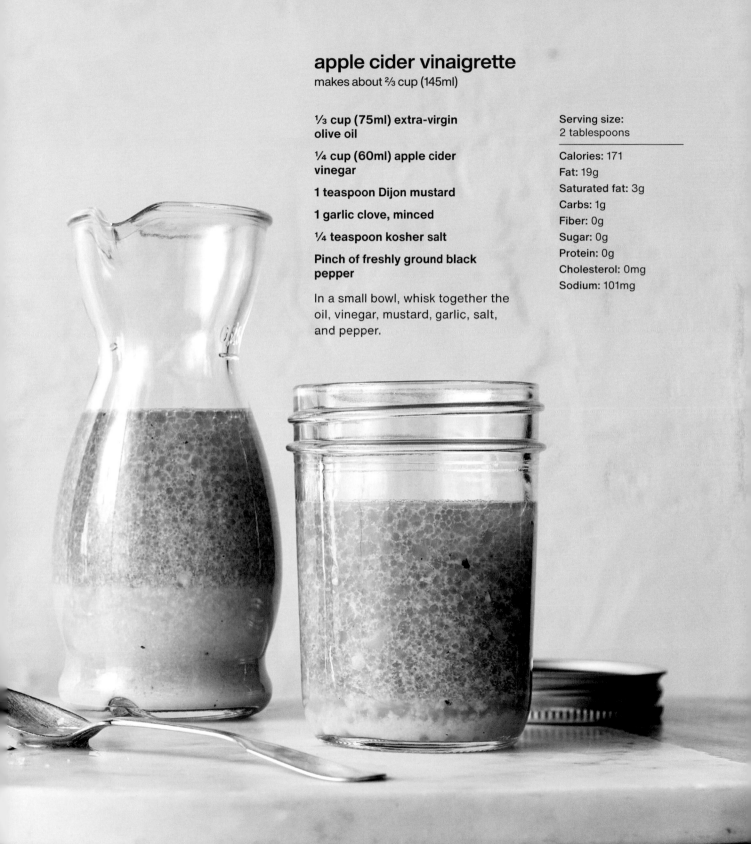

apple cider vinaigrette

makes about ⅔ cup (145ml)

⅓ **cup (75ml) extra-virgin olive oil**

¼ **cup (60ml) apple cider vinegar**

1 teaspoon Dijon mustard

1 garlic clove, minced

¼ **teaspoon kosher salt**

Pinch of freshly ground black pepper

In a small bowl, whisk together the oil, vinegar, mustard, garlic, salt, and pepper.

Serving size:
2 tablespoons

Calories: 171
Fat: 19g
Saturated fat: 3g
Carbs: 1g
Fiber: 0g
Sugar: 0g
Protein: 0g
Cholesterol: 0mg
Sodium: 101mg

garlic sautéed beet greens

While bulby beet roots get all the attention, don't let the leaves go to waste! Beet leaves have a mild, delicate flavor, similar to Swiss chard, and can be sautéed just like any other leafy green. Make sure to wash the leaves well (remember, these aren't prewashed greens like bags of baby spinach), then sauté them with a little garlic and oil. And don't forget to finely dice and toss in the stems too—there are lots of nutrients in them! **serves 2**

1 bunch of beet greens, rinsed well

1 tablespoon extra-virgin olive oil

3 garlic cloves

Zest and juice of ½ lemon (about ½ tablespoon zest + 1½ tablespoons juice), zest reserved for garnish

¼ teaspoon kosher salt

Freshly ground black pepper

1. Remove the beet leaves from the stems. Finely dice the stems and roughly chop the leaves.

2. In a large pan, heat the oil over medium heat. Add the garlic and stems and sauté for 1 to 2 minutes, until tender. Add the leaves, lemon juice, salt, and pepper and sauté for another 2 to 3 minutes, until the leaves have wilted. Garnish with lemon zest.

storage
Store in an airtight container in the fridge for 3 to 4 days.

to reheat
Sauté in a pan or heat in the microwave for 30 seconds, until warmed through.

helpful tip
Beet stems, no matter if they're from red beets or golden beets, are high in fiber and minerals. They're also full of betalains (the natural red and yellow pigment), which is a powerful antioxidant and anti-inflammatory. Translation: Beet greens are most definitely not kitchen scraps!

Serving size:
½ cup (65g)

Calories: 91

Fat: 7g

Saturated fat: 1g

Carbs: 7g

Fiber: 4g

Sugar: 1g

Protein: 2g

Cholesterol: 0g

Sodium: 357g

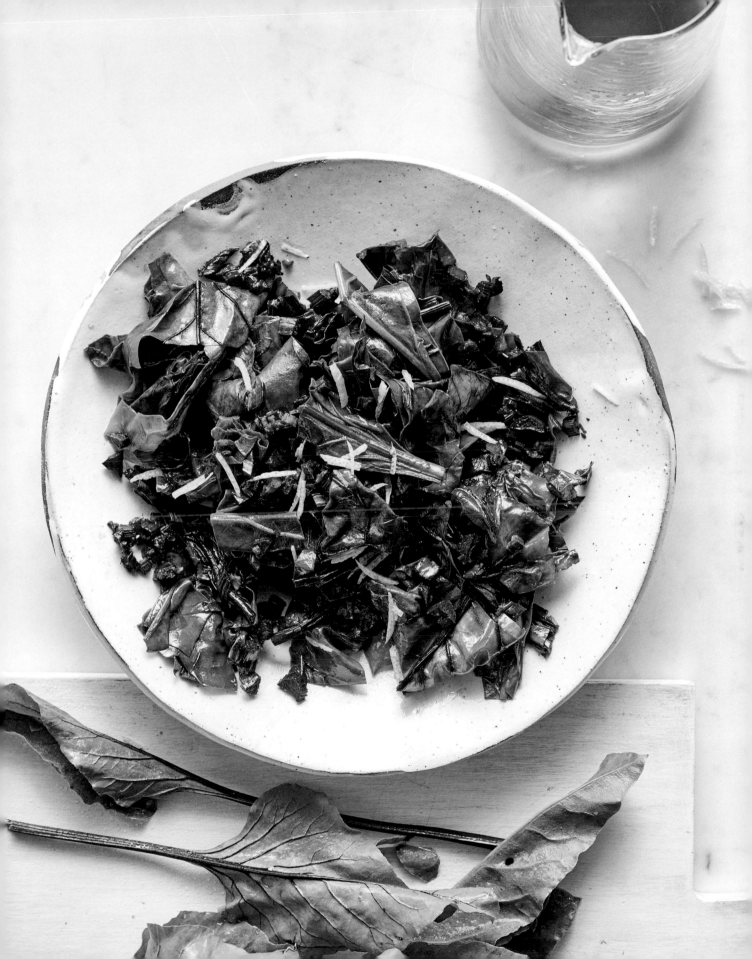

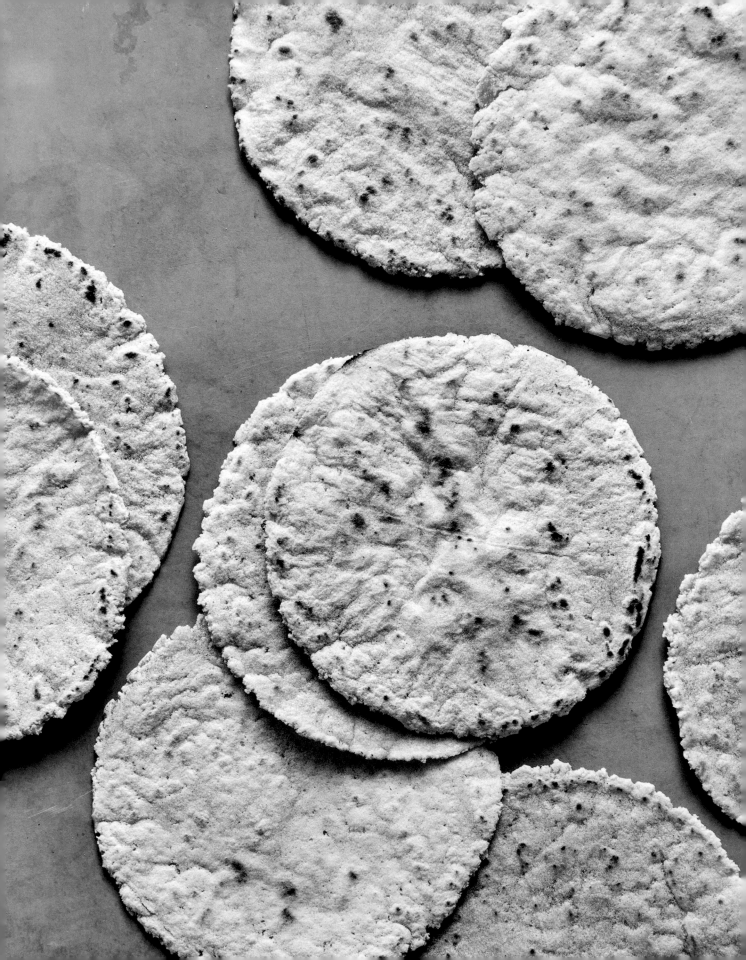

cassava flour tortillas

storage

Store in an airtight container (with parchment paper between the tortillas) in the fridge for 4 to 5 days, or in the freezer for up to 3 months.

helpful tips

The dough should have the texture of soft Play-Doh. If it's too sticky, add more flour. If it's too dry and crumbly, add more water. I've also found that the brand of cassava flour can make a difference in achieving the perfect texture. I always use Otto's Cassava Flour.

One of the many things I love about traveling the world is the inspiration I get with food. Years ago, I was fortunate to spend two months in Bali. I shopped in farmers' markets, explored the countryside, chatted up the neighbors, and learned from a little bakery in Canggu all the amazing things you can make with cassava flour—including breads, muffins, pancakes, and, yes, even tortillas. Upon my return home, I whipped up this recipe for cassava flour tortillas, and it's been a staple recipe ever since. Back then, store-bought cassava flour tortillas didn't exist, and while they do today, I still prefer this homemade version for everything from tacos to my Portobello Mushroom Sheet Pan Fajitas (page 225), quesadillas, wraps, and more. The tortillas are pliable, and stretchy—they'll almost fool you into thinking there's gluten in them! **makes 6 tortillas**

1 cup (150g) cassava flour

½ teaspoon cream of tartar

¼ teaspoon baking soda

¼ teaspoon kosher salt

2 tablespoons extra-virgin olive oil

⅔ cup (160ml) warm water

1. In a large bowl, stir together the flour, cream of tartar, baking soda, and salt.

2. Add the oil and knead it with your hands into the dry ingredients for a minute. The mixture will be dry and crumbly.

3. Add the warm water and knead for 2 to 3 more minutes. The dough will be sticky at first, but as the flour absorbs the water, it will become more pliable.

4. Divide the dough into 6 parts, then roll each piece into a ball. If you have an 8-inch tortilla press, press each ball of dough flat into a tortilla between two sheets of parchment paper. Without a tortilla press, place each ball of dough between two pieces of parchment paper and roll out into an approximate 6-inch (15cm) circle.

5. Heat a skillet or flat griddle on medium-high heat. Place one tortilla in the dry pan and cook for approximately 1 minute, until it starts to bubble and turn golden. Flip and cook the other side for an additional minute. Continue cooking all tortillas.

Serving size: 1 tortilla

Calories: 126
Fat: 5g
Saturated fat: 22g
Carbs: 2g
Fiber: 2g
Sugar: 0g
Protein: 1g
Cholesterol: 0mg
Sodium: 99mg

maple orange glazed carrots

Not going to lie, these almost taste like candy to me! Roasting carrots not only caramelizes the natural sugars in the vegetable, but it also reduces the maple orange marinade into a glossy, syrupy coating. They're sure to impress even your pickiest veggie eaters. **serves 6**

2 pounds (908g) carrots, sliced

¼ cup (80ml) pure maple syrup

3 tablespoons freshly squeezed orange juice

1 tablespoon extra-virgin olive oil

2 garlic cloves, minced

½ teaspoon ground ginger

½ teaspoon kosher salt

¼ teaspoon freshly ground black pepper

1 teaspoon orange zest

1. Preheat the oven to 425°F (220°C).

2. In a large mixing bowl, toss the sliced carrots with the maple syrup, orange juice, oil, garlic, ginger, salt, and pepper.

3. Pour the carrots and glaze into a 13 x 9-inch (33 x 23cm) casserole dish or a rimmed quarter sheet pan, and spread them out into a single layer. Roast the carrots for 35 to 40 minutes, tossing halfway through. You can also broil for an extra 2 to 3 minutes to caramelize the edges.

4. Remove the carrots from the oven, add the orange zest, and toss again. Transfer to a serving plate and pour any excess liquid from the baking sheet over the top of the carrots.

storage

Store in an airtight container in the fridge for 3 to 4 days, or in the freezer for up to 3 months.

to reheat

If frozen, thaw in the fridge overnight. Sauté in a pan for 2 to 3 minutes, or heat in the microwave for 1 minute, until warmed through.

Serving size:
½ cup (80g)

Calories: 122

Fat: 3g

Saturated fat: 0g

Carbs: 25g

Fiber: 4g

Sugar: 16g

Protein: 2g

Cholesterol: 0mg

Sodium: 199mg

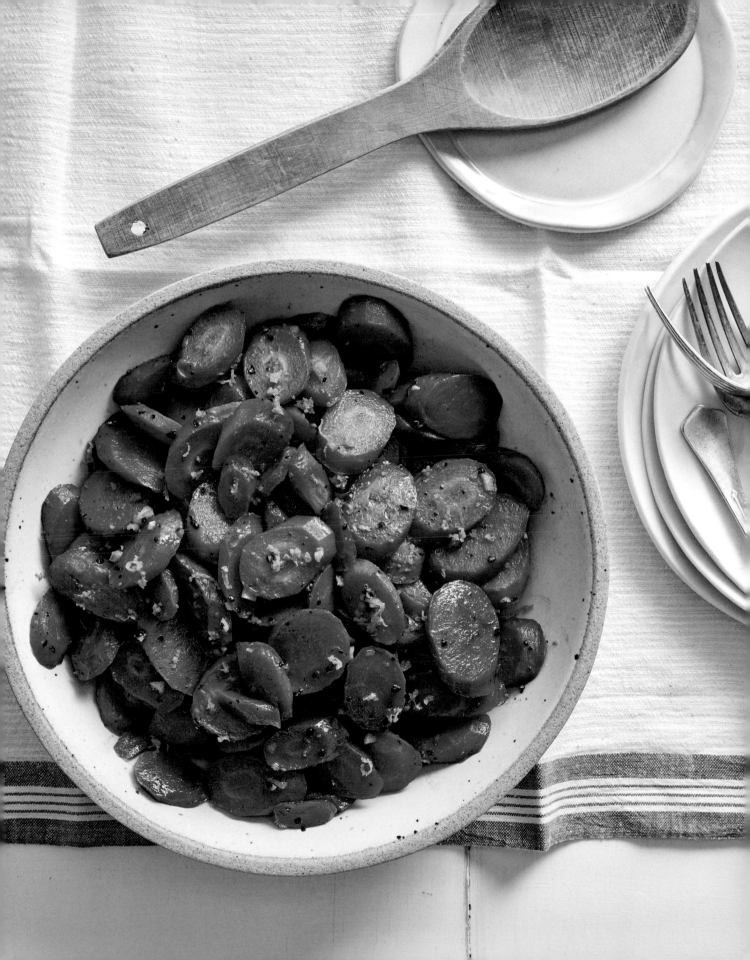

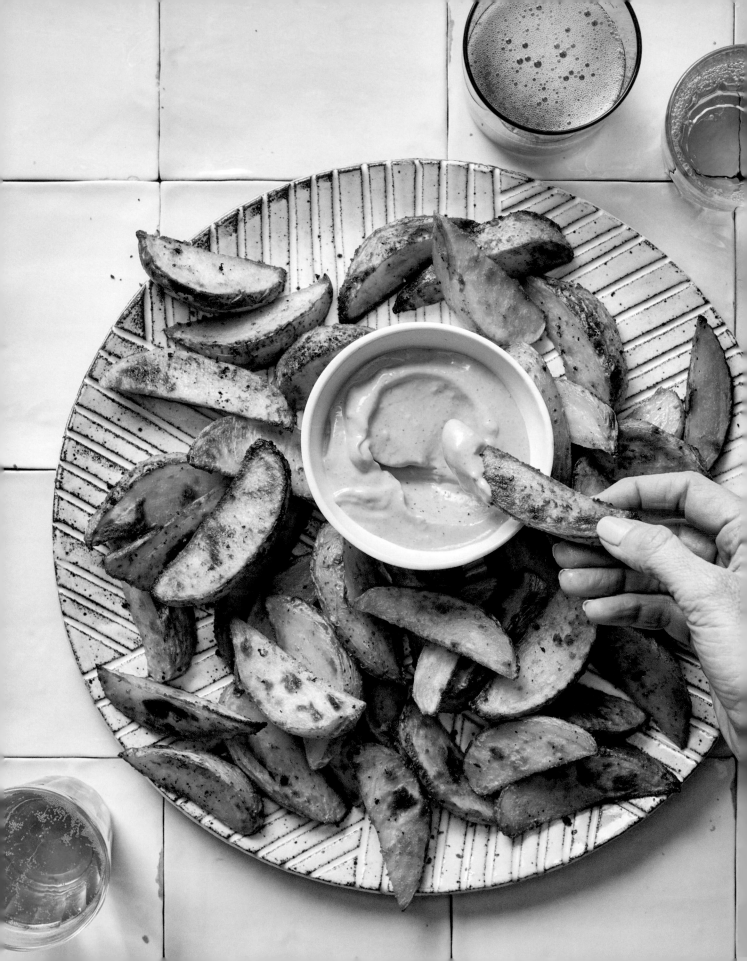

roasted potato wedges with sriracha aioli

storage

Store the potatoes and aioli in separate airtight containers in the fridge. The potato wedges will keep for 3 to 4 days; the aioli, for up to 1 week.

to reheat

Place wedges on a rimmed baking sheet and reheat in a 350°F (180°C) oven for 5 to 8 minutes, or until warmed through.

helpful tip

If you have leftover aioli, drizzle it on tacos and fajitas, use it as a veggie dip, or slather it on lettuce-wrapped burgers.

Serving size: About 5 potato wedges + 2½ tablespoons aioli

Calories: 409

Fat: 32g

Saturated fat: 5g

Carbs: 28g

Fiber: 2g

Sugar: 2g

Protein: 4g

Cholesterol: 15mg

Sodium: 589mg

All my friends go crazy for these perfectly crispy and seasoned potato wedges. So much so, I often double this recipe because I know they'll disappear as soon as they're plated up. The key to their addictive nature is their golden and crispy edges—make sure a cut edge is always flat against the sheet pan. There's just something about that crispy outside and pillowy soft inside that's highly addictive. Plus, if you like a little spicy kick, the sriracha aioli is ultra dippable. **serves 6**

FOR THE POTATOES

2 teaspoons garlic powder

1 teaspoon onion powder

1 teaspoon smoked paprika

1 teaspoon kosher salt

¼ teaspoon freshly ground black pepper

2 pounds (908g) waxy potatoes, such as Yukon Gold or Red Bliss

2 tablespoons extra-virgin olive oil

FOR THE SRIRACHA AIOLI

1 cup (220g) mayonnaise

2 tablespoons sriracha

1 tablespoon fresh lime juice

2 garlic cloves, minced

1. Preheat the oven to 425°F (220°C).

2. To make the potatoes: In a small bowl, stir together the garlic powder, onion powder, paprika, salt, and pepper. Set aside.

3. Cut each potato into 8 even wedges. Place the potatoes in a medium bowl, drizzle with the oil, and add the seasoning. Toss together to thoroughly coat.

4. Spread the potato wedges out on a rimmed baking sheet in a single layer, making sure one cut side is lying flat for extra crispy edges. Roast for 25 minutes, then flip and roast an additional 15 to 20 minutes, until crispy on the outside and tender on the inside.

5. To make the sriracha aioli: In a small bowl, stir together the mayonnaise, sriracha, lime juice, and garlic. Serve alongside the potato wedges.

room for dessert

As I mentioned in the introduction, I want this to be a realistic cookbook. And in reality, I do eat desserts—yes, it's true! While I don't cook with any processed sugars (I default to maple syrup, honey, and coconut sugar most of the time), I have zero guilt in indulging in healthier sweet treats when the mood strikes. Because healthy eating and life—well, it's all about a little thing called balance.

So in this chapter I've assembled some decadent nibbles and bite-size desserts that will help you satisfy those sweet cravings in healthier ways. Just one bite of my Chocolate Hazelnut Thumbprint Cookies (page 284) or Chocolate Espresso Shortbread Bars (page 288) is enough to tick the box on that chocolate craving. And for cooling desserts on hot, sunny days, you can't beat an incredibly easy Banana Berry Nice Cream (page 280) or Pineapple Coconut Whip (page 283)—no funky thickeners or emulsifiers, just whole fruit goodness!

maple meringue and pecan cookies

Meringue cookies are light and airy, perfectly sweet, and delightfully crunchy. I always get this visual that I'm biting into a crunchy, fluffy cloud when I'm eating them. Traditional meringue cookies use processed white sugar, but I've swapped that for maple syrup, which gives them a rich, distinctive flavor. A light sprinkle of chopped pecans on top adds to the crunch. If you're feeling ambitious, you can use a piping bag to add some flair. But feel free to just dollop them with a spoon into mounds. Either way, they'll be impressive little cookies that make for a perfect holiday (or everyday) treat. **makes about 50 cookies**

2 **large egg whites**

½ **teaspoon cream of tartar**

Pinch of kosher salt

½ **cup (160ml) pure maple syrup**

⅓ **cup (39g) finely chopped pecans**

1. Preheat the oven to 200°F (100°C) and set two oven racks in the middle. Line two baking sheets with parchment paper and set aside.

2. In the bowl of a stand mixer (or using a separate bowl with an electric hand mixer), combine the egg whites, cream of tartar, and salt. Beat on low speed until frothy, then increase the speed to medium-high until soft peaks form. With the mixer running, gradually add the maple syrup until the mixture is stiff and glossy.

3. Dollop the mixture into small rounds, about 2 tablespoons in size, or use a piping bag to pipe the cookies onto the prepared baking sheets. Sprinkle with chopped pecans. Bake the cookies for 1½ to 2 hours, until dry and light beige in color. Turn off the oven and leave the meringue cookies in the oven for another hour to cool.

storage

Store in an airtight container at room temperature for up to 2 weeks.

helpful tip

If the cookies are left out, they're likely to absorb moisture and humidity and become sticky. If that happens, you can dry them out in the oven again at 200°F (100°C), until the moisture has evaporated.

Serving size: 4 cookies

Calories: 14
Fat: 1g
Saturated fat: 0g
Carbs: 2g
Fiber: 0g
Sugar: 2g
Protein: 0g
Cholesterol: 0mg
Sodium: 5mg

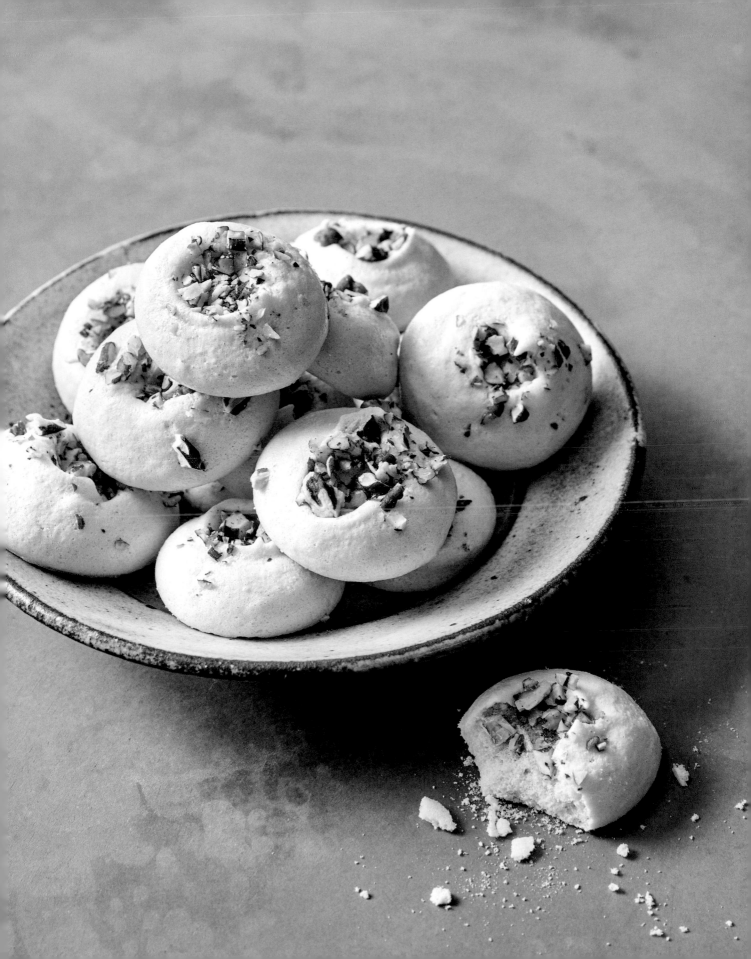

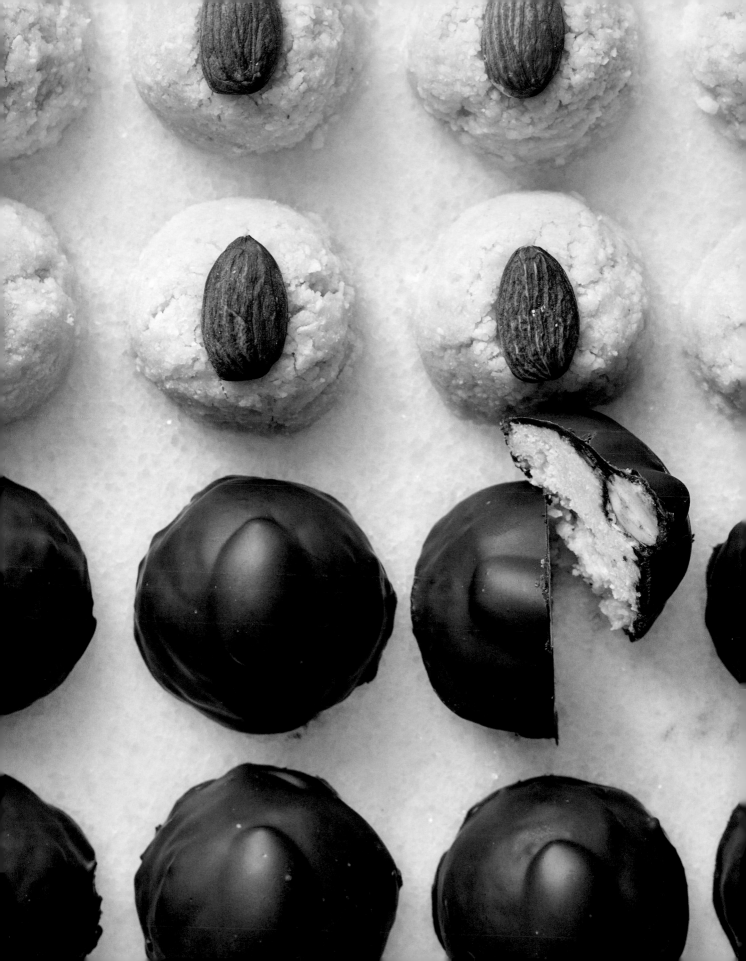

almond joy bites

storage

Store in an airtight container in the fridge for several weeks, or in the freezer for up to 3 months.

helpful tip

If you use a 1-tablespoon cookie scoop, it's as easy as scooping, packing the mixture, and releasing on the parchment paper to get that perfect dome shape. If you're not so particular about the dome shape, you can also press the coconut mixture into a silicone mini cupcake pan or Souper Cubes mini tray, cover with chocolate, and then pop them out when firm.

Little mounds of chocolate, coconut, and almond—what's not to love? This healthier version of your candy bar favorite is made with just a handful of kitchen staples, and—bonus—they're corn-, dairy-, and soy-free (unlike the store-bought version). They're perfect for Easter or Halloween, but you know what I love most? That I can freeze them for months, then thaw, and pop one in my mouth to satisfy those run-of-the-mill late-night chocolate cravings! **makes 20 bites**

2½ cups (200g) unsweetened shredded coconut

¼ cup (80ml) pure maple syrup

2 tablespoons + 1½ teaspoons melted coconut oil

1 teaspoon vanilla extract

20 raw almonds

1 cup (180g) dark chocolate chips

1. In a food processor, blend the shredded coconut, maple syrup, 2 tablespoons of the oil, and the vanilla extract for about 1 minute, until mostly smooth and starting to clump together but before turning into coconut butter.

2. Using a spoon or small cookie scoop, scoop 1 tablespoon of the mixture to create a compressed mound (you can also roll it in your hands), then place it on a quarter baking sheet or plate lined with parchment paper. Lightly press one almond into the top the mound. Repeat with the remaining mixture. Freeze for 15 minutes to firm up the bites.

3. In a medium heatproof bowl over simmering water, melt the chocolate chips with the remaining 1½ teaspoons oil. Alternatively, microwave the chocolate chips in a microwave-safe bowl in 20-second increments. Stir together until smooth. Drop the bites into the chocolate and spoon melted chocolate over the top. Use a fork to lift the bites out and allow any excess chocolate to drip off, then place them back on the parchment paper. Continue until all bites are chocolate covered, then return them to the freezer for 5 to 10 minutes to firm up.

Serving size: 1 bite

Calories: 164
Fat: 13g
Saturated fat: 10g
Carbs: 11g
Fiber: 2g
Sugar: 7.5g
Protein: 1g
Cholesterol: 1mg
Sodium: 6mg

almond butter stuffed dates

The great thing about this treat is that I almost always have these ingredients in my pantry, so I can satisfy a sweet craving on a whim. It's the perfect salty-sweet combo with just four ingredients! **makes 12 dates**

12 Medjool dates

⅓ cup (85g) almond butter

2 tablespoons roughly chopped dark chocolate

Flaked sea salt

1. Use a knife to make a cut lengthwise down the date, but don't cut all the way through. Remove the pit and use your fingers to create a small cavity.

2. Add 1 teaspoon of the almond butter to the center of the date. Top with chopped chocolate and a pinch of sea salt.

storage
Store in an airtight container at room temperature if you prefer them soft and drizzly, or in the fridge for a firmer texture. Either way, they'll keep for up to 2 weeks.

helpful tips
For a slightly less messy and oozy stuffed date, chill the almond butter in the fridge for 30 minutes to firm it up a little. Then spoon it into the date.

get creative
You can use any type of nut or seed butter in this recipe, so feel free to switch it up with peanut butter, cashew butter, sunflower seed butter, and more!

Serving size: 1 date

Calories: 120

Fat: 5g

Saturated fat: 1g

Carbs: 21g

Fiber: 3g

Sugar: 18g

Protein: 2g

Cholesterol: 0mg

Sodium: 49mg

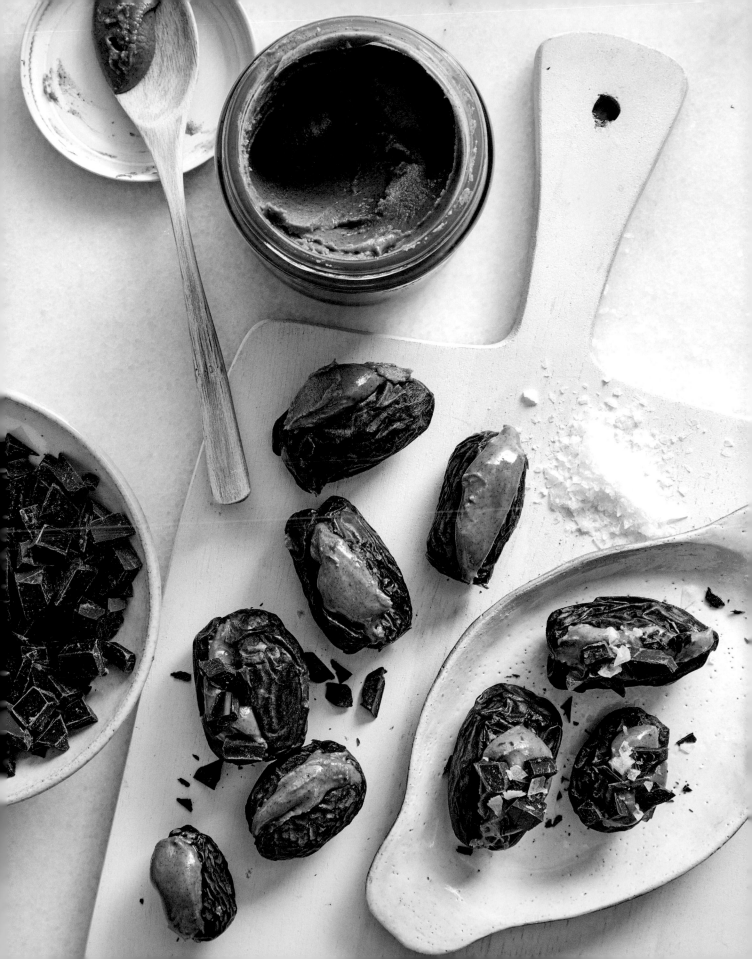

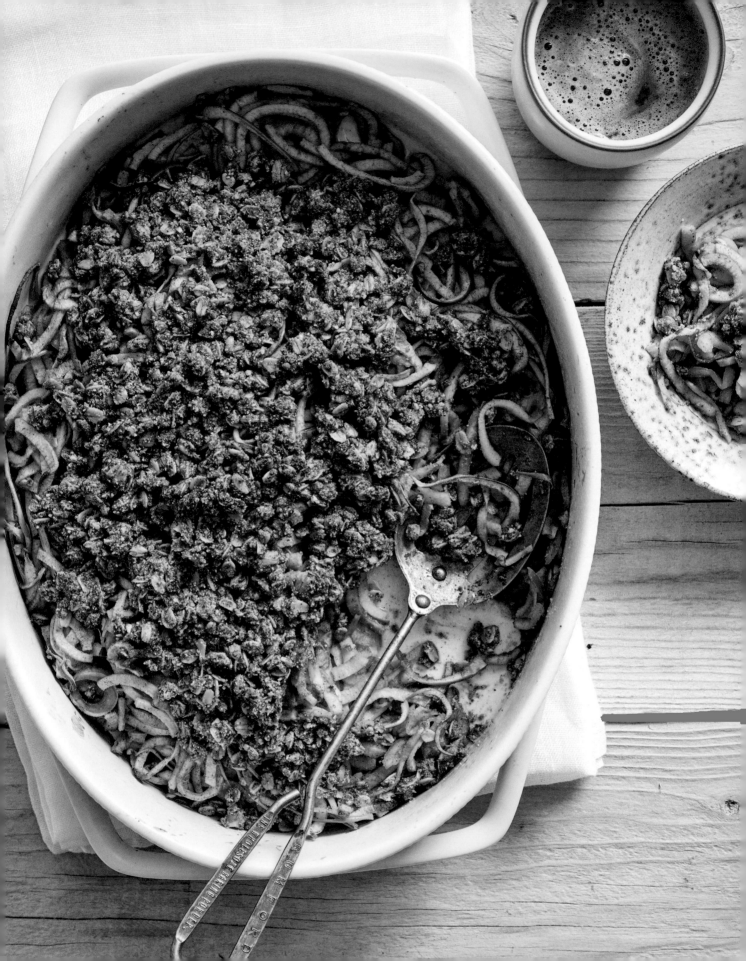

spiralized apple crisp

Apple pie is about as classic as they come. But when you don't want to slice a whole bunch of apples or roll out dough, make this incredibly easy apple crisp instead! Spiralizing half a dozen apples takes less than a minute—and you don't even have to peel the apples. Just toss them with a little sweetener and spices, then bake with a crunchy, crumbly, cinnamon streusel oat topping. For a fun flavor twist, spiralize pears instead of apples! **serves 8**

FOR THE FRUIT BASE

6 Granny Smith apples, spiralized

¼ cup (80ml) pure maple syrup

1 tablespoon arrowroot powder

1 tablespoon fresh lemon juice

1 teaspoon ground cinnamon

FOR THE APPLE CRISP TOPPING

1 cup (108g) old-fashioned rolled oats

1 cup (120g) almond flour

⅓ cup (53g) coconut sugar

½ teaspoon ground cinnamon

¼ teaspoon kosher salt

½ cup (113ml) melted butter or coconut oil

1 teaspoon vanilla extract

1. Preheat the oven to 350°F (180°C).

2. To make the fruit base: In a large bowl, toss together the apples, maple syrup, arrowroot powder, lemon juice, and cinnamon until well combined. Transfer the apple mixture to a 13 × 9-inch (33 × 23cm) baking dish and bake for 20 minutes.

3. To make the topping: While the apples are baking, in a medium bowl stir together the oats, flour, sugar, cinnamon, and salt. Add the melted butter and vanilla to the bowl and stir until clumpy.

4. Remove the apples from the oven, give them a toss with tongs, then spread the topping evenly across the apple filling. Place the baking dish back in the oven and bake for 25 to 30 minutes more, or until the fruit is soft and the topping is golden brown. Serve warm with a dollop of ice cream or whipped cream (dairy or dairy-free).

Serving size: 1 cup (155g)

Calories: 394
Fat: 21g
Saturated fat: 8g
Carbs: 50g
Fiber: 8g
Sugar: 30g
Protein: 6g
Cholesterol: 30.5mg
Sodium: 41mg

banana berry nice cream

Nice cream is a luscious sugar-free, dairy-free dessert made from blending frozen pieces of fruit in a high-powered blender or food processor. Years ago my mom bought one of those Yonanas machines, and I may have laughed at the gimmicky contraption. But what's *not* gimmicky is the end result: a creamy, all-natural, fruit-based "ice cream." And the good news is, you don't need a specialty machine to make it! This vegan ice cream has the consistency of sorbet, and it's highly adaptable with a variety of fruit. Choose a single seasonal fruit or make a mixed-berry blend. A few flavors I love are peach, cantaloupe, cherry, and mango. Just make sure to always include bananas for the creamiest texture. **serves 4**

3 large ripe bananas, sliced and frozen

1½ cups (210g) frozen mixed berries

¼ cup (60ml) almond milk or other nondairy milk

1 teaspoon vanilla extract

In a high-powered blender on high speed, blend the frozen banana slices, berries, milk, and vanilla for 1 minute, or until smooth. If your blender has a tamper, use that (see Helpful Tips). The nice cream will be a soft texture at this stage and you can serve immediately, but if you'd like it firmer, place in a storage container and freeze for 1 to 2 hours.

storage

Store in an airtight container in the freezer for up to 3 months. Once frozen, the berry nice cream will be quite hard. Let it thaw on the counter for 25 to 30 minutes before scooping and serving.

helpful tips

Remember that you need a certain amount of ingredients in a high-powered blender to properly blend with the tamper, so if you want to reduce the quantity of this recipe, I recommend using a food processor instead. Nice cream by definition doesn't usually include a sweetener. But if you want to add maple syrup, by all means feel free to add it.

Serving size:
¾ cup (184g)

Calories: 125

Fat: 1g

Saturated fat: 0g

Carbs: 31g

Fiber: 4g

Sugar: 17g

Protein: 1g

Cholesterol: 0mg

Sodium: 18mg

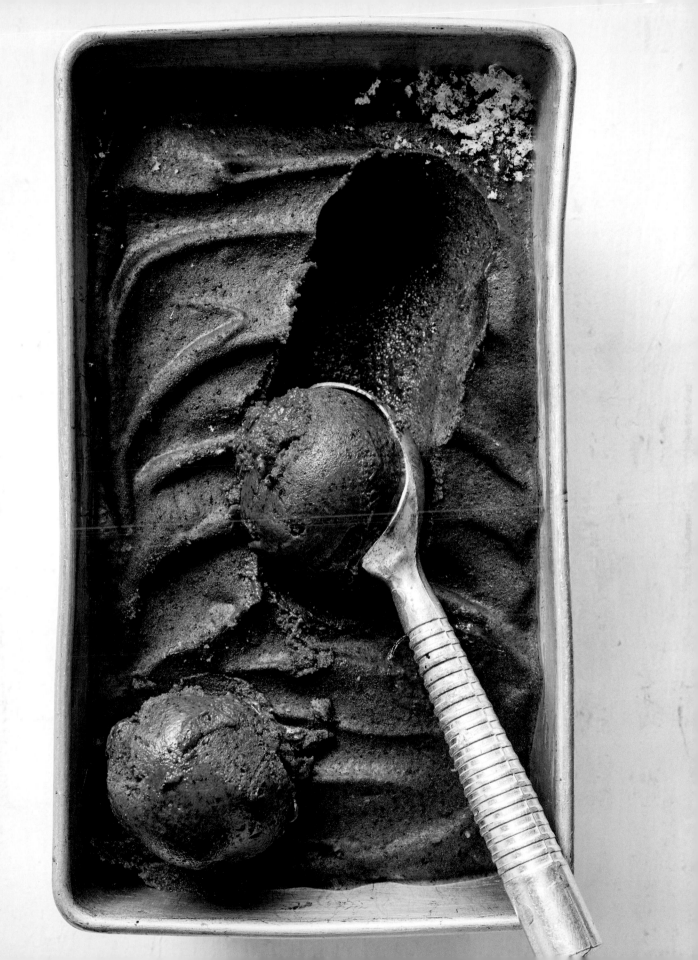

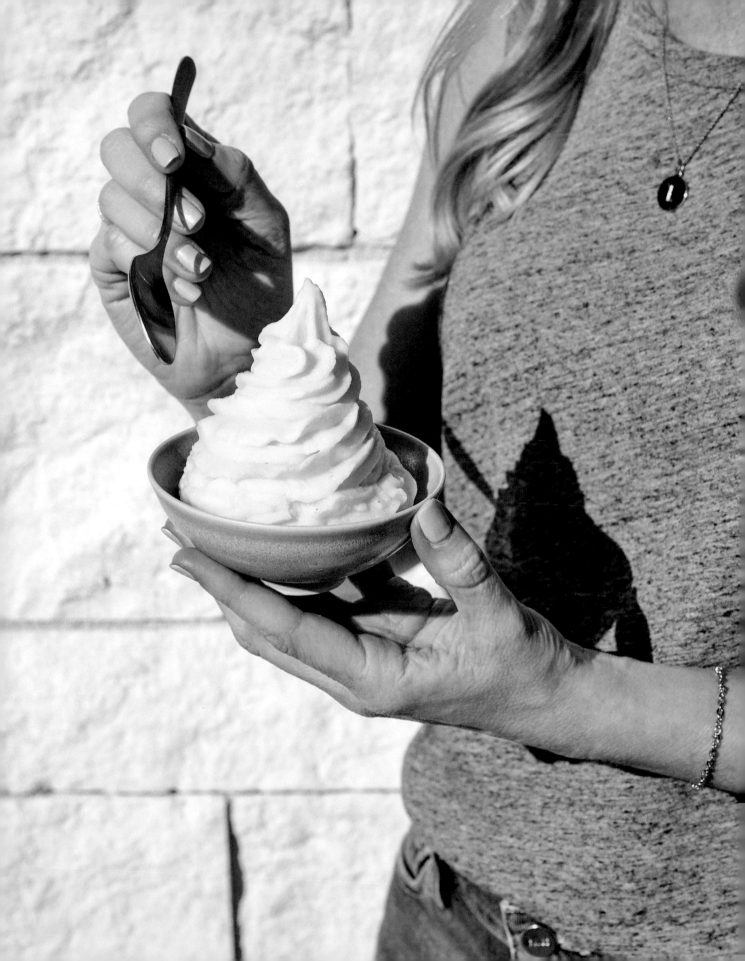

pineapple coconut whip

storage

Store in an airtight container in the freezer for up to 3 months. Once frozen, it will be quite hard. Let it thaw on the counter for 25 to 30 minutes before scooping and serving.

dietary swaps

If you're not a fan of coconut, you can swap that with a large scoop of your favorite dairy or dairy-free ice cream. You can also use almond milk, cashew milk, oat milk, or another nondairy milk, but it won't be quite as creamy.

get creative

If you really want to replicate your Disneyland favorite, just add the blended pineapple coconut whip to a piping bag with a large tip and swirl it around in a small glass—it'll look just like soft serve!

When you live in SoCal, virtually in the backyard of Disneyland, it's hard not to be obsessed with Dole Whip, an iconic Magic Kingdom treat that's the equivalent of a creamy pineapple soft serve. It's perfectly refreshing on hot days, puts a little pep back in your step, and makes your inner child grin from ear to ear. The authentic version is simply pineapple juice, frozen pineapple, and ice cream, but it's easy to make dairy-free with coconut cream. Plus, it tastes more like a frozen piña colada whip, and I'm 100 percent okay with that!

serves 4

4 cups (560g) frozen pineapple chunks

½ cup (120ml) pineapple juice

½ cup (120ml) canned coconut cream

1. In a high-powered blender or food processor, blend the pineapple chunks, pineapple juice, and coconut cream for 1 minute or until smooth. If your blender has a tamper, use that (see Helpful Tips on page 280) and scrape down the sides as necessary.

2. Scoop the blended whip into individual serving glasses.

Serving size:
¾ cup (188g)

Calories: 146
Fat: 6g
Saturated fat: 5g
Carbs: 22g
Fiber: 2g
Sugar: 7g
Protein: 1g
Cholesterol: 0mg
Sodium: 11mg

chocolate hazelnut thumbprint cookies

Soft and chewy, these hazelnut thumbprint cookies are filled with a simple chocolate ganache for a healthier Nutella-esque vibe. I'm using store-bought hazelnut flour (also called hazelnut meal), but you can also grind your own at home with a blender or food processor (see Helpful Tips). This recipe is entirely vegan, as I've swapped an egg with ground flaxseed for a naturally chewy texture, and the rich chocolate ganache is just melted chocolate chips and coconut milk. These cookies have a luxurious texture and pastry shop-fancy look to them, but they're incredibly easy (and fun) to make! **makes 24 cookies**

FOR THE CHOCOLATE GANACHE

1 cup (180g) semi-sweet chocolate chips (Pascha brand is vegan)

½ cup (120ml) full-fat coconut milk

1 teaspoon vanilla extract

FOR THE HAZELNUT COOKIES

2 cups (224g) hazelnut flour

2 tablespoons ground flaxseed

½ teaspoon baking soda

¼ teaspoon kosher salt

½ cup (160ml) pure maple syrup

3 tablespoons coconut oil, melted

storage

Store in an airtight container at room temperature or in the fridge for up to 2 weeks, or in the freezer for up to 3 months.

helpful tips

If you can't find hazelnut flour you can make your own. Add hazelnuts to a food processor or high-speed blender and pulse until finely ground. That's it! For a more neutral flavor, substitute almond flour for the hazelnut flour. If you're transporting these cookies and don't want the chocolate center oozing out, you can simply fill the cookies with melted chocolate and omit the coconut milk and vanilla for a hard chocolate filling.

1. Preheat the oven to 350°F (180°C). Line a baking sheet with parchment paper.

2. To make the ganache: In a medium heatproof bowl over a pot of simmering water, melt the chocolate. Alternatively, microwave the chocolate in a microwave-safe bowl in 20-second increments. Add the coconut milk and vanilla to the chocolate and stir until smooth. Place this chocolate ganache in the fridge for about 20 minutes to cool and slightly firm up.

3. To make the cookies: In a large mixing bowl, stir together the flour, flaxseed, baking soda, salt, maple syrup, and coconut oil until well combined. Drop tablespoon-size balls of dough, evenly spaced, onto the prepared baking sheet. Use your thumb to press an indentation in the cookie's center. Bake the cookies for 13 to 15 minutes, until lightly golden. Remove the cookies from the oven and let them cool on the baking sheet.

Serving size: 1 cookie

Calories: 142

Fat: 11g

Saturated fat: 4g

Carbs: 11g

Fiber: 2g

Sugar: 9g

Protein: 2g

Cholesterol: 0mg

Sodium: 68mg

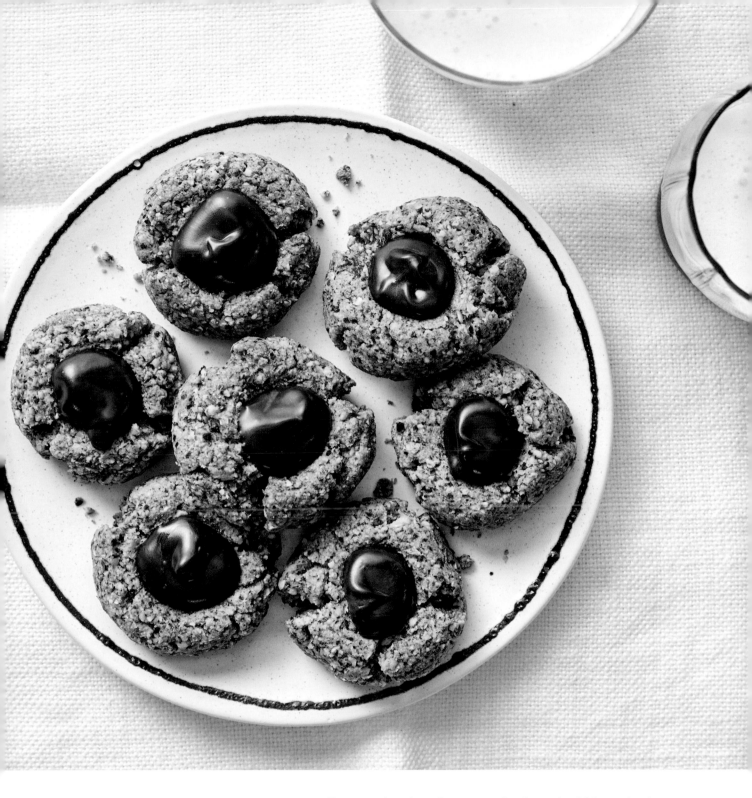

4. Remove the chocolate ganache from the fridge, give it a stir, and spoon a dollop into the center of each cookie. The ganache will continue to firm up and set at room temperature. Alternatively, you can place the cookies in the fridge for about 30 minutes to firm up the chocolate center faster.

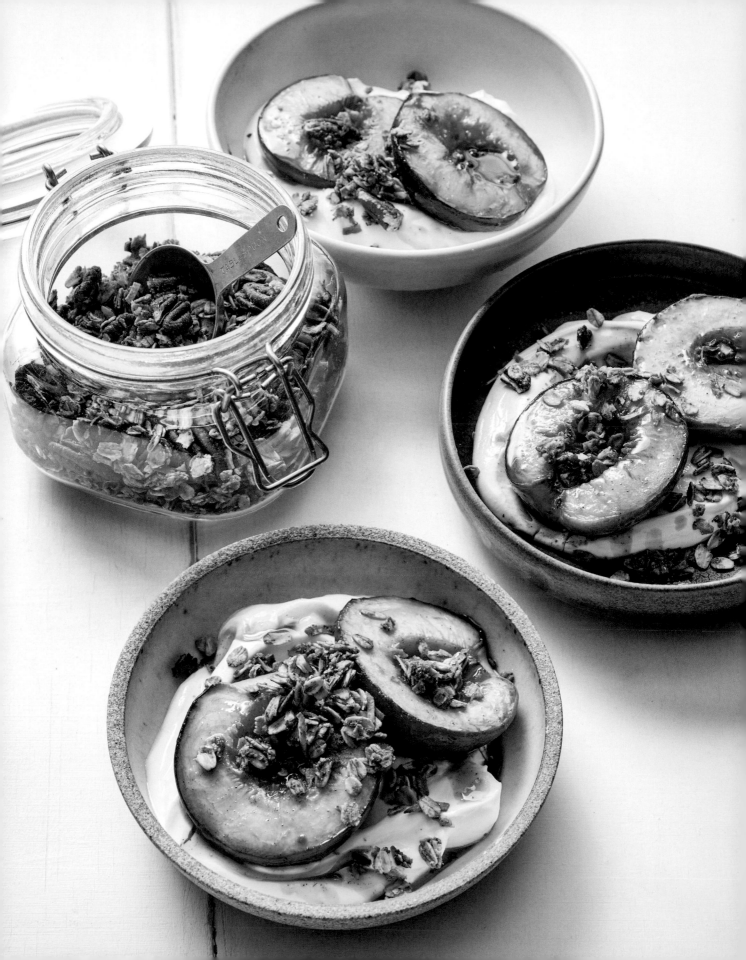

ginger roasted stone fruit with yogurt and granola

storage

Store in an airtight container in the fridge for 3 to 4 days, or in the freezer for up to 3 months.

to reheat

For the easiest method, reheat in the microwave in 30-second increments, or warm them up in a pan on the stove.

When it comes to easy desserts, it's hard to beat this one. Perfectly ripe stone fruit is infused with warming spices, and after a quick pop in the oven they become syrupy sweet. I serve them with a dollop of vanilla yogurt and crunchy granola, but you can opt for a scoop of ice cream if you're feeling indulgent. **serves 6**

1½ pounds (680g) nectarines, peaches, plums, or other stone fruit, halved and pitted

½ teaspoon ground ginger

¼ teaspoon ground cardamom

2 tablespoons honey

1½ cups (342g) vanilla yogurt

1½ cups (135g) Homemade Granola (page 106)

1. Preheat the oven to 375°F (190°C).

2. Place the fruit halves cut side up in a single layer in a 9 × 9-inch (23 × 23cm) baking dish.

3. Sprinkle the fruit with the ginger and cardamom, then drizzle the honey on top. Roast for 25 to 30 minutes, gently tossing halfway through, until the fruit is soft and tender. Serve with a dollop of yogurt and a sprinkle of granola.

Serving size: 2 stone fruit halves + ½ cup yogurt + ¼ cup granola

Calories: 286
Fat: 8g
Saturated fat: 4g
Carbs: 48g
Fiber: 4g
Sugar: 39g
Protein: 9g
Cholesterol: 6mg
Sodium: 101mg

chocolate espresso shortbread bars

I need all the adjectives to describe these bars—decadent, ultra-rich, scrumptious, irresistible, fabulous, and exceptionally delicious. Trust me, it will be hard to stop at just one bar! The base is a flaky, buttery (if you so choose) almond flour crust, and the chocolate espresso top is a riff on the chocolate cake and brownie recipe from my website. Both the espresso powder and coconut sugar deepen the richness of the chocolate layer, and the shortbread crust is just divine. This is a recipe that's sure to garner oohs and ahhs. **makes 16 bars**

FOR THE SHORTBREAD BASE

⅓ cup (75ml) melted butter or coconut oil

⅓ cup (107ml) pure maple syrup or honey

1 teaspoon vanilla extract

2 cups (240g) almond flour

⅓ cup (40g) coconut flour

¼ teaspoon kosher salt

FOR THE CHOCOLATE ESPRESSO TOPPING

½ cup (113ml) melted butter or coconut oil

½ cup (90g) chocolate chips

1 cup (160g) coconut sugar

1 tablespoon instant espresso powder

1 teaspoon vanilla extract

3 large eggs

¼ cup (30g) tapioca flour

1. Preheat the oven to 350°F (180°C). Line an 8 × 8-inch (20 × 20cm) baking pan with parchment paper, with paper going up the sides.

2. To make the crust: In a large bowl, whisk together the butter, maple syrup, and vanilla. Add the almond flour, coconut flour, and salt. Stir or use your hands to mix everything together until you have a crumbly dough.

3. Scrape the dough into the prepared baking pan. Use your hands to press the dough firmly and evenly in the pan. Bake the shortbread crust for 13 to 15 minutes, or until lightly golden on top and slightly darker around the edges, then remove and set aside. If the center puffs up slightly, gently press it down as it cools to flatten.

4. To make the topping: In a heatproof medium bowl set over a saucepan of simmering water, melt the butter with the chocolate

storage

Store in an airtight container at room temperature or in the fridge for up to 5 days, or in the freezer for up to 3 months.

get creative

If you want to make this recipe even more indulgent, serve it with a dollop of ice cream while it's still slightly warm from the oven.

helpful tips

You can use dark chocolate or milk chocolate chips in this recipe. I typically use semi-sweet chocolate chips in the 50% to 60% cacao range. Espresso powder is much more concentrated and rich than instant coffee, but you could substitute instant coffee in a pinch. Just don't use ground coffee beans, which won't dissolve and will create a gritty texture.

Serving size: 1 bar

Calories: 298

Fat: 21g

Saturated fat: 9g

Carbs: 26g

Fiber: 3g

Sugar: 20g

Protein: 5g

Cholesterol: 50mg

Sodium: 35mg

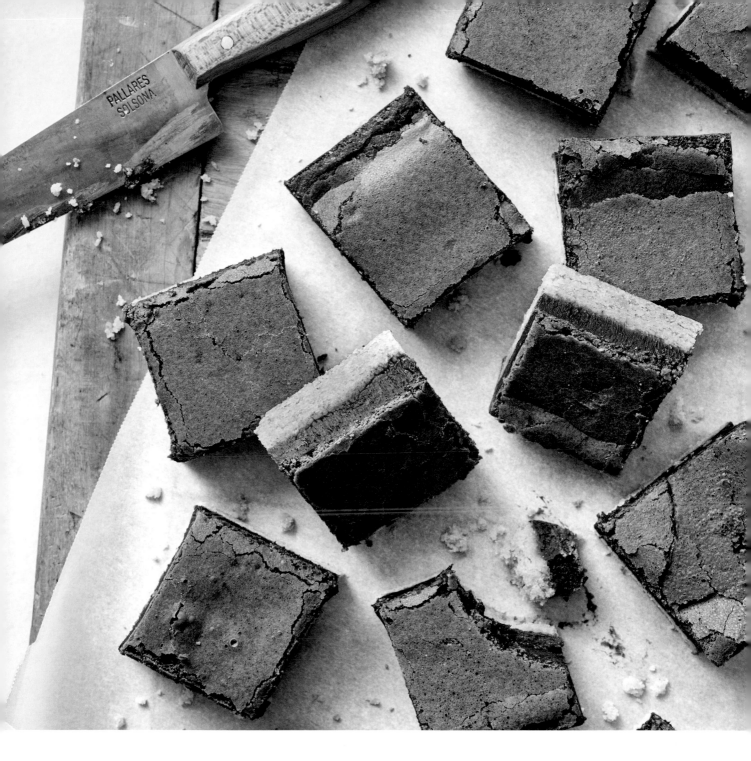

chips, stirring occasionally until smooth. Remove the bowl from the heat and whisk in the sugar, espresso, and vanilla until fully blended. Whisk in the eggs, one at a time, until incorporated. Add the tapioca flour and stir until just combined.

5. Pour the chocolate mixture on top of the crust and bake for 25 to 30 minutes, until the center is set. Remove from the oven and let cool at room temperature, then slice into bars.

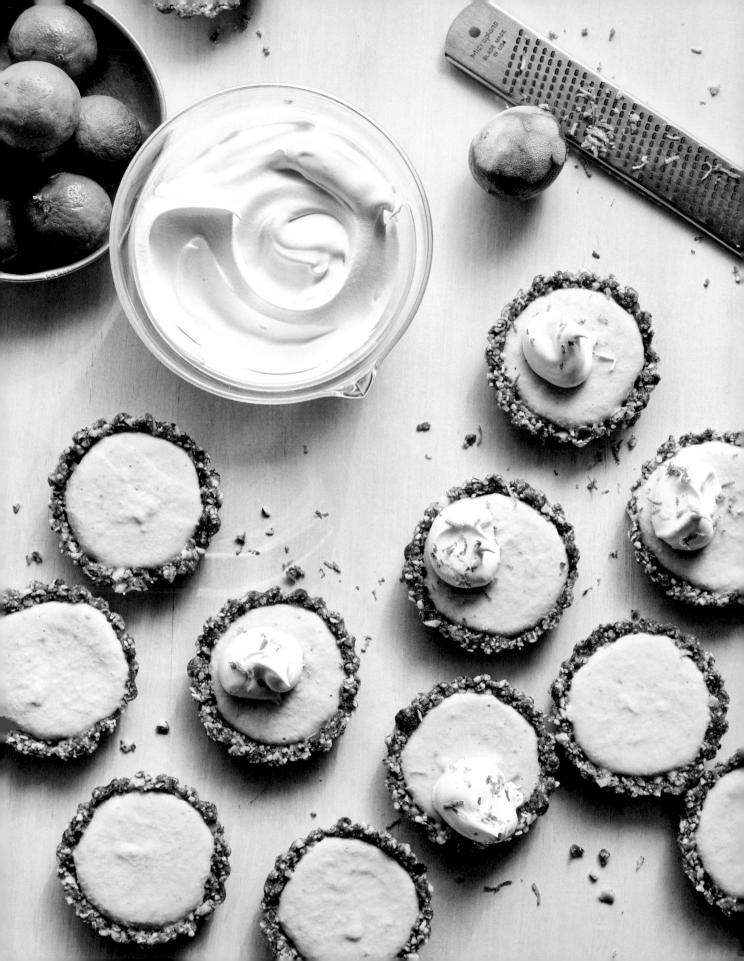

key lime tartelettes

These adorable key lime tartelettes are everything you love about a classic key lime pie but in smaller, healthier form. The filling is entirely vegan and made from soaked and blended cashews, which makes it ultra-creamy! Of course, there's plenty of lime juice and lime zest, and if you can find key limes, great, but if not, regular limes work just as well. Together, the creamy lime filling plus nutty coconut crust delivers up a winning bite-size dessert. **serves 12**

FOR THE CRUST

1 cup (140g) raw almonds

1 cup (120g) raw pecans

1 cup (80g) unsweetened shredded coconut

4 Medjool dates, pitted

2 tablespoons pure maple syrup

½ tablespoon melted and cooled coconut oil

FOR THE FILLING

1½ cups (210g) raw cashews, soaked overnight and drained

Zest and juice of 4 or 5 key limes (about 2½ tablespoons zest + ½ cup/120ml juice), plus more zest for garnish

¼ cup (57ml) melted and cooled coconut oil

⅓ cup (107ml) pure maple syrup

¼ cup (60ml) water

½ teaspoon vanilla extract

Whipped cream, for serving (optional)

1. To make the crust: In a food processor, pulse the almonds, pecans, shredded coconut, dates, maple syrup, and coconut oil until finely ground with a little bit of texture. Don't overprocess the mixture or it may turn into nut butter. Wipe out the food processor for the filling.

2. Divide the mixture into a 12-cavity mini tart pan (with individual removable bottoms so you can pop them out easily) or a 12-muffin pan with liners. Use your fingers to press the mixture flat on the bottom and up the sides a little to make the tartelette crusts.

3. To make the filling: In the food processor, blend the cashews, lime zest and juice, coconut oil, maple syrup, water, and vanilla for 2 to 3 minutes, until creamy.

4. Pour the filling into the crusts, and chill in the fridge until firm, about 2 hours. Sprinkle with a little lime zest and, if desired, serve with whipped cream.

Serving size: 1 tartelette

Calories: 401
Fat: 30g
Saturated fat: 11g
Carbs: 32g
Fiber: 5g
Sugar: 20g
Protein: 7g
Cholesterol: 0g
Sodium: 6g

acknowledgments

People weren't kidding when they said a writing a cookbook is a labor of love (a nice way of saying it's an insane amount of work) and that it seriously takes a village. I had no idea until I started this process just how true those words were. Yet, three years later, I'm now flipping through this cookbook, beaming with gratitude for the entire community of downshifters who motivated me to write it, and for the rock-star team who helped me bring it to life—it's been a dream come true!

First and foremost, to the Downshiftology community. You're simply amazing. I'm humbled by your kindness and eternally appreciative of your trust in my recipes. Chatting with you online every single day and watching you make my recipes in your own homes brings me so much joy. I get to do what I do every day because of you, so from the bottom of my heart, thank you! I look forward to one day giving you oxytocin hugs in real life.

To my social media manager, Emily Liao (aka work-wife, sister, daughter, friend, hype-girl, and all-around right-hand woman), there's no way this cookbook would have ever crossed the finish line without you working tirelessly beside me. Thank you for your never-ending positivity and can-do attitude, and for making me laugh when I was losing my marbles and overwhelmed. I appreciate you more than words.

To my agent, Janis Donnaud, who is the best of the best. Thank you for guiding me along this journey, answering my gazillion questions, and championing my vision from day one. There's no one else I'd rather have in my court.

To the entire Clarkson Potter team—what a talented bunch! Raquel Pelzel, Susan Roxborough, Ian Dingman, Jan Derevjanik, Stephanie Davis, Windy Dorrestyn, Kate Tyler, Erica Gelbard, Chris Tanigawa, Kim Tyner, and Joyce Wong. Thank you for your wordsmithing, editing, design, marketing, and all-around expertise in helping me create one gorgeous looking cookbook.

To my photographer, Ren Fuller, and the entire photo, video, and stylist team—David Peng, Marian Cooper Cairns, Natalie Drobny, Alicia Buszczak, Stephanie Hanes, and Sam Fuller. Not even a pandemic rescheduling or caravan to OC could deter this rock-star team from getting the perfect shot.

And last, but certainly not least, to my mom, Karen, and brother, Alan. Thank you for your constant love and support of my hairbrained ideas . . . like oh, ditching the corporate world and starting a blog. Downshiftology is what it is today because you "liked" and "shared" every single one of my recipes in those very early days, before there even was a community. You guys are my rock and my biggest cheerleaders—I love you with all my heart.

I also know my dad would be so proud—boastfully telling everyone his daughter's book is being sold at bookstores everywhere and just thinking about that brings a smile to my face.

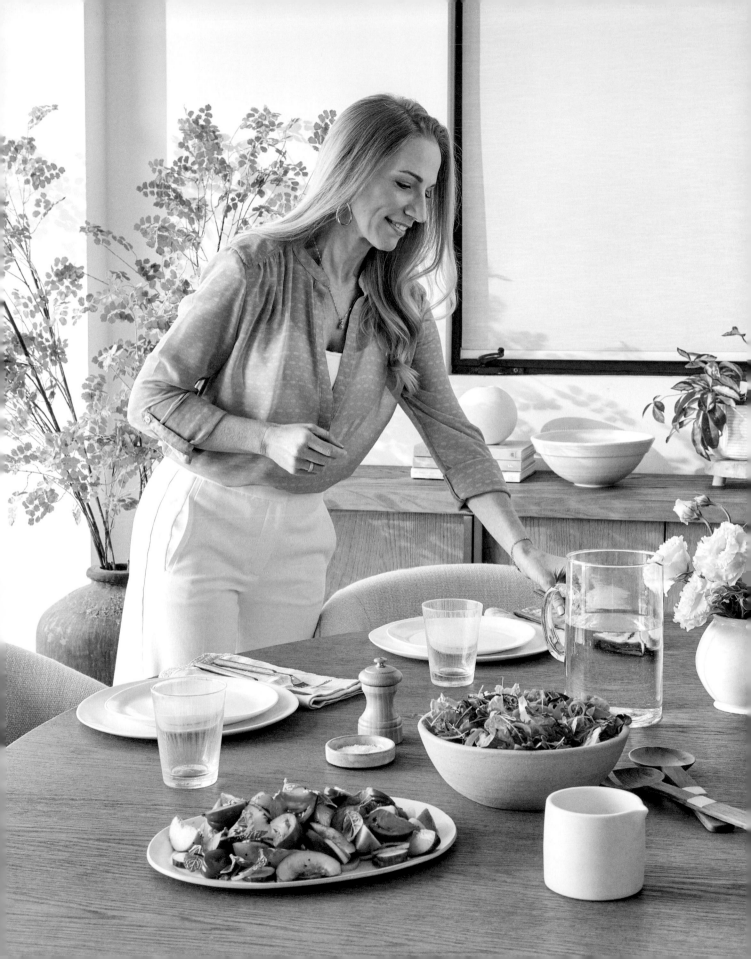

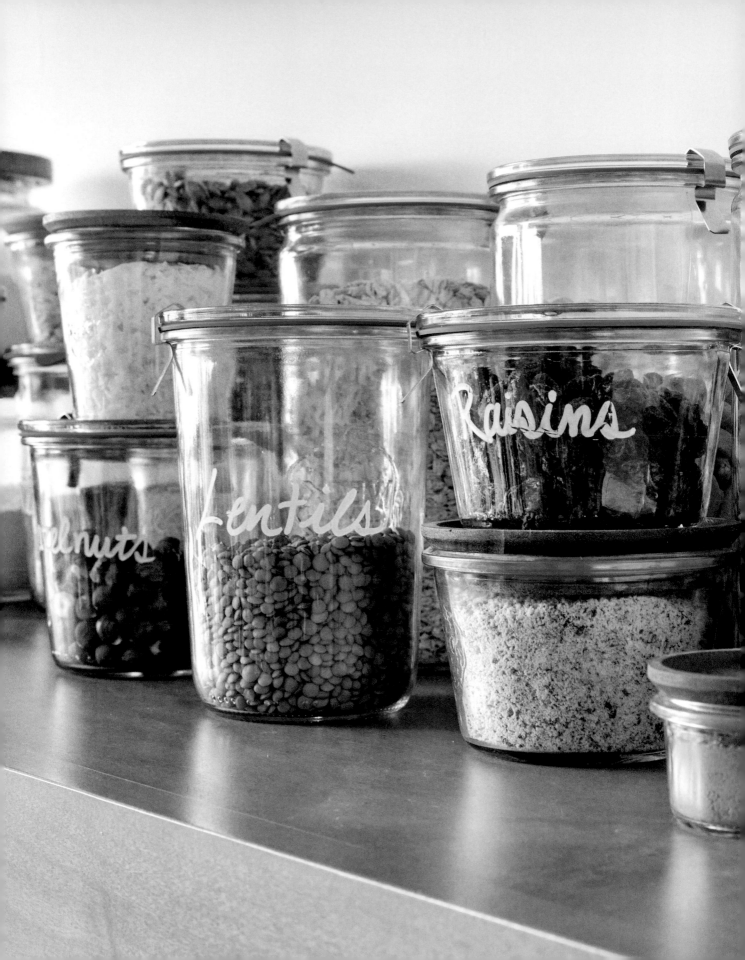

universal conversions

Fahrenheit to Celsius

200°F \ 100°C	350°F / 180°C
250°F / 120°C	375°F \ 190°C
275°F \ 140°C	400°F / 200°C
300°F / 150°C	425°F \ 220°C
325°F \ 160°C	450°F / 230°C

Liquids

Note that honey and maple syrup weigh slightly more and oil is slightly lighter.

Cup	Imperial	Metric
⅛ cup	1 fl oz	30ml
¼ cup	2 fl oz	60ml
⅓ cup	3 fl oz	80ml
½ cup	4 fl oz	120ml
⅔ cup	5 fl oz	150ml
¾ cup	6 fl oz	180ml
1 cup	8 fl oz	240ml
2 cups	16 fl oz	480ml
3 cups	24 fl oz	720ml
4 cups	32 fl oz	1 liter

Common Ingredients

1 cup almond flour	120g
1 cup raw almonds	140g
1 cup almond butter	256g
1 cup coconut sugar	160g
1 cup chocolate chips	180g
1 cup shredded coconut	80g
1 cup raw cashews	140g
1 cup dry lentils	200g
1 cup dry white rice	180g
1 cup old-fashioned rolled oats	108g
1 cup yogurt	228g

Inches to Centimeters

Imperial to Metric

½ inch \ 1.3cm		9 inches \ 23cm	
1 inch / 2.5cm		10 inches / 25cm	
2 inches \ 5cm		12 inches \ 30cm	
8 inches / 20cm		13 inches / 33cm	

Nutrition Note

Nutrition information is calculated using an online database and should be considered an estimate. Garnishes and optional ingredients are not included. Accuracy may vary based on precision of measurements, brands, and ingredient size. To obtain the most accurate representation of nutritional information in any given recipe, you should calculate the nutritional information with the actual ingredients used in your recipe.

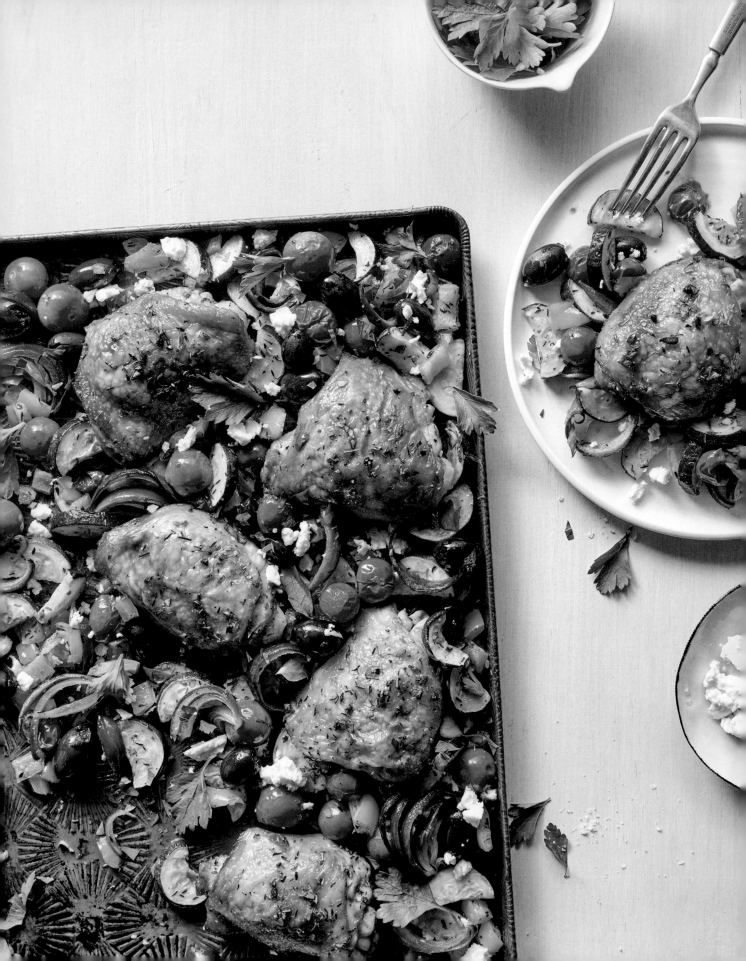

index

Published in the United States by Clarkson Potter/
Publishers, an imprint of Random House, a division of
Penguin Random House LLC, New York.
ClarksonPotter.com
RandomHouseBooks.com

CLARKSON POTTER is a trademark and POTTER with
colophon is a registered trademark of Penguin Random
House LLC.

Library of Congress Cataloging-in-Publication Data
Names: Bryan, Lisa, author. | Fuller, Ren, photographer.
Title: Downshiftology healthy meal prep / Lisa Bryan,
    Ren Fuller.
Description: New York : Clarkson Potter, 2022. |
    Includes index.
Identifiers: LCCN 2022000130 (print) | LCCN
    2022000131 (ebook) | ISBN 9780593235577
    (hardcover) | ISBN 9780593235584 (ebook)
Subjects: LCSH: Gluten-free diet—Recipes. | Sugar-
    free diet—Recipes. | Celiac disease—Diet therapy. |
    LCGFT: Cookbooks.
Classification: LCC RM237.86.B79 2022 (print) | LCC
    RM237.86 (ebook) | DDC 641.5/639311—dc23/
    eng/20220121.
LC record available at https://lccn.loc.
    gov/2022000130
LC ebook record available at https://lccn.loc.
    gov/2022000131

ISBN 978-0-593-23557-7
Ebook ISBN 978-0-593-23558-4

Printed in China

Book and cover design by Jan Derevjanik

10 9 8 7 6 5 4 3 2 1

First Edition

PHOTOGRAPHER: Ren Fuller
PHOTOGRAPHY ASSISTANT: David Peng
FOOD STYLIST: Marian Cooper Cairns
FOOD STYLIST ASSISTANT: Natalie Drobny
PROP STYLIST FOR FOOD: Alicia Buszczak
PROP STYLIST FOR LIFESTYLE: Stephanie Hanes
EDITOR: Susan Roxborough
EDITORIAL ASSISTANT: Bianca Cruz
DESIGNER: Jan Derevjanik
PRODUCTION EDITOR: Joyce Wong
PRODUCTION MANAGER: Kim Tyner and Heather Williamson
COMPOSITORS: Merri Ann Morrell and Hannah Hunt
COPY EDITOR: Jude Grant
INDEXER: Elizabeth Parson
MARKETER: Stephanie Davis
PUBLICIST: Erica Gelbard